ORDINARY MAGIC

DATE DUE

1 11 / 2 8			

ORDINARY MAGIC

Resilience in Development

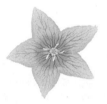

ANN S. MASTEN

THE GUILFORD PRESS
New York   London

To the memory of Ruth,
a natural protective factor in the lives of children

Library of Congress Cataloging-in-Publication Data

Masten, Ann S.
    Ordinary magic : resilience in development / Ann S. Masten.
       pages cm
    Includes bibliographical references and index.
    ISBN 978-1-4625-1716-9 (hardback)
    ISBN 978-1-4625-2371-9 (paperback)
    1. Resilience (Personality trait) in children.   2. Child psychology.
3. Child welfare.   I. Title.
    BF723.R46M37 2014
    155.4′1824—dc22
                                                        2014017571

ABOUT THE AUTHOR

Ann S. Masten, PhD, is a Regents Professor and the Irving B. Harris Professor of Child Development in the Institute of Child Development at the University of Minnesota. She is former president of the Society for Research in Child Development, a Fellow and former Division President (Division 7: Developmental Psychology) of the American Psychological Association (APA), and a Fellow of the Association for Psychological Science. She co-chairs the Forum on Investing in Young Children Globally for the U.S. National Academies. Dr. Masten is an internationally known expert on resilience in human development, with over 170 publications in scientific journals and books. She is a recipient of the 2014 Urie Bronfenbrenner Award for Lifetime Contribution to Developmental Psychology in the Service of Science and Society from the APA.

PREFACE

Nearly four decades ago, I was drawn into the newly emerging science of resilience as I embarked on doctoral studies in clinical psychology at the University of Minnesota. A group of pioneering investigators who studied children who were, for various reasons, at risk had noticed the striking variation among individuals exposed to adversity, with some young people thriving or at least holding their own despite their high-risk background or hazardous experiences. We were curious about the roots of this observable resilience: How do some individuals fare so well while others struggle? Would it be possible to foster resilience in other young people at risk if we understood more about this phenomenon?

Three waves of research followed as scientists and their students tried to understand resilience in human development, initially describing the variation in adaptation observed in risky or stressful circumstances and later advancing to studies of processes that might account for the variation, particularly the pathways to positive outcomes. Ultimately the goal was to inform efforts to promote resilience. A new century and new technologies—including brain imaging, genetic assessment, and statistics for modeling complex systems—ushered in the fourth wave of resilience science, marked by efforts to integrate knowledge across system levels to predict or promote positive adaptation in the context of adversity.

In 2001, I published an essay called "Ordinary Magic: Resilience Processes in Development," which briefly summarized conclusions I had reached after 25 years of work in the field, beginning as a student. This essay would become my most cited paper, and I soon realized that I wanted to elaborate on those conclusions. I began to plan this book, but ongoing research, teaching, and administrative responsibilities slowed the process of producing it. With time, I felt a growing urgency to integrate the ideas and findings on resilience in children and youth. I had witnessed three major waves of resilience science and knew that a major new wave was coming. I also knew that the science would keep evolving and improving but with the fourth wave rising, the time was ripe for a book-length summation of progress to date.

Internationally, resilience science is burgeoning in many different fields as scientists study the variation in the responses of complex systems to challenges. Global catastrophes in the form of terror attacks, natural disasters, climate change, pandemics, economic crisis, and warfare are motivating action at many levels of policy and intervention in an effort to protect life, promote global well-being, and improve the odds of resilience in populations threatened by adversities. There is growing recognition that resilience in children is interconnected with the resilience of families, communities, governments, economies, and ecologies.

APPROACH AND ORGANIZATION

My goal in this volume is to describe the progress in research on resilience in children and youth to date from the vantage point of an early participant–observer. In this volume, I discuss the origins and progress of developmental resilience science, the research models and strategies that evolved, exemplary findings from illustrative lines of work, and the implications of what we know so far for practice and future science. Fundamental concepts are carefully defined and illustrated with both case material and empirical examples. Three major domains of research are highlighted, including longitudinal studies of child adaptation in relation to stress and adversity, research on socioeconomically disadvantaged children, and studies of mass trauma related to war and disaster.

Diverse studies from many different places and kinds of adversities point to a fundamental set of adaptive systems that account for much of the capacity for doing well or recovering well in the context of adversity exposure. This set, which I have called the "short list," provides important clues to key protective factors in the lives of young people with implications for preventive interventions.

The focus of the book is on individual resilience observed at a behavioral level, but even in the initial waves of research, studies that included other system levels have played an important part in accounting for resilience. Chapters of the book highlight the rapidly emerging science on the neurobiology of resilience and research on three contexts of child development that are central to the lives and resilience of children: families, schools, and culture. Wherever possible, I have tried to provide international perspectives and research examples. Though relatively neglected in early waves, global research is expanding rapidly with ever greater attention to cultural context and resilience in the economically developing parts of the world.

Resilience science has transformed multiple fields of practice, shifting models and intervention strategies toward strength-focused models and goals. A resilience framework for action is delineated in one of the closing chapters. The book concludes with a discussion of enduring controversies and where I see the study of resilience headed.

Long a believer that complex ideas can be described in straightforward language, I have attempted to write in a style accessible to diverse readers while simultaneously doing justice to the ideas and provocative findings. Compelling case examples are included, some of which are drawn from non-Western cultures and countries, such as Sierra Leone and Cambodia. These individual life examples serve the dual purpose of illustrating important points in the resilience literature and bringing the phenomenon of resilience to life. A glossary of terms is provided in Appendix

A, as well as a list of abbreviations in Appendix B and suggestions for further reading grouped by topic in Appendix C.

AUDIENCE

This book is written both for scholars who already study resilience and for those who may want to get involved in this expanding domain of research, including students, and also for those who want to improve the lives of children at risk as a result of trauma exposure or adverse rearing conditions. Professionals in psychology, psychiatry, social work, education, sociology, nursing, pediatrics, public health, applied economics, humanitarian assistance, and disaster planning should find useful ideas and background for their work. Promoting resilience is a multidisciplinary endeavor.

ACKNOWLEDGMENTS

My pathway to research on resilience was shaped by many people and experiences over the years. Growing up in the military undoubtedly influenced my personal interests in adaptation, mobility, and the effects of war on children. Academically, I had the good fortune to be mentored by a sequence of great scholars, each connecting me to the next. At Smith College, I wrote my first serious term paper in psychology on Robert White's theory of competence for a seminar I took with Professor Elsa Siipola. She referred me to David Shakow for a job when I was finishing college and I became his research assistant for 3 years at the National Institutes of Health (NIH). David was a renowned researcher on schizophrenia who was 73 when I began to work for him, already a Scientist Emeritus, the first, I believe, with that status at NIH. David was one of the founding fathers of modern clinical psychology and he inspired me to go on to graduate school in this field. One of David's frequent visitors was Norman Garmezy, who also had studied schizophrenia for many years but later turned his attention to studying the origins of mental illness in childhood. Garmezy, who had a contagious passion for research, told me about his new work on children at risk who nonetheless do well, his studies of "stress-resistant children." I was hooked and for many years during and beyond my PhD, his enthusiastic support would be invaluable to my thinking and my persistence in the study of resilience. Moreover, through

Garmezy, I met and learned from other pioneers in psychology and psychiatry who were shaping the emerging science of risk and resilience, most particularly Michael Rutter, Arnold Sameroff, and Emmy Werner.

At Minnesota, I benefited from both an outstanding faculty and a remarkable set of fellow graduate students. Irving Gottesman, Alan Sroufe, and Auke Tellegen were particularly influential teachers. Other students on Garmezy's team included my long-term collaborator, Margaret O'Dougherty Wright, and Patricia Morison. Dante Cicchetti was both a fellow student and a precocious mentor who would influence me and many others in the decades to come in regard to developmental psychopathology and resilience.

Once I became a faculty member and moved down the block to the Institute of Child Development, I learned a great deal from the students I mentored at Minnesota, as well as my colleagues. As all decent mentors know, this relationship is a dynamic exchange in which the mentor usually learns more than the mentored. These students have honed my thinking and gone on to do great work on risk and resilience in their own right. Their work is cited throughout this volume. I also gleaned most of what I know about developmental theory from my brilliant and feisty colleagues in the "Tute."

My thinking about resilience was enriched along the way by many other national and international colleagues, including Frosso Motti-Stefanidi and Joy Osofsky. I am also grateful for the illuminating interactions over the years with Jack Block, Tom Boyce, Emory Cowen, Ron Dahl, Glenace Edwall, Glen Elder, Vivian Faden, Xiaojia Ge, Lance Gunderson, Stuart Hauser, Mavis Hetherington, Elizabeth Hinz, Rich Lerner, Jeff Long, Pat Longstaff, Suniya Luthar, Michael Maddaus, Danny Pine, Rainer Silbereisen, and Joe White. The writing of this book benefited from the insightful comments of Dante Cicchetti, Catherine Panter-Brick, and Michael Rutter, as well as my editors at The Guilford Press, including Rochelle Serwator, Kristal Hawkins, and C. Deborah Laughton. Zoe Jacobson was an enthusiastic and astute editor and assistant as I finished this volume.

The work described in this book would not have been possible without the generous contributions and trust of many participants, teachers, and other professional staff in schools and community agencies who gave their time so that others could learn about resilience. I also am grateful to the funders who supported my own and all the other research on resilience discussed in this volume, particularly the funders of longitudinal data collection. I especially want to thank the William T. Grant Foundation, the National Institute of Mental Health, the National Science Foundation, the National Institute of Child Health and Human Development, the Center for Urban and Regional Affairs, the Institute of Education Sciences, the Jacobs Foundation, the John D. and Catherine T. MacArthur Foundation, and the University of Minnesota for their support of work included in this volume. The opinions expressed in this book, of course, are solely my own, and not necessarily shared by any of these funders or other investigators.

This volume is dedicated to the memory of my mother, Ruth, who showed me and many others the magic of an adult who believes in you and laughter in the worst moments. She, along with my father, Charlie, and a small army of resourceful relatives, taught me the power of protective people in your life. And last, but most important, I want to thank my husband, Steve, and our daughters, Carrie and Madeline, for all their support during the years of research and writing that eventually became this book.

CONTENTS

PART IV. MOVING FORWARD: IMPLICATIONS FOR ACTION AND FUTURE RESEARCH

PART I

INTRODUCTION AND CONCEPTUAL OVERVIEW

CHAPTER 1

INTRODUCTION

Probably as long as humans have told stories to one another, there have been tales of individuals who overcame difficulties to succeed in life. Traditional folktales and fairytales portray themes of struggle and transformation, persistence and heroic deeds in the face of adversity, and young people of humble origins who rise in life through their wits and actions, sometimes assisted by a guide or magical figure. These traditional stories have proven to be "irresistible" over the centuries to people around the world (Zipes, 2012). In the 21st century, when it is possible to share stories in many different ways—through social media, in books or newspapers, in films or television shows, through e-mails or blogs, on various digital communication devices—people remain intrigued with stories of youth who face grave danger or grow up in poverty and nonetheless turn out well. Humans are fascinated by such accounts, and I believe that these stories capture a fundamental truth about human resilience that is the theme of this book: *Resilience arises from ordinary resources and processes.*

Interest in resilience also seems to rise in troubled times. If so, then we should not be surprised by the current levels of attention to resilience readily observable on the Internet, and in books, conferences, and articles. The beginning of the 21st century has witnessed an extraordinary sequence of global calamities stemming from natural disasters, political conflicts and war, virus outbreaks, economic crises, and industrial accidents, with fears of

3

climate change looming. The lives of children and youth around the world today are threatened in staggering numbers by war, terrorism, natural disasters, poverty, starvation, disease, neglect, dislocation, and many other hazards to life and development.

It is not possible to prevent all the known threats to child development. Thus, it is imperative to understand how to protect children from the worst ravages of adversity and how to promote positive development when rearing conditions are not optimal. Research on resilience in child development can illuminate what makes a difference, for whom, and when, providing guidance for efforts to improve the chances for healthy development among children at risk for problems related to negative life circumstances. This premise motivated the scientists who initiated the systematic study of resilience phenomena in children in the 1960s and 1970s.

The scientists who pioneered the study of resilience in human development were profoundly influenced by World War II. The war brought global attention to the plight of children exposed to bombs, death, starvation, genocide, displacement, and other adversities on a massive scale. The war motivated multiple waves of research on the effects of adversity on children and adults, including long-term follow-ups of those who experienced concentration camps, radiation, starvation, loss of parents, and other challenges. A number of the key individuals who would subsequently initiate influential studies of resilience in children were directly impacted by the war. Norman Garmezy, for example, participated in the war as a young American soldier and he was present at the Battle of the Bulge. Emmy Werner was one of the many children and adolescents who experienced the bombing of Europe firsthand, and efforts after the war by UNICEF, founded in the wake of World War II, and other organizations to prevent millions of children from starving in the aftermath of the devastation. Michael Rutter was one of the "seavacuees," British children who were sent across the ocean to safety in North America to escape the bombing. Eventually, each of these individuals became a leading scientist studying resilience in children at risk.

After World War II, there was a rapid expansion of research in psychology, psychiatry, and related fields seeking to advance knowledge about the causes of mental health and behavioral problems, with the goal of better treatments or prevention. Scientists aiming to understand causes of psychological and behavior problems followed a public health strategy. They began by identifying *risk factors* associated with the negative outcomes of interest. The public health model addressed three questions (Gruenberg, 1981, p. 8):

1. Who gets sick, and who doesn't get sick?
2. Why?
3. What can we do to make the sickness less common?

It was too expensive in resources to follow the development of a general population of children over time to observe who may or may not develop problems, particularly in the case of uncommon disorders or problems. Risk factors were a way to choose groups of children with higher than usual probabilities of developing a particular problem of concern. Many risk factors or predictors of mental and behavioral problems were identified and these fell into three major categories: genetic risk or being related to people with serious mental disorders (e.g., child of a parent with schizophrenia), exposure to stressful life experiences (e.g., war, maltreatment, divorce), and status indicators of precarious life circumstances (e.g., premature birth, low socioeconomic status [SES], low maternal education, unwed teenage parents). By studying the development of children in high-risk groups, risk researchers hoped to learn in an efficient way about the processes that lead to disorders, with the ultimate goal of informing prevention and treatment. Garmezy, Rutter, and Werner were among these risk researchers.

When investigators began to study high-risk children over time, it became clear that there was tremendous variability in the course of their unfolding lives (Masten, 1989; Sameroff & Chandler, 1975). A small but influential group of risk researchers was struck by the observable fact that numerous children in the risk groups were thriving in the face of formidable odds. They began to ask a somewhat different set of questions:

1. Who stays well and recovers well?
2. How?
3. What can we do to promote and protect health and positive development?

Leading scholars in psychology and psychiatry, including E. James Anthony, Emory Cowen, Norman Garmezy, Lois Murphy, Michael Rutter, George Vaillant, and Emmy Werner, began to talk and write about the importance of these questions and their observations on positive development among high-risk children and youth. These investigators would propagate the first wave of resilience research.

FOUR WAVES OF RESILIENCE SCIENCE

Over the past half-century, there have been four major waves of resilience science (Masten, 2007; Wright, Masten, & Narayan, 2013). The first wave was descriptive, as scientists began systematically to define, measure, and describe the phenomenon of good function or outcomes in the context of risk or adversity and attempt to identify the predictors of resilience. Wave 1 is characterized by these types of questions: What is resilience? How do we measure it? What makes a difference? With clues from Wave 1 work, investigators in the second wave shifted their attention to the *processes* of resilience and to *how* questions: What are the processes that lead to resilience? How do protective, promotive, or preventive influences work? How is positive development promoted in the context of risk? Wave 2 set the stage for the third wave, focused on promoting resilience through interventions, while simultaneously testing theories from the first two waves about what matters for resilience and how: Can resilience be promoted? Are theories about the processes leading to resilience on target? Advances in technology and knowledge—in genetics, statistics, neuroscience, and neuroimaging—gave rise to the fourth wave of resilience science, which is characterized by dynamic, systems-oriented approaches, with a focus on interactions of genes with experience, persons with contexts, connecting levels of analysis, and multidisciplinary integration. Fourth-wave questions are just emerging: How do genetic differences play a role in resilience? Do individuals have differential sensitivity to traumatic experiences? Are the same individuals also sensitive to positive interventions? How is brain development protected from high levels of stress and stress hormones? Is it possible to influence important human adaptive systems to foster resilience? How do communities and societies nurture resilience? The evidence, controversies, and lessons learned from each of these waves to date will be examined further throughout this volume.

The great insight of the early pioneers in resilience science was in recognizing the potential significance of understanding positive outcomes among high-risk children and youth for practice and policy as well as for scientific theory. They inspired their students and other investigators to study and understand the positive as well as the negative influences in children's lives, with the ultimate goal of tilting the odds toward positive development. Now, after half a century of research, it is time to take stock of what has been learned from research on resilience in young people: the evidence and the surprises, the conclusions and the controversies, the gaps and the future goals, and the implications to date for practice and policy.

Ordinary Magic

The biggest surprise that emerged from the study of children who overcome adversity to become successful youth and adults in society was the *ordinariness* of the phenomenon (Masten, 2001). Captivating stories of resilient individuals may have created misleading perceptions that resilience is rare and results from extraordinary talents or resources (symbolized by magic powers and helpers in myths and fairytales). Evidence strongly suggests, on the contrary, that resilience is common and typically arises from the operation of basic protections. There are exceptional cases, where children overcome heavy odds because of extraordinary talents, luck, or resources, but most of the time, the children who make it have ordinary human resources and protective factors in their lives. Resilience emerges from commonplace adaptive systems for human development, such as a healthy human brain in good working order; close relationships with competent and caring adults; committed families; effective schools and communities; opportunities to succeed; and beliefs in the self, nurtured by positive interactions with the world. Studies of resilience repeatedly point to the same factors associated with positive adaptation or development in the context of risk, representing clues to what really matters for resilience. These findings highlight the power of human and social capital for development and suggest priorities for those who aim to shift the odds in favor of good outcomes among children threatened by a variety of negative life circumstances.

The study of resilience has had transformative effects on the guiding frameworks for interventions and policies designed to help children at risk for academic and behavioral problems. Deficit models are being replaced by more balanced models that include assets, strengths, and protective factors along with risks, problems, and vulnerabilities. It turns out that many of the most strategic ways to prevent and ameliorate problems in development may be to promote competence and success, which is also far more appealing as an objective to parents and the public than programs focused on reducing problems (Masten, 2011; Masten & Coatsworth, 1998).

Resilience research is also quintessentially developmental in nature. The science of resilience grew out of research on children at risk for mental disorders, and longitudinal studies played a key role in its history. Resilience science emerged from the same roots that gave rise to *developmental psychopathology*, an integrative and multidisciplinary approach to mental health theory and practice that emphasizes the full range of individual differences in adaptation and development over the lifespan (Cicchetti, 2006, 2010; Masten, 2006a, 2012a). The study of resilience in children at risk for mental health problems is one of the core domains of work under the broad umbrella of developmental psychopathology.

WHAT EXACTLY DOES *RESILIENCE* MEAN IN DEVELOPMENTAL SCIENCE?

The word *resilience* stems from the Latin verb *resilire* (to rebound). In colloquial English, the word *resiliency* retains a similar meaning, referring to the property of elasticity or springing back, much as a rubber band does after it is stretched and then released. In engineering science, materials are said to be resilient when they resist cracking or breaking under stress or return to original form after distortion by stress or load. In ecology, resilience refers to "the capacity of a system to absorb disturbance and reorganize and yet persist in a similar state" (Gunderson, Folke, & Janssen, 2006). The conceptual similarity among resilience concepts in multiple fields likely stems in part from shared origins in general systems theory (von Bertalanffy, 1968). Resilience refers to the adaptation and survival of a system after perturbation, often referring to the process of restoring functional equilibrium, and sometimes referring to the process of successful transformation to a stable new functional state. As a living system, a human individual could be described as resilient when showing a pattern of adaptation or recovery in the context of potentially destabilizing threats.

With each wave of research on resilience in children, the definitions and models of resilience became more dynamic. In early work, resilience often was defined in terms of doing well or avoiding mental illness in the context of risk or adversity. In the behavioral sciences of psychology, psychiatry, and related fields, the concept of resilience continues to refer generally to *positive adaptation in the context of risk or adversity*. It is a very broad term that encompasses a range of phenomena, including the capacity for doing well under adversity, the processes of coping with challenges, recovery from catastrophe, posttraumatic growth, and the achievement of good outcomes among people at high risk for failure or maladaptation. In developmental studies, resilience refers to positive development in a context of high risk for problems or maladjustment. In more recent work, resilience is defined in terms of processes or systems, with an eye toward achieving a terminology that could work across disciplines that focus on different systems and levels of analysis and thus would facilitate integrative research and application that requires this type of integration, such as disaster response. Currently, I would define resilience as follows:

> The capacity of a dynamic system to adapt successfully to disturbances that threaten system function, viability, or development.

This book is focused on resilience in individual young people, but the concept of resilience can be applied to any dynamic system, including a family, a school, a community, an organization, an economy, or an ecosystem.

From a general systems theory perspective, resilience does not necessarily connote "good" outcomes from the viewpoint of human rights or individual child well-being. It is possible for a "resilient" organization or government, for example, to commit atrocities against children. However, in developmental science, the concept of resilience does carry the connotation of good outcomes, requiring definitions and judgments about what constitutes positive or desirable outcomes for children.

Patterns and Pathways of Resilience

The meaning of resilience can also be expressed in terms of life-course patterns of functioning or development. Figure 1.1 illustrates a sample of basic life pathways or patterns encompassed by the construct of resilience. In all cases, there is sufficient adversity experienced to potentially derail the normal course of development or functioning.

For youth on Path A, a relatively steady course of good functioning is maintained, even though there is an acute trauma experienced at time x, or there is a history of chronic ongoing adversity before and after time x, such as growing up in poverty, with domestic violence, or in a war-torn community. The adaptation of these young people may fluctuate but their function stays in the

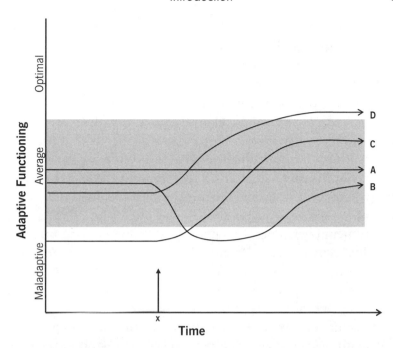

FIGURE 1.1. A sample of resilience pathways: (A) stress resistance in the context of either acute trauma occurring at time *x* or chronic adversity before and after time *x*; (B) recovery following acute, overwhelming trauma at time *x*; (C) normalization after marked *reduction* of adversity beginning at time *x*; (D) posttraumatic growth following trauma at time *x*.

zone of normal adaptation, meeting the general expectations for healthy development as they move through life. It was often cases like these that captured the attention of pioneering scientists who were studying children at risk for psychopathology and other problems. School teachers often know of such children, growing up in chaotic households or poverty, who nevertheless do well at school, succeeding academically and socially. Initially, such children were described as "invulnerable" or "stress resistant," as scientists wondered what could account for their positive functioning in the midst of extremely challenging circumstances. As research accrued, the secrets of their success looked less mysterious; powerful protective forces appear to be operating on behalf of such children.

Path B represents a different kind of resilience, character-ized by trauma and recovery. These individuals are developing normally until they encounter overwhelming adversity. Adaptive functioning declines, as one would expect in the face of disaster, but then improves as the individual recovers to normal function-ing. This pattern can unfold relatively quickly, with an acute crisis and rapid recovery, or over more extended periods of time, when it takes longer for individuals to recover as often happens follow-ing a major disaster. Children do recover from the loss of parents, terrifying experiences, and other major blows in life.

Path C shows a major shift in the quality of adaptation or development over time, from poor functioning to good function-ing. This "normalization" pattern is what one hopes to see if rear-ing conditions or resources substantially improve in the lives of individuals living in conditions of extreme deprivation or chronic adversity. One of the most dramatic examples in modern times of this situation occurred after the fall of the Ceauşescu regime in Romania, when many children were moved out of orphanages ill suited to the developmental needs of children into adoptive homes. Though there have been lingering problems for some of these children, particularly those who lived for long periods in the worst situations, many internationally adopted Romanian orphans showed marked improvements in development following improved rearing conditions (e.g., Rutter, 2006; Rutter & the Eng-lish and Romanian Adoptees Study Team, 1998; Rutter, Sonuga-Barke, Beckett, 2010; Rutter, Sonuga-Barke, & Castle, 2010).

Path D represents posttraumatic growth, where adaptive function improves following trauma or adversity. This pattern has been reported in the literature, although research on post-traumatic growth, particularly in children, is limited (Masten & Narayan, 2012).

Resilience is a broad concept and many other pathways toward or away from resilience could be illustrated. Given the complexity of human life and myriad influences on adaptation and development, one would expect that there would be many roads to resilience. Examples of the diverse paths of resilience are discussed throughout this book.

TWO JUDGMENTS:
THE CRITERIA FOR RESILIENCE

Identifying resilience in a person's life requires two kinds of evaluation: judgments about exposure to adversity and judgments about how well a person is doing in the midst or aftermath of the adversity. In other words, resilience is inferred from two sets of evaluations, one concerning the nature of threat posed by their life experiences (has there been risk?) and a second one about the quality of adjustment or a person's development (is this person doing okay?). People make these judgments all the time in the course of daily life and most, when asked, can think of a person from their own experience who has manifested resilience.

If there is little or no threat in an individual's life, or if there is not (yet) evidence of recovery or good outcome, then there is no observed resilience (at least not yet). This sounds obvious and straightforward, but the devil is in the details of defining risk and good outcome, and who gets to decide on these criteria. It has become clear in the study of resilience that these decisions can be complex and controversial (Luthar, 2006; Masten 2007, 2012a; Rutter, 2012b).

Judging Threats to Child Development and Adaptation

Over the past century, many forms of risk to child development and functioning have been studied, ranging from premature birth to war (Evans, Li, & Sepanski Whipple, 2013; Garmezy, 1974; Kopp, 1983; Obradović, Shaffer, & Masten, 2012; Sameroff & Seifer, 1983). Risk factors are established predictors of undesirable outcomes, where there is evidence suggesting a higher-than-usual probability of a future problem. There are numerous well-documented risks for specific and general problems in the developmental sciences, including attributes of the environment, family, or child, and a wide variety of potentially stressful experiences. Examples include low birth weight, family violence, low SES, divorce, harsh or neglectful parenting, natural disasters, terrorism, cognitive difficulties, malnutrition, poverty, homelessness, and other forms of family displacement. A risk factor could be highly specific to a particular outcome, but many of the most common risk factors of childhood (e.g., poverty, maltreatment, or birth to a very young, single parent) predict multiple problems of behavior, health, and growth. There are several likely explanations for this observation. First, risk factors are often related to one another: risk predicts risk. Poverty, malnutrition, exposure to lead, low birth weight, low maternal education, and child neglect co-occur. Thus, when one risk factor is measured, there are likely to be a number of other unmeasured risk factors that also are present. Second, risk factors may reflect underlying processes that are so fundamental that they undermine more than one aspect of adaptation and development. Normal development requires basic nutrition; malnutrition can produce a broad array of problems in growth, brain development, and cognition (Fiese, Gunderson, Koester, & Washington, 2011; Walker et al., 2011). And third, it is likely that one problem leads to another, so that over time, the same risk factor could account for snowballing problems in multiple domains. A risk factor that negatively influences the development of self-regulation skills in the preschool years, representing essential tools for attention and impulse control, can have profound consequences for subsequent success at school, interfering with learning, friendships, and relationships with teachers (Diamond & Lee, 2011; Masten, Herbers, et al., 2012).

Almost immediately after risk research began, investigators realized that risk factors rarely appear in isolation in the lives of children, but often occur in batches or pile up over time. Investigators described this phenomenon in terms of *cumulative risk* (Masten, Best, & Garmezy, 1990; Rutter, 1979; Sameroff, Seifer, & Bartko, 1997). Moreover, it became clear that the likelihood of problems increased as the number of risk factors increased. Behavioral and emotional problems in children were much more common among those with multiple risk factors as compared with children who had few or no major risk factors (Evans et al., 2013; Obradović et al., 2012). Further, investigators also recognized that most of the major risk factors (predicting very broadly or with large effects) were actually markers of much more complex processes embedded with many threats and stressors. Divorce, for example, is a general risk factor for a variety of child and adult problems, over both the short and long term, but it is not a simple experience (Hetherington, 1979; Kelly & Emery, 2003). Years of interparental conflict may precede and follow divorce, and there may be many additional threats associated with family breakup, including financial strains and disruptions in housing, schooling, and relationships with family and friends, as well as the stresses of parental dating or reconstituted families.

In the resilience literature, there have been two major approaches to the study of cumulative risk. One is focused on tabulating the number of known risk factors present in a person's life. The second approach calculates the level of exposure to stressful events and experience, either by summing negative life events in a given time period or otherwise quantifying the severity of cumulative exposure to potentially damaging life experiences. Cumulative risk scores are then related to outcomes of interest, as discussed in more depth in Chapter 2, on models of risk and resilience. As cumulative risk levels increase, more problems typically are observed on average in a group of people (see discussion on *risk gradients* in Chapter 2).

Judging How Well Life Is Going: Developmental Tasks, Competence, and Cascades

To determine or study resilience, one must also judge how well an individual person (or system) is doing in terms of adaptive function or development, either in the short term or in the long term. In complex, living organisms like human beings, positive outcomes can be judged in many ways and at multiple levels of analysis (Cicchetti, 2010; Masten, 2007; Masten, Burt, & Coatsworth, 2006). Over the years, there has been some controversy about the criteria for defining positive adaptation for resilience studies, including debates about whether to include internal well-being along with external achievements, who should define the criteria, and whether to use global or specific criteria (see Chapter 12; Luthar, 2006; Luthar, Cicchetti, & Becker, 2000; Masten, 1999, 2007, 2012a, 2013b; Schoon, 2006).

In behavioral studies of resilience, two popular kinds of criteria for judging outcomes focus on positive or negative function in terms of (1) competence or success in age-salient developmental tasks or (2) symptoms of psychopathology. Whether one focuses on desirable or undesirable outcomes or both, evaluations are made about how a person's life is going in relation to established norms or expectations grounded in developmental, historical, cultural, and/or situational contexts.

It is not surprising that the absence of symptoms related to mental health problems has been popular as a criterion for defining good adaptation, given that the study of resilience arose from efforts to understand and prevent the development of mental illness. If children at risk for mental disorders are studied, then it would be reasonable to define good outcomes in terms of avoiding mental health problems. However, if one were to ask ordinary adults in society to think of a person whose life is going well, it is unlikely they would respond, "She is not mentally ill." It is much more likely that they would describe positive qualities or achievements. Similarly, if one asks parents what outcomes they desire for their children, parents will describe achievements or happiness rather than the absence of problems. Parents typically want their children to succeed in relationships, in school, in jobs, and also in finding happiness, though implicitly they may want their children to avoid mental illness, teen pregnancy, drugs, or dropping out of school.

Developmental studies of resilience often define good adaptation in relation to success in age-salient developmental tasks (Masten, 2001; McCormick, Kuo, & Masten, 2011; Roisman, Masten, Coatsworth, & Tellegen, 2004; Sroufe, 1979). Developmental tasks are the expectations for behavior and accomplishments shared by members of a community or society for people of different ages. The idea of developmental tasks has deep roots (see Masten, Burt, et al., 2006) but it was popularized in education and human development by Robert Havighurst (1974) when he was a professor at the University of Chicago. Some of these expectations for the behavior of children and youth are so widely held among human societies as to be labeled "universal." All societies expect children to learn to walk and talk and follow the rules of the society. Other tasks are common among societies of similar industrial development or culture. For example, many communities worldwide expect children to attend school and to learn something useful there. Still, there are developmental tasks that are much more specific to a given region or cultural group, such as the expectation to learn weaving or fishing. Also, there are optional developmental tasks at some periods of life, when individuals in a particular society or culture have some leeway to choose alternatives (e.g., focus on a job or focus on child rearing).

Developmental tasks typically include observable achievements, such as talking or academic achievement, but they also may include internal achievements, such as happiness or a sense of identity. Erik Erikson (1963, 1968), for example, viewed identity formation as the key developmental challenge of adolescence. Examples of common developmental tasks in many industrialized nations are provided in Table 1.1. In a given period of development, there tends to be a group of salient developmental tasks that are particularly important for judging how a person is doing. These salient tasks reflect both the capabilities of typical human individuals of a given age or level of experience, and also the collective wisdom of the culture as to important milestones and predictors of success in the future in that culture. As people mature, some tasks wane in importance while others emerge. During the toddler years, for example, crawling becomes less important as walking is achieved. Similarly, as children become adults, success in school becomes less salient and success in work or parenting becomes more salient.

Young children have little awareness of these developmental task expectations of their parents and society, but are judged by such criteria nonetheless. Older children and youth become quite aware of these criteria and may evaluate their own success, failure, or self-worth according to how well they perceive themselves to be doing on these tasks, or how they perceive others are judging their progress or success. Youth who become alienated from their families or society may pursue paths through life that are

**TABLE 1.1. Common Age-Salient
Developmental Tasks**

Infancy period

Forming attachment bonds with primary caregivers
Learning to sit and crawl
Emerging: learning to communicate by gesture and language

Toddler and preschool period

Waning: crawling
Learning to walk and run
Learning to speak the language of the family
Obeying simple commands
Learning to play with other children
Emerging: self-control of attention and impulses

Early school years

Attending school and behaving appropriately
Learning to read and write the language of the community
Getting along with other children
Respecting and obeying elders
Emerging: making close friends

Adolescence

Adjusting to physical maturation
Successful transitioning to secondary schooling
Following the rules and laws of society
Committing to a religion
Forming close friendships
Emerging: exploring identity, romantic relationships, work

Early adulthood

Waning: academic achievement
Achieving a cohesive sense of self
Forming a close romantic relationship
Contributing to family livelihood through work in the home
    or community
Establishing a career
Establishing a family
Emerging: civic engagement

deliberately at odds with the developmental task expectations of the larger society. Erikson (1968) described this phenomenon in terms of "negative identity" formation.

Why do societies, parents, other stakeholders, and eventually children themselves care about competence in developmental tasks? I think it is because societies and families have observed over generations that these developmental milestones signify that a child is on track to do okay in the future. There is a popular belief that *competence begets competence* in these developmental tasks and this tenet also is central to developmental theories of competence and its development. The science on competence in development strongly supports this core idea (Heckman, 2006; Masten, Burt, et al., 2006; McCormick et al., 2011).

The thesis that how well one does in one developmental task domain can spill over to affect other domains of adaptation has been examined most broadly in research on *developmental cascades*. Cascading, progressive, or snowball effects generally refer to spreading consequences over time from one domain of function to another, one level of function to another, one system to another, or even one generation to another (Masten & Cicchetti, 2010c). There can be positive or negative cascades in a child's life. Cascades are discussed further in later chapters on models, research findings, and interventions to promote positive or interrupt negative cascades.

Children or youth who are doing well in all the ways that children might be judged in the community and family in which they live could be said to be well-adjusted, competent, successful, or adaptive. However, such children would not meet the criteria for resilience unless they also had a history of high risk or adversity exposure. By definition, resilience requires evidence of risk as well as positive adaptation.

WHAT MAKES A DIFFERENCE?

The study of resilience ultimately has a practical goal, to inform efforts to change the odds in favor of positive adaptation and development. From its inception, resilience research has been driven by this broad question: What makes a difference for children whose lives are threatened by disadvantage or adversity? The pioneers believed that understanding resilience processes—how it is that some children successfully overcome severe life challenges to grow up competent and well-adjusted—would provide important strategies for intervening to prevent or ameliorate the effects of adversity on child development and well-being. The first step on the road to understanding resilience was to identify the differences between those who made it and those who did not, searching for clues to what matters. There are a number of ways to do this, but the simplest is to compare people from the same background or with the same risk factors who turn out very differently. These groups often differ in ways that suggest adaptive processes at work.

The characteristics that distinguish resilient from maladaptive children and youth—differences in the children, their families, their relationships, or other aspects of their lives—are so consistent across diverse studies worldwide that it is possible to compile a "short list" of commonly observed resilience factors (described in Chapter 6). These factors, including individual, family, and community qualities, are generally associated with better outcomes among young people who have experienced adversity. This list has important implications for uncovering adaptive processes that explain much of the resilience observed across diverse people and situations. At the same time, these general protections would not be expected to account for all cases of observed resilience. Undoubtedly, there are circumstances when unique configurations of individual risks and protections combine in a particular instance to yield resilience.

THE ORGANIZATION OF THIS BOOK

In the next chapter, I describe key models of risk and resilience that have guided research on resilience in human development. Part II of the book provides a concise overview of key evidence about resilience in children and youth, highlighted with case and research examples. It is not an exhaustive review that would require multiple volumes, but rather provides an overview of three major kinds of resilience studies with illustrative research examples. In these chapters, I selectively review literature on resilience in children exposed to common negative life events, poverty and homelessness, and disaster and war, focusing on illustrative findings from my own and related studies of children exposed to both common and extraordinary adversities. In Part III, I describe the short list of factors implicated in resilience research and discuss what these factors suggest about the adaptive systems and processes behind resilience. Additional chapters in this section further discuss research on resilience from the perspective of multiple levels of analysis. One chapter examines the emerging neurobiology of resilience. Additional chapters consider resilience in relation to three important contexts of development: families, schools, and culture. Part IV summarizes the implications and lessons of research on resilience, both for efforts to promote resilience in practice and policy and also for future research. In Chapter 11, I present a resilience framework and guidelines for practice and policy that aim to promote positive adaptation and development in children at risk due to adversity or disadvantage. The concluding chapter summarizes the lessons learned to date about resilience in development and also discusses enduring controversies in resilience science as well as new research horizons. Resilience models and research are just beginning to encompass exciting advances in the neurobiological sciences. At the same time, investigators are beginning to test resilience theories about specific protective processes through intervention experiments aiming to create resilience and alter the course of human development in more positive directions. A glossary of terminology as used in this book can be found in Appendix A.

This book is focused on the development of individual resilience, rather than the resilience of larger systems, such as family or community resilience, though clearly the resilience of the systems in which the lives of children are embedded influence the resilience of the children connected to these systems. Thus, I do address the roles of families, schools, communities, and culture in the resilience of individual young people. This book also focuses on resilience in the early decades of life, from childhood into early adulthood, when foundations for resilience are established. There is growing interest and research on resilience in adulthood, but much of the initial research was focused on the years from birth to maturity, rather than adult development or aging. Resilience in the middle and late years of life is a rapidly growing area of research (see Hayslip & Smith, 2012; Reich, Zautra, & Hall, 2010). I give special attention to developmental transitions (e.g., into school, into adolescence, into adulthood), because these are crucial windows of vulnerability and opportunity for children at risk. I also discuss late bloomers, who shift developmental direction dramatically in the transition to adulthood.

The thesis of this book is a simple one: Resilience arises from "ordinary magic" and it is possible to understand where it comes from and how to foster it. However, this does not mean that resilience is a simple phenomenon. Human adaptation and development are highly complex and the worlds in which children grow up are diverse and ever changing. As a result, the path to understanding resilience is not an easy journey. Nonetheless, there is progress. Moreover, there are children who cannot wait for scientists to understand the whole story. The purpose of this book is to consider what we know now that could guide efforts to help children unlikely to make it on their own.

CHAPTER 2

MODELS OF RESILIENCE

The systematic study of resilience required models, measures, and strategies of analysis. Resilience research has taken many forms as investigators attempted to understand naturally occurring resilience and to mobilize resilience in intervention studies. These diverse approaches can be categorized into two distinct groups and a hybrid group, each encompassing a variety of analytical models (Masten, 2001). *Person-focused studies* are characterized by the identification of individuals who have a life history suggesting resilience. Their lives are examined for clues to the resources or protective processes that may account for their manifested resilience. The person-focused approach includes single-case studies and aggregated-case studies of passively observed resilience, studies of individuals as they change or respond over time, and research on interventions to produce resilience among individuals at risk for serious adaptation problems. *Variable-focused studies* are characterized by empirical efforts to examine and statistically test patterns among variables in groups of individuals, linking measured characteristics of people, their relationships, and their environments with their experiences, again with the goal of identifying what matters for resilience and how it works. Variable-focused approaches usually test models linking threats to specific outcomes of interest, taking into account potentially influential attributes or processes in the person, his or her relationships, resources, or interactions with the environment that could account for differential outcomes. More recently, with the advent of sophisticated statistical tools to study similarities in the patterns that individuals show in function over time, hybrid approaches have emerged that combine features of person- and variable-focused methods.

Each of these approaches to resilience has strengths and limitations (Luthar, 2006; Masten, 2001). Person-focused studies provide powerful and compelling case examples of resilience and capture the configural nature of resilience, in keeping with the commonsense perspective that the whole person must be adaptive, in multiple ways, to be considered resilient, though not necessarily successful in equal measure across domains. A trauma survivor who succeeds at school or at work but abuses family members usually would not be described as resilient. Person-oriented approaches also respect the empirical evidence that key features of resilience or protections associated with resilience often co-occur in ways that do not appear to be random and may reflect the operation of complex systems of adaptation where the whole is greater than the sum of the parts or inseparable from the components or processes that constitute it.

Variable-focused strategies are better suited to testing specific processes or protective influences for particular aspects of adaptive functioning. Until recently, the statistical techniques available for testing resilience models favored the variable-focused approach, which relies on powerful and well-established, long-available multivariate techniques. Now, advances in person-oriented research and tools that address the complexity of human behavior in context have given rise to exciting new methods for person-centered analysis. These methods keep the whole person together in time and yet also allow for finer-grained analysis of what makes a difference when and for whom and utilize more of the information from individual variation that once gave the variable-focused approaches their statistical power (Bergman & Magnusson, 1997; Nagin, 1999).

PERSON-FOCUSED MODELS OF RESILIENCE

The Single Case

Often in the history of resilience science, investigators reported that they were motivated to study these phenomena because they were inspired by life stories of young people who overcame great adversity to succeed. The early resilience scientists were typically psychologists and psychiatrists studying children at risk (for maladaptation or mental health problems due to adversity or disadvantage) who became intrigued by such cases. One of those pioneers, Norman Garmezy (1982), was moved to write an article on "The Case for the Single Case," which lays out the heuristic value of single-case studies.

Most single-case accounts of resilience consist of biographical or autobiographical accounts that include an extraordinary variety of adversities endured and successes achieved by real people, with the rich complexity of human life detailed over time. Resilience as recounted in these profiles is rarely portrayed as a straight or simple road. In a series of autobiographies, beginning with *I Know Why the Caged Bird Sings* (1971), Maya Angelou tells the complex story of her down-and-up journey through life in luminous prose, growing up as an African American female in the United States, enduring abandonment, discrimination, rape, and poverty. Oprah Winfrey, among the most successful and influential people in the entertainment media of our time, similarly overcame a history of childhood deprivation and adversity. The story of a teenager's experiences during the Cambodian holocaust perpetrated by Pol Pot is told by JoAn Criddle (1998) in the book *To Destroy You Is No Loss*, the title referring to a slogan of the Khmer Rouge. This harrowing tale begins with the fall of Phnom Penh to the Khmer Rouge and chronicles 5 years in the life of Thida Butt Mam and her family as they try to survive the war and eventually escape to Thailand. Antwone Fisher's memoir *Finding Fish*, which inspired a popular film, tells the moving story of a child raised in institutions and foster care, suffering repeated losses and abuse, who turned his life around after he enlisted in the navy, aided by an effective therapist (Fisher & Rivas, 2001). *Homeless to Harvard*, a 2003 Lifetime Television movie, portrayed the story of Liz Murray, daughter of drug-abusing parents, destitute and orphaned by age 15, who won a *New York Times* scholarship to attend Harvard. Murray published her memoir *Breaking Night* in 2010 after her graduation from Harvard. Kidnap victim Elizabeth Smart recounted her story of 9 months in captivity, often living in rustic camps, repeatedly chained and raped, hungry, living in constant fear, before she was rescued (Smart & Stewart, 2013). Ten years after this traumatic experience, she also describes the reunion with her family, readjusting to life at home, and dealing with the later trial of her kidnappers. Smart is now married and heads a foundation she created to address issues of crimes against children.

Norman Garmezy, the pioneer who was my mentor, believed such cases held value both for illustrating the phenomenon of resilience and generating ideas for research. He enjoyed telling students about resilient individuals, some famous and others known only to a few. One of his favorite stories of spunky resilience was drawn from a 1978 local newspaper account of an 11-year-old girl who was abducted and locked inside the trunk of a car. The child, a big fan of the fictional detective Nancy Drew, kept her cool under terrifying circumstances and escaped by taking apart one of the car's taillights (Garmezy, 1982). He also enjoyed telling the story of a more famous girl in history whose father killed her mother and whose half-sister imprisoned her in the Tower of London. She was subsequently crowned Queen Elizabeth I.

Garmezy (1985) also wrote about the case of Vreni, the resilient daughter of a patient treated by Manfred Bleuler, son of Eugen Bleuler, a founding father of psychiatry. Bleuler described Vreni as a "paradoxical case" in a 1984 chapter of a volume summarizing many of the early risk studies (Watt, Anthony, Wynne, & Rolf, 1984). Vreni endured a difficult childhood and adolescence with many responsibilities related to caring for her younger siblings and her substance-abusing and unhealthy parents. Bleuler stayed in touch with her as she became a happy, healthy wife and mother. According to Bleuler, Vreni did not possess special talents; he believed that she was called to fulfill responsibilities that she felt were important, found enjoyable, and was able to do well.

In 2003, reading the alumni magazine of the University of Minnesota, I learned about the life story of Michael Maddaus (Broderick, 2003). Mike endured a childhood in a chaotic family marked by alcoholism and violence, headed down a delinquent road in adolescence, and grew up to be a highly successful surgeon. Dr. Maddaus represents a classic case of a "late bloomer." He turned his life around in the transition to adulthood, during a period of development that may offer a window of opportunity for the emergence of resilience in young people whose lives are offtrack (Masten, Obradović, & Burt, 2006). During emerging adulthood, new planning capacity, motivation, and orientation to the future emerge in many young people, in conjunction with late-maturing aspects of brain development and function. These capabilities coincide with opportunities that many societies provide during this age period to scaffold positive growth in the transition to adulthood, including military service, advanced schooling or technical training, and the legal freedom to move and direct one's own life (Masten, Obradović, et al., 2006; Masten et al., 2004).

Maddaus began to realize in his late teens that he needed to change his life, which is consistent with the accounts of other late bloomers and also consistent with the maturing of self-reflection skills that accompany brain development during these years. He joined the military and after an honorable discharge took advantage of the GI Bill to return to school. Subsequently, mentors encouraged him to go into medicine. However, his path from juvenile delinquent to physician was not a smooth or straight one. He describes military service as one of several major steps in the right direction, yet he continued to have occasional problems and setbacks. Not long after he left the military, Maddaus had a car accident while driving drunk. Waking up on a gurney in the emergency room, he resolved to head down a new road.

Despite the bumps along the way, the Maddaus story is a compelling tale of resilience. With the goal of inspiring others, he has chosen to share his story with different groups of young people, including teenagers headed down dangerous roads and young physicians setting out on the road to a surgery career. Maddaus's story was featured in the PBS Nova program, *This Emotional Life*, shown on public television in 2010.

More recently, Mike's life has taken new turns, including major stumbles. It is evident to him and to me as he recounts his life story, through the ups and downs, that his capacity for resilience persists but fluctuates. He also may have vulnerabilities that date back to experiences in his childhood. As his life illustrates, resilience does not mean invulnerability or smooth sailing through life. Maddaus continues to share his life story with young people, sharing the mistakes and struggles along with the successes and triumphs. Not long ago, he visited one of my large undergraduate classes to speak. The students were fascinated by his journey and his honesty in recounting the highs and the lows of his life. When asked to write about the protective influences that might account for his past and future resilience, they identified his intelligence, ability to connect with people, determination, key mentors, opportunities, and optimism.

It is interesting to consider the significance to individuals of "sharing the story" of resilience, whether in motivational talks to young audiences or in art forms, such as books, paintings, or film. This kind of sharing appears to be a potentially transformative or therapeutic form of gaining some control or mastery over traumatic experiences.

In the biography of Thida Butt Mam by JoAn Criddle (1998), there is a vivid passage where this survivor of the Khmer Rouge reached a turning point from despair to hope in the dark days when Pol Pot ruled Cambodia. After one of her teenage friends in the work camp disappeared, she and her friends learned that the girl had been raped to death. Thida Butt Mam described to Criddle how they lived in terror of the same thing happening again and vowed to kill themselves rather than become victims. She became depressed, with a sense of impending doom. She and her friends began to carry poison: "I felt dead inside, and found myself fingering the little bottle several times a day" (p. 156). The following passage describes the epiphany that ensued, as this young girl realized that the brutal soldiers of the Khmer Rouge did not control everything that happened in the world. Angka Loeu in this passage refers to the supreme leadership of the Khmer Rouge.

> Then, unexpectedly, on my way to the rice fields one morning, I glanced up, just as the sun rose over the paddies. The sheer beauty of heavy ripening rice silhouetted against the glorious orange sky took my breath away. A massive, plodding buffalo moved across the scene, giving a sense of the continuity of life from former times to now—an instant lesson in patience and perseverance. All nature affirmed that some things were beyond Angka Loeu's power to control. Neither sunrise nor storm, neither cloud nor wind nor bamboo, nor I, would be controlled by Angka. Angka Loeu was not omnipotent. I felt—for the first time in months—that life might still hold something worthwhile. (pp. 156–157; reprinted by permission of JoAn D. Criddle)

Viktor E. Frankl, in *Man's Search for Meaning*, also described the intense appreciation of natural beauty shared among prisoners in a concentration camp as they clung to life:

> One evening, when we were already resting on the floor of our hut, dead tired, soup bowls in hand, a fellow prisoner rushed in and asked us to run out to the assembly grounds and see the wonderful sunset. Standing outside we saw sinister clouds glowing in the west and the whole sky alive with clouds of ever-changing shapes and colors, from steel blue to blood red. The desolate grey mud huts provided a sharp contrast, while the puddles on the muddy ground reflected the glowing sky. Then, after minutes of moving silence, one prisoner said to another, "How beautiful the world *could* be." (2006, p. 40; copyright ©1959, 1962, 1984, 1992 by Viktor E. Frankl. Reprinted by permission of Beacon Press, Boston and Penguin Random House, London)

In contrast to the many anecdotal accounts of resilience, there are only a few case studies of individual resilience published in scientific journals. The case of "Sara" (a pseudonym) provides one example (Masten & O'Connor, 1989). Sara was hospitalized at the age of 30 months in total growth failure, after her height, weight, and head circumference fell below the second percentile. She was admitted for a comprehensive assessment and disposition planning for her future. The presenting question for this case was whether Sara should be adopted or institutionalized, a profound charge for the evaluation team. It was quickly apparent that Sara had experienced traumatic losses followed by an unsuitable foster care placement. Sara's biological mother was mentally ill and frequently homeless and Sara was taken into protective custody the day after she was born. Her records indicated normal growth and development her first year, with problems arising early in her second year following the death of her foster father. At age 15 months, at the request of her grieving and overwhelmed foster mother, Sara was abruptly moved to a new foster home. She was picked up by a stranger and brought to a new home to live with more strangers. For a child of this age, these events constituted a major calamity. Adding to the trauma, the second home was not well suited to the needs of this devastated toddler. Sara responded with profound developmental regression: she stopped talking, walking, and reportedly sat in the window crying and waiting for her parents to come get her. Soon her pediatrician was worried about her growth rate, which slowed dramatically. Over the following year, she barely grew at all, and a decision was finally made to hospitalize her for assessment. It was clear to the assessment team that Sara's life had reached a crossroads, where life-altering decisions would be made on her behalf. After a month of diagnostic observation and stimulating age-appropriate interactions in a therapeutic environment, the interdisciplinary team made their recommendation. Concluding that Sara's growth and other developmental problems were not caused by a medical disorder; the team recommended adoption by a family well matched to her needs.

Sara's evaluation team had the rare opportunity to prescribe a new environment for a child in the hope of producing resilience. They believed that "tender loving care" was the core requirement, but careful thought went into the team's "family prescription" for Sara. A motivated social worker found an ideal family to fill the prescription: they were very stable, with two older children and an optimistic attitude about Sara's future. Sara moved from the hospital straight into this adopting home and over the following year, her development rebounded across all domains. Her physical growth was the easiest to document (shown in Figure 2.1) and she was soon back on a normal developmental trajectory.

There was a formal follow-up assessment when Sara was 6 years old, with assessments on standardized instruments by professionals blind to her history. Though there were some signs of vulnerability in the form of sad themes in her responses, Sara appeared to be flourishing in multiple domains. Her physical and cognitive development were normal, she was obviously happy in her family, and she was doing well in all the developmental tasks of her age, at school and with friends.

The Limitations of Single-Case Studies

Single-case reports, no matter how compelling, always raise questions about generalizability. Certainly, there are familiar themes across single-case examples that suggest clues to what may make a difference, such as the presence of competent and caring adults, door-opening opportunities, a talent for figuring things out, an appealing personality, resolution to survive, or hope for the future. Yet it is impossible to know whether the individual case or the particular situation is unique. Thus, investigators have turned to the power of numbers in the search for clues to resilience, aggregating cases into larger groups that are likely to be more representative of larger populations and that also make it possible to test hypotheses about resilience.

Aggregated Cases

There are several person-focused models of resilience that group people together to examine what accounts for those who manifest resilience in comparison to those who flounder or those who never experience significant adversity. The *classic model* of resilience begins with a sample of people known to have high risk for some reason; they have experienced adversities severe enough to

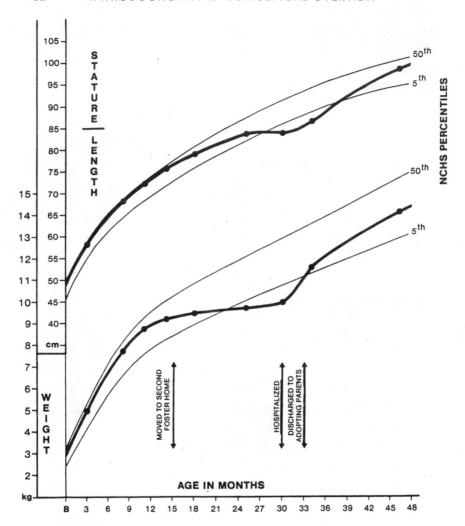

FIGURE 2.1. Growth chart from the case report on "Sara" showing a marked slowdown in growth following the death of her first foster father and abrupt separation at age 15 months from her first foster mother, with dramatic recovery following adoption by a family well matched to her needs. From Masten and O'Connor (1989, p. 276). Copyright 1989, published by Lippincott Williams & Wilkins. Reprinted with permission from Elsevier.

derail development or have one or more risk factors associated with maladaptive development. Then a subgroup of people who are doing well or "okay" on the outcome(s) of interest is identified within the risk group (see Figure 2.2). The resilient subgroup can be compared with the rest of the risk group to search for clues to their resilience.

One of the most important examples to date of a classic person-focused approach is provided by the Kauai Longitudinal Study of resilience (Werner, 1993; Werner & Smith, 1982, 1992, 2001). The Kauai study comprised a birth cohort (initially 698 babies) born in 1955 on the Hawaiian island of Kauai and followed over time. This study initially focused on vulnerability and risk, but became a study of resilience when the investigators shifted their attention to understanding how some of the highest-risk children were flourishing. In their landmark 1982 volume *Vulnerable but Invincible: A Study of Resilient Children*, Werner and Smith highlighted the differences between two subgroups of children classified as high in risk based on cumulative risk score tabulating biological and environmental risks present before age 2. These included the risk factors of being born into poverty, chronic family discord, parental mental or physical illness, and moderate to severe perinatal stress. About one third (201) of the surviving children in this birth cohort were classified as high risk due to scores of 4 or more on this risk index. The majority of children in this high-risk

High-Risk Group

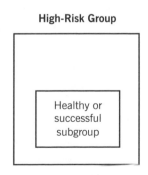

Healthy or successful subgroup

FIGURE 2.2. Classic aggregated case model of resilience: identifying members of a high-risk group who are doing well.

group (about two-thirds) had developed significant problems by ages 10 or 18. However, one-third (72 children) appeared to be doing well at the time of initial classification in many of the developmental tasks commonly assessed as criteria for adjustment. They were successful in school, socially competent, law-abiding, engaged in the community, and mentally healthy.

These two groups, the resilient and the troubled, were compared on a host of variables that had been collected over the years in this longitudinal study. These comparisons revealed many differences, beginning early in life and persisting between the children who would manifest resilience as they grew up and those who would not. There appeared to be many promotive and protective influences along the way: higher-quality caregiving from early in childhood; more positive and supportive relationships with relatives, teachers, and other mentors; better cognitive skills and appealing personalities; greater self-efficacy, optimism, and motivation to succeed; and, as they grew older, more faith and religious connections.

When the cohort was followed up in adulthood (around age 32), the youth originally classified as resilient generally continued to thrive. In addition, a substantial portion of the high-risk youth (particularly the troubled teenage girls) had "staged a recovery" (Werner & Smith, 1992, p. 193), with their lives showing marked changes for the better. Werner (1993) attributed the change in these late bloomers to an "opening of opportunities" afforded in the transition to adulthood by higher education, work opportunities, military service, positive/stable romantic relationships or marriages, or active involvement in a religious community.

The classic model of resilience is focused on a group of people who all have been exposed to one or more factors known to pose significant risks to adaptation or development. Researchers examine differences between the subgroup that does well on the outcome(s) of interest and the subgroup that does not do well. If a researcher finds a difference on some factor, however, it will not be clear whether this factor is important only when risk is high or is generally associated with better outcomes regardless of risk status, because the range on risk is restricted to high-risk individuals. To address this issue, a variation on the classic model added low-risk groups to the comparison (e.g., Masten et al., 1999).

The *expanded classic model* classifies groups according to both risk/adversity and adjustment/adaptation. Groups are formed by cross-classifying people into categories of risk (e.g., high, medium/ mixed, or low on a criterion of risk or adversity) and adaptation (e.g., good, medium/mixed, or poor on the criterion for desired outcome). The addition of low-risk groups makes it possible to compare resilient people with people who are doing just as well by the relevant outcome criteria but who have not experienced high risk or adversity. It is also possible to consider people who are not doing well, even though they were not exposed to the risk, a situation that suggests great vulnerability or a non-normal individual. Adding low-risk people into the analysis provides the means to distinguish protective factors or influences that either operate only during threat or become especially important under risky conditions from influences that are good for nearly everyone no matter what the life circumstances. Children with good parents or quick-learning brains may have the developmental edge on many outcomes, regardless of adversity or risk exposure. Nonetheless, there may be certain adaptive tools or advantages that matter only under risky conditions or that matter much more than usual when adversity is high.

The Project Competence Longitudinal Study has included person- as well as variable-focused strategies (Masten & Tellegen, 2012; see Chapter 3). An extended classic model was used in the person-centered analyses, in which the cohort was classified according to their cumulative adversity exposure and their competence in multiple domains of age-salient developmental tasks. The categories are shown in Figure 2.3. Comparative analyses focused on testing differences among the low-risk competent, the high-risk resilient, and the high-risk maladaptive groups (findings are discussed in the next chapter). The low-risk maladaptive group proved to be so small in a normative school cohort that it could not be analyzed statistically. This nearly "empty cell" has been observed in other studies and we believe it signifies an evolution-based bias toward adaptive functioning (Masten et al.,

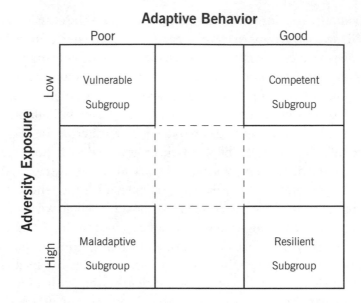

FIGURE 2.3. Expanded classic aggregated case model of resilience: identifying low-risk as well as high-risk subgroups of individuals based on their function on one or more criteria of adaptive function, typically using cutoff scores. Mixed or middle levels of adversity and/or adaptive functioning often are excluded to compare relatively pure or strongly contrasting subgroups (i.e., the four corner subgroups in the figure).

1999). There are not many people who do poorly in life without exposure to risks and adversities. Humans are equipped through biological and cultural evolution to adapt reasonably well under usual conditions. Doing poorly under benign conditions suggests that the individual is unusual in some way, perhaps not equipped for the usual challenges of human development. Of course, it is also possible that there are unknown, unmeasured, or hidden adversities in this group.

Updated Classic: Resilient Trajectories

With the emergence of statistical methods to study patterns of growth and change over time within individuals (Bergman & Magnusson, 1997; Fitzmaurice, Laird, & Ware, 2004; Grimm,

Ram, & Hamagami, 2011; Nagin, 1999), the classic model of resilience has been updated to accommodate individual differences in growth over time. For example, it is feasible to examine individual patterns of behavior over time in a group of individuals who share a common risk factor, such as homelessness. As an example, Figure 2.4 shows achievement test scores for individual second graders in a school district who were identified by federal guidelines as "homeless or highly mobile" (HHM; see Obradović et al., 2009). Most of these children were identified as HHM when they

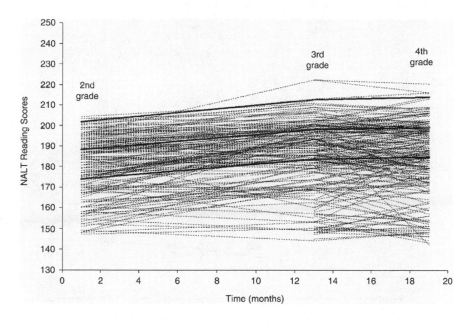

FIGURE 2.4. Sample of observed individual reading scores on a standardized test in a cohort of children identified as homeless or highly mobile (HHM) by federal guidelines, tested in the spring of second and third grade and again in the fall of fourth grade in an urban school district. The national mean on the test and one standard deviation above and below this mean are shown by solid lines to approximate the "average" range on the test. Although the average score of HHM children is substantially below the mean on the test and well below their more advantaged classmates, with numerous individuals having very low scores (in the bottom 5% on the test), many homeless children nonetheless show reading levels and growth over time in the average range. From Obradović et al. (2009, p. 511). Reprinted with permission from Cambridge University Press.

entered a family emergency shelter. Individual scores on a widely used and nationally normed test are shown for three test points over time in second to fourth grade. The national average and average range on this test are indicated by solid lines. One could classify the children who consistently maintain test scores near or above the national average over time as a "resilient group" and compare them with homeless children who clearly are struggling over time. With appropriate data, one could use multiple criteria to classify the resilient group, such as patterns of good conduct in the classroom as well as good academic achievement.

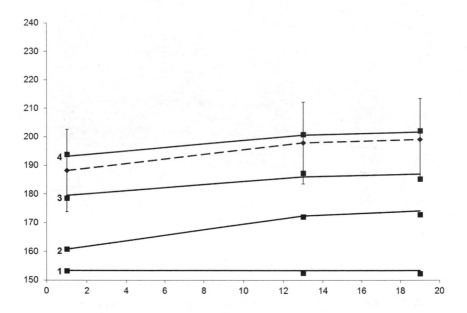

FIGURE 2.5. Four trajectories of reading achievement empirically derived from the reading scores of the same cohort of individuals plotted in Figure 2.4, using semiparametric mixture modeling (PROC TRAJ of SAS version 9.1; Jones, Nagin, & Roeder, 2001; Nagin, 1999). The dashed line represents the national mean on the test, with brackets representing one standard deviation above or below this national average. Data suggested four trajectories for the HHM students: (1) an extremely maladaptive group with no observable improvement in reading over time, (2) a maladaptive but improving group, (3) a low-resilient group, and (4) a high-resilient group. Reproduced with permission from Jelena Obradović.

It is also possible to empirically identify subgroups in such data of individuals who follow similar trajectories, using methods developed by Nagin (1999). Figure 2.5 shows trajectory patterns extracted from the data in the same cohort of HHM second graders. The analysis suggested there were four groups, including a higher-resilient group, a lower-resilient group, a maladaptive but improving group, and a persistently maladaptive group. Similarities and differences among these groups could be compared. However, schools do not routinely collect data on the kind of differences that intrigue most resilience researchers, such as parent involvement, motivation to learn, or connections to competent and caring adults. Moreover, children who share the risk factor of homeless status also may differ dramatically in other life experiences. It is likely that the children grouped together in a broad risk category have had different life experiences that might explain why some are doing better than others. Some homeless children have experienced maltreatment or malnutrition, while others have not. Models designed to explain individual trajectories by variables that measure exposure to risks or adversities, as well as resources and potential protective factors, offer a blend of person- and variable-centered approaches that is discussed at the end of this chapter. More clues to risk and resilience in homeless children are discussed in Chapter 4.

VARIABLE-FOCUSED MODELS OF RESILIENCE

Resilience research in human development is fundamentally concerned with variation in the lives of people and the processes that explain patterns of adaptation in the context of experiences that threaten development in different ways. Capitalizing on the power of multivariate statistics, variable-focused methods and models ultimately aim to understand patterns in variation, the processes that may account for covariation, and what covariation may signify for predicting the future or for designing interventions. The striking variation observed by resilience research pioneers in the lives of children at risk for mental disorders inspired subsequent generations of work to identify the correlates and predictors of child outcomes and then to understand the underlying causes of good versus poor adaptation in the context of varying risk. Important models emerged from this effort, initially to describe naturally occurring resilience and later to describe intervention designs. Basic variable-focused models of risk and resilience are described in this section; intervention models are described in Chapter 11.

Risk and Asset Gradients

Early in the history of resilience research investigators recognized that risk often varied along a continuum, whether the risk measure was a single variable of SES, a cumulative count of risk factors in a child's life, or a composite score from a measure of life events. Sameroff (2006) chronicled the history of such risk scores in the medical and social sciences dating back to the Framingham heart study. In this famous study of risk for heart disease, the investigators concluded that no single risk factor was important for everyone, but rather that it was a composite of varying risk factors that predicted heart problems. In a series of articles, Sameroff and his colleagues have shown that psychosocial risk factors for behavioral outcomes work in a similar way (Sameroff, 2006; Sameroff, Seifer, Barocas, Zax, & Greenspan, 1987). Investigators using this approach typically have counted the number of risk factors present from a set of factors with well-established links to the outcome of interest. Common risk factors included child status indicators (such as minority racial/ethnic status), parent factors (lacking a high school diploma, young age of mother at first child's birth, mental illness, substance use, criminality), family factors (single-parent household, crowded household, welfare status, homelessness), and neighborhood factors (high crime, high poverty). When the outcome variable (e.g., behavior problems, symptoms, school achievement, child IQ score) was plotted as a function of the cumulative risk variable, a *risk gradient* often emerged, reflecting the association between the composite risk variable and the outcome variable. The average level of problems rose as risk level increased or, in the case of a positive outcome, the average level of competence fell as risk level rose. A simple risk gradient is illustrated in Figure 2.6.

There are numerous examples of risk gradients across different areas of research in the social and health sciences. "Dose gradients" have been widely observed in the literature on disaster and trauma (see Chapter 5), indicating that the risk for stress reactions and disorders generally rises as exposure severity increases (Masten & Narayan, 2012). Similarly, research on the linkage of SES or poverty to health has repeatedly revealed "SES gradients," where the risk of mortality or morbidity is related to the degree of socioeconomic disadvantage (Adler & Ostrove, 2006; see Chapter 4).

The association of cumulative risk or adversity and positive adaptation or health need not be linear. Indeed, there are data suggesting exponential effects and asymptotic effects. Rutter (1979), for instance, published an often-cited example linking aggregated

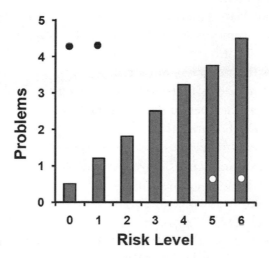

FIGURE 2.6. Risk gradient illustrating a general linear rise in the average level of problems as a function of higher risk level or exposure to trauma or adversities. White dots represent individuals who are doing much better than average for a given level of risk (suggesting resilience) and black dots represent individuals who are doing much worse than average for a given level of risk (suggesting vulnerability). From Masten and Narayan (2012, p. 236). Copyright 2012. Reprinted with permission from *Annual Reviews.*

family risk to child psychiatric symptoms where problems in the child appeared to jump substantially when a combination of any four or more risk factors were present. More recently, in studies of children exposed to extreme trauma, such as war atrocities, there is evidence suggesting ceiling effects—where a level of exposure effects is reached beyond which additional trauma does not increase symptoms (Masten & Narayan, 2012).

Graphs linking cumulative risk to outcomes can be compelling in showing the overall association of cumulative risk with child problems or competence. However, two key points pertinent to resilience are obscured by such gradients. First, the risk variable is likely to represent assets or resources as well as risk. As noted in Chapter 1, many "risk" scores are arbitrarily labeled negatively, while in reality many risk variables are continuous in nature, with low scores reflecting more assets or resources and high scores reflecting both low resources and high risk. There are two reasons for this. One is that many so-called risk factors for child outcomes are actually dimensional in nature, varying along a continuum from positive to negative poles (high to low income or parental education, good to poor parent function), hence a high score means that one has more risk but also less of a key asset. The second reason is that risk factors (even those that are only negative when they occur, such as traumatic life events) tend to co-occur not only with other risk factors but also with reduced resources. Low-income children are exposed to more environmental hazards and tend to have less-educated parents and fewer community resources (Kiernan & Mensah, 2011; Luthar, 1999; McLoyd, 1998). Many risk gradients could be inverted and labeled as "asset gradients."

Investigators at the Search Institute in Minneapolis, Minnesota, have generated asset gradients based on a measure they developed for large community surveys, which includes 40 "Developmental Assets" for youth (e.g., Scales, Benson, Leffert, & Blyth, 2000; Scales, Benson, Roehlkepartain, Sesma, & van Dulmen, 2006). The 40 assets include individual, family, and community resources that can be counted (e.g., "Young person is motivated to do well in school" or "Family life provides high levels of love and support"). When school achievement or alcohol problems are plotted as a function of such assets, striking gradients are observed. Achievement rises and problems fall as a function of the sum of assets. Many of the variables that Search Institute investigators term assets could be viewed as inverted risk factors (e.g., "Young person is unmotivated to do well in school" or "Family life provides high levels of rejection and hostility"). The Developmental Assets measure focuses on the positive side of many variables that could be viewed either way and therefore yields asset gradients that could reflect the opposite of risk gradients, a point readily acknowledged by this group (Benson, Scales, Hamilton, & Sesma, 2006; Sesma, Mannes, & Scales, 2013). Their positive focus on assets emphasizes the importance of the presence of positive resources in the lives of youth, in part with the goal of motivating communities to engage in asset building as a strategy for promoting positive development in youth.

The second key aspect of resilience obscured in risk gradients is the variation in function of children at each risk level. Gradients reflect statistical averages or estimates across a group of individuals. If one plots each person on the graph in a scatter plot, then the variation becomes salient. One of the important contributions of resilience pioneers was recognizing this variability and its significance. Even at high levels of risk, they noticed children who were doing better than expected, or "off-gradient" children. Similarly, there can be children who are doing much worse than expected for their risk level. The outcomes of such children are not predicted very well by their risk scores. Some part of the story is missing. The white and black dots in Figure 2.6 illustrate individuals who are off the risk gradient, doing better (white dots) or worse (black dots) than expected for the level of risk There are a number of explanations for off-gradient children. True risk on the measured risk variable may not have been measured accurately, or an important risk factor may have been left out of the risk assessment. But other factors may play a role. Resilience investigators are particularly interested in factors that may compensate for risk or moderate its effects because these variables have implications for intervention. The basic resilience models described in the next section attempt to account for more of the story than risk and outcome variables alone can offer.

Resilience Models Linking Risks, Assets, Mediators, Moderators, and Outcomes

What could explain the variation in outcome among children exposed to risk at varying levels? Resilience models were developed to address this question, to organize and link variables in an effort to advance understanding of resilience (see Garmezy, Masten, & Tellegen, 1984; Luthar et al., 2000; Luthar, Shoum, & Brown, 2006; Masten, 2001, 2013b). These models represent basic theoretical frameworks and also research designs for testing hypotheses. Each of these models also serves as a guide to intervention, discussed further in Chapter 11.

Compensatory or Main Effect Models

The most basic model of resilience includes some combination of risks and assets that contribute directly to positive outcomes, as shown in Figure 2.7. The risk factor here could be a negative experience (e.g., child abuse) and the asset could be a talent (e.g., musical or artistic) or resource that is positive when it is present in some degree. The bipolar variable represents a dimensional variable, such as attention skills or parenting quality, that is distributed along a

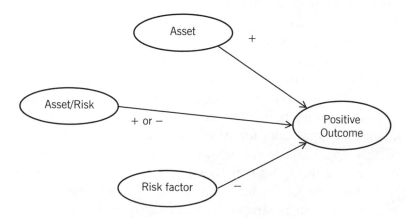

FIGURE 2.7. Compensatory (main effects) model of resilience showing direct effects of a risk factor (negative influence), an asset or resource (positive influence), and a bipolar variable (positive or negative influence along a continuum) on a positive outcome of interest.

continuum and predicts a particular child outcome (e.g., reading achievement). Interventions related to this model include preventing the risk factor from occurring (e.g., preventing child abuse), adding assets that may compensate for the presence of risk (e.g., adding a reading tutor), or shifting the continuous variable toward the positive end (e.g., improving attention skills or parenting).

Mediator Models

There was good reason to believe early in the study of risk that some kinds of adversity damaged the lives of children *indirectly*, through their effects on key assets in a child's life. Figure 2.8 illustrates a mediating effect of this kind. A classic example of risk mediation is provided by the studies of Iowa farm families that were affected by the economic crisis in the latter part of the 20th century. In their research program, Rand Conger, Glen Elder, and their colleagues tested mediating models, whereby economic hardship affected the parents in the family (via alterations in mood and marriage quality) that in turn was hypothesized to undermine effective parenting and lead to increased problems among their adolescent children (Conger & Conger, 2002; Elder & Conger, 2000). Cross-sectional and longitudinal results supported their ideas that the farm crisis affected adolescents in part indirectly, through such effects on their parents. Work conflicts or bereavement in parents could have similar spillover effects on children, by undermining parenting quality. Interventions conceptualized in a mediational model are designed to shore up or

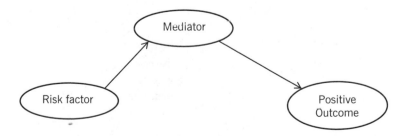

FIGURE 2.8. Mediator model showing an indirect negative effect of a risk factor on a positive outcome through its influence on a third variable.

protect the mediator if the risk factor cannot be prevented, for example, by providing support to parents in crisis. Investigators have tested the efficacy of interventions focused on parents and parenting to help children faced with divorce, bereavement, and other difficult family situations (Brody et al., 2006; Forgatch & DeGarmo, 1999; Patterson, Forgatch, & DeGarmo, 2010; Wolchik et al., 2002). Results of such work, discussed further in Chapters 8 and 11 of this book, corroborate the positive effects of supporting parents through such crises to protect child development.

Moderator Models

Resilience investigators also have been intrigued with the possibility of variables that serve to buffer, ameliorate, or in some other way protect children from the full effects of a potential risk factor or adversity. Two kinds of moderators are shown in Figure 2.9. One is a risk-activated protective factor, while the other reflects various potential moderators of risk that are not triggered by the threat but nonetheless alter the effects of a risk factor in either direction (worsening or ameliorating the impact of the threat).

The risk-activated moderator is analogous to an airbag (protective factor) in an automobile that is triggered by an accident (the risk factor) and reduces damage (moderates impact) to the

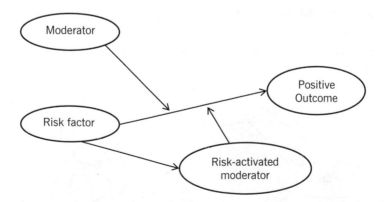

FIGURE 2.9. Model of moderated effects, one triggered by the threat itself (like antibodies or airbags) and the other not. Both moderators alter the impact of the risk factor on the outcome.

passenger in the car. Until there is an accident, the airbag has little or no influence on the individual (except perhaps affording peace of mind), thus there is little or no main effect at a low level of risk (when there is no accident or a very low-impact accident). Human antibodies operate in a similar fashion, having no role until the specific agent of harm (infection) is present. Emergency services are designed to function this way, including fire and rescue services, as well as child protection and crisis nurseries. Parents also may be said to function in this way if they take specific action to protect children in the presence of threat. For instance, a parent can step between an attacker and a child or mobilize help for a child. Vaccines are interventions designed on this model, boosting immunity of the host to a specific agent. Other kinds of interventions might focus on the availability of services or the efficiency of activation. One of the most effective risk-activated, "protective factor" interventions of the 20th century in the United States was the widespread adoption of 911 emergency services.

It is worth noting that protective systems can malfunction or fail, either because they don't deploy or function effectively when needed, they deploy when they are not needed (a danger of airbag systems), or they overreact in damaging ways. The immune system, for example, can go awry by failing to mount a sufficient response (suppression due to illness, medication side effects, etc.), by turning against the self (autoimmune disorders), or by overreacting (allergic reactions that can cascade to anaphylactic shock).

In contrast, the independent moderator alters the impact of the threat on outcome by its nature, but is not explicitly activated by threat. Individual differences in personality are construed to work this way, by moderating the effects of stressors and other experiences on outcomes. Some people are more stress reactive, while others are more easygoing when exposed to the same situation. Similarly, there are individual differences in sensitivity or susceptibility to experience at many levels, from genes to neural function. An analogy is provided by phenylketonuria (PKU), a gene-based susceptibility to the effects of phenylalanine in the diet, which can lead to mental retardation and other severe developmental problems. PKU is caused by inheriting a recessive gene from each parent. At some point, gene therapy may be feasible. At present, however, preventive intervention takes the form of testing for this genetic problem shortly after birth and then avoiding exposure to phenylalanine in susceptible individuals. More generally, in the case of independent moderators, interventions can be designed to prevent exposure, improve the fit of person to context, alter or counter a susceptibility to a risk factor, or change the moderator in a more favorable direction.

Research on the interplay of genes, biology, and experience in resilience and risk moderation has burgeoned in recent years. There is growing attention to the role of genes as moderators of environmental risk and experiences as moderators of expressed genotype, as well as the moderating roles of genes or experience on human stress regulation (Cicchetti, 2010, 2013; Kim-Cohen & Gold, 2009; Kim-Cohen & Turkewitz, 2012; Sapienza & Masten, 2011). These moderating effects all involve interactions across level of analysis, with a focus on integrating genetic and neurobiological processes into the science of resilience. There is emerging research on risk-potentiating and risk-mitigating genes, and also on sensitivity genes that appear to index greater susceptibility to experiences (good or bad). Highlights of recent work on the neurobiology of resilience are discussed in Chapter 7.

One of the most intriguing possibilities raised by recent research on risk moderators in children is the idea that greater susceptibility to stress could arise from exposure to severe adversity or "toxic stress" during early development, particularly during periods when individual differences in personality and self-regulation are forming. Investigators are particularly interested in the impact of adversity on the development and function of stress-response systems and cognitive-control systems (see Belsky & Pluess, 2009; Blair & Raver, 2012; Boyce, 2007; Boyce & Ellis, 2005; Gunnar & Vazquez, 2006; Loman & Gunnar, 2010; McEwen & Gianaros, 2011; Meaney, 2010; Obradović & Boyce, 2009; Shonkoff, 2011; Shonkoff, Boyce, & McEwen, 2009). In other words, a child who might have developed normal, healthy stress reactivity and good self-regulation skills in a benign rearing environment might develop maladaptive stress reactivity and poor regulatory skills in an adverse rearing environment. Subsequently, this experience-related combination could function to exacerbate the effects of exposure to adversity on child outcomes. If adversity experiences in children can exacerbate vulnerability to subsequent adversities, it becomes imperative to prevent these toxic stress exposures or to bolster capacity for responding effectively or both. This kind of research, discussed further in Chapter 11, is profoundly altering models of how resilience develops and how to promote it.

THE BEST OF BOTH WORLDS: PEOPLE AND VARIABLES

Resilience investigators often included multiple approaches in their studies in order to take advantage of the different strengths of various person- and variable-focused methods. Multiple methods also have been employed in a number of early resilience studies, including the Kauai Longitudinal Study (Werner & Smith, 1982, 1992, 2001), the Project Competence Longitudinal Study (Masten & Tellegen, 2012; see Chapter 3), the Rochester Child Resilience Studies (Cowen, Wyman, Work, & Parker, 1990; Wyman 2003), and Luthar's (1991) study of resilience among inner-city youth. More recently, elegant new approaches for combining the strengths of person- and variable-focused strategies have become available with the emergence of growth curve modeling and related strategies in the social sciences, particularly in developmental research (Grimm et al., 2011; Muthén & Muthén, 2000; Nagin, 1999). These methods have been uncommon in the study of resilience in the past, but hold great promise for future research focused on delineating and explicating different resilience pathways and trajectories among individuals studied over time.

SUMMARY

Research on resilience required models and analytical strategies. This chapter highlights some of the most influential approaches that emerged to guide the science described in this volume. Person-focused approaches consider similarities and differences among people who show resilience compared with those who experience similar adversities and who do not fare as well or those who show similarly positive outcomes but have experienced far less adversity. These contrasts often provide clues to resources or protective processes that may help to explain resilience. The most basic person-focused approach is a case study of a person viewed as resilient; case studies are often highly compelling but lack generalizability. Aggregated case studies move beyond the single case to identify and compare groups of individuals who show good or poor adaptation under high- or low-adversity conditions in an effort to learn about common rather than unique factors that may account for resilience.

Variable-focused methods examine patterns of variation among the characteristics of individuals—their experiences, relationships, and contexts—in search of consistencies that might explain how some people or families or other systems fare so much better than others in the context of risk or adversity. Multivariate statistical strategies can be used to test different models of direct, mediated, and moderating effects, reflecting hypothesized processes of risk or competence promotion, and vulnerability or protection. In theory, the effects of adversity can be counteracted or moderated (exacerbated or mitigated) by individual differences (e.g., in genes or cognitive abilities or personality); quality of relationships; socioeconomic, civic, or cultural resources and protections; and other influences that can be modeled in multivariate analyses.

Investigators also combine person- and variable-focused strategies to gain the benefits of both approaches, either by including both strategies or by using hybrid models. The Project Competence Longitudinal Study (Masten & Tellegen, 2012), discussed in the next chapter, combined both approaches. The advent of growth-modeling techniques has made it feasible to study variations among individuals or groups in the trajectories of intraindividual behavior or neurobiological function measured over time, looking for different patterns of positive or negative adaptation. Growth modeling requires longitudinal data with repeated measures. Examples of this approach are provided in subsequent chapters (especially Chapters 4 and 5).

PART II

STUDIES OF INDIVIDUAL RESILIENCE

CHAPTER 3

RESILIENCE IN A COMMUNITY SAMPLE

The Project Competence Longitudinal Study

The study of competence and resilience that evolved into the Project Competence Longitudinal Study (PCLS) began shortly after I began graduate studies in clinical psychology with Norman Garmezy at the University of Minnesota. I was drawn to Minnesota and the Project Competence research team by Garmezy's ideas and personality, intrigued by his interest in studying high-risk children who succeed. I met Garmezy while working at the National Institutes of Health as a young research assistant to his long-time colleague and friend David Shakow. Garmezy was an engaging scientist, renowned for his wit and warmth as well as his scholarship. When he visited, he told me about his plans to study the phenomenon of "stress-resistant" children who achieved competence despite adversity and recruited me to join his team when I applied to Minnesota for doctoral training in clinical psychology. In 1976, I set off for Minnesota, with little awareness that I was headed into an extraordinary convergence of people and ideas that would influence a generation of scholars concerned with the development of competence and psychopathology. Their ideas were transformative for theory and practice, giving rise to the integrative approach known as "developmental psychopathology," as well as research on resilience in the context of adversity or risk (Cicchetti, 2006; Masten, 2006a, 2007).

Garmezy's own career reflects the historical origins of resilience research. After serving in World War II, he studied competence in veterans while he was a graduate student at the University of Iowa (Garmezy & Crose, 1948). Subsequently, his early work at the Worcester State Hospital and later at Duke University with mentor Elliott Rodnick was focused on adults with schizophrenia, where he had a particular interest in what they termed "premorbid competence" (Garmezy & Rodnick, 1959). Clinicians and scientists studying serious mental disorders had observed that a positive life history prior to mental illness was related to better prognosis for recovery. Soon this group of investigators would begin searching for the origins of serious mental illness by use of the "high-risk" method. As noted above, it was too expensive to follow a general population to observe the emergence of psychopathology, so the risk investigators focused on identifying groups of individuals with elevated probabilities of mental illness. Eventually, a risk consortium formed to study groups of children believed to be at risk for developing psychopathology, aimed at discovering causal processes (Watt et al., 1984). Garmezy had a leading role in this group, and also began studies of high-risk children and youth with his own graduate students and colleagues after a move to the University of Minnesota. In the volume reporting on the results of studies from the risk consortium, it is noteworthy that the chapter on their work is called "Project Competence: The Minnesota Studies of Children Vulnerable to Psychopathology" (Garmezy & Devine, 1984).

In the research on children presumed to be at risk for psychopathology, including children with a family history of mental illness, poverty, or violence, and many other kinds of risk factors, Garmezy was impressed by the variable outcomes of individuals in the risk groups. With his history of interest in competence, Garmezy in particular was attending to positive as well as negative indicators of adaptation, particularly in terms of the life tasks of love, work, and play.

The revolutionary insight of the pioneers like Garmezy was in recognizing the significance of understanding positive adaptation, particularly in risky contexts, for both preventing or treating psychopathology and promoting competence or resilience. They observed variability in pathways of adaptation or development and realized that many important roads and clues for intervention had been left unexamined.

The design of the PCLS was influenced by Garmezy's own research history, and numerous collaborators and students at Minnesota, their colleagues in the nascent field of resilience, and also by the emergence of developmental psychopathology itself, especially at Minnesota (Masten & Tellegen, 2012). The most unique aspects of this study at the time it began were its focus on competence as well as adversity and the study of a normative (rather than high-risk) school-based sample.

In this chapter, I highlight concepts and findings from this study, which in multiple ways reflect the evolution, decisions, and issues confronted by many first-wave resilience researchers. The main findings of this study are highly congruent with other longitudinal studies of the first wave, and the conclusions continue to hold up surprisingly well.

CONCEPTUAL FRAMEWORK

The conceptual framework for this study evolved over time as did the design, often benefiting from theoretical or methodological advances as well as numerous interactions among investigators interested in resilience. The study began as a cross-sectional investigation of competence and adversity in a normative school population. With subsequent follow-ups of the participants, it became a long-term longitudinal study. Despite the normal evolution one might expect for any study that spans more than 20 years, many of the guiding principles and core concepts remained essentially the same. With benefit of hindsight, it is easy to see mistakes and wrong turns in this and other studies of the time. I hope that investigators looking back will appreciate the challenges we faced at the time, studying a complex topic like resilience with very little in the way of developed concepts and tools. These early studies were groundbreaking in the most laborious sense of this term.

Defining Resilience

The overarching goal of the Project Competence research over the years, like other early efforts to study resilience, was to understand the observable phenomenon of variation in the adaptation of individuals at risk for maladaptation. Resilience was conceptualized as an inferential concept, referring to positive adaptation in the context of risk or adversity. Because of Garmezy's long-term interest in competence, it is not surprising that this research team focused on the concept of competence for defining and measuring positive adaptation in their studies of resilience. In a 1971 paper, Garmezy described the "hallmarks of competence" in children and youth as follows: "good peer relations, academic achievement, and commitment to education and to purposive life goals, early and successful work histories" (p. 114). In the early planning for what would become the PCLS, resilience was conceptualized in terms of manifested competence despite exposure to stressful life experiences (Garmezy, 1981; Garmezy et al., 1984). The research team set out to operationalize and measure multiple domains of competence as well as exposure to stressful life experiences.

Garmezy and his early collaborators became intrigued with the observation of manifest competence among individuals in their "high-risk" studies. Garmezy and his colleagues also realized that little was known about the people who did well in such risk research, even though their lives might provide key insights for prevention or treatment. Clinical researchers at that time were preoccupied with a medical model that focused on measuring symptoms and treating psychopathology. Resilience in some of their studies was defined in terms of escaping mental illness or "not manifesting symptoms." Project Competence investigators were interested in the full range of adaptation, spanning psychopathology and competence, and they were early advocates of a positive definition of adaptation in resilience, defined by the

presence of good adaptation and not simply by the absence of psychopathology.

With respect to the other essential component of resilience, the concept of risk, the Project Competence investigators over the years have studied a wide range of potential threats to adaptation. Many traditional risk factors were included among the PCLS assessments, such as low maternal education. However, in defining and operationalizing resilience, the focus of the PCLS was on the concept of adversity or exposure to stressful life experiences in a normative, school-based sample of children. We assumed that adversity exposure would vary across the population and also change over time. By the time the study began, there also was growing recognition that risks and adversities tend to co-occur so that it was misleading to define risk in terms of a single risk factor.

How does adversity exposure vary in a normative group of urban school children? How is adversity related to competence? When children exposed to severe adversity manifest competence, how can we account for such resilience? These basic questions are typical "first-wave" questions in resilience science. To address these questions, the research team worked over the years to refine and measure the core components in resilience—the concepts of competence, adversity, and resources or protective factors—and to develop models and analytical strategies for testing the connections among these components for clues to adaptive processes in resilience. The next section summarizes the overall design of the PCLS, with a particular focus on how these core concepts were developed and operationalized.

OVERVIEW OF THE DESIGN

Participants

The design of the PCLS evolved from a larger study of competence and life events conducted in collaboration with the Minneapolis Public Schools. All families with third to sixth graders attending two schools in the same large catchment area were invited to complete a Life Events Questionnaire (LEQ; Masten et al., 1988), while at the same time, the competence of the children was assessed at school, based on academic data, teacher reports, and peer assessment methods. This was intended as a broad, preliminary survey of life events and how such events might be related to children's success at school. Data were obtained for up to 612 children attending those grades in school, including measures adapted specifically for this study, including the Revised Class Play (see Masten, Morison, & Pellegrini, 1985) and the LEQ. Some of these measures were repeated over time to ascertain the stability of the measures of life events and competence based on peer or teacher ratings (e.g., Masten et al., 1985).

When additional funding became available, we invited all families that had returned LEQs for the initial survey (59% of all the third to sixth graders who were sent these questionnaires) to join a more intensive study of competence and resilience. Willing families were subsequently interviewed multiple times in their homes and their children participated in a series of assessments spanning multiple school years. These participants became the core sample of the PCLS, followed up after 7, 10, and 20 years to date. The core sample of 205 children included 91 boys and 114 girls, with 26 sibling pairs. They were socioeconomically diverse, much like the large catchment area for the schools, predominantly lower-working to middle class but with some extremely poor families on welfare and some well-off professional families. On the Duncan Socioeconomic Index (Hauser & Featherman, 1977), this cohort had an average initial score of 43 (the level of skilled labor and clerical positions), with a range from 7 (e.g., household worker) to 92.3 (e.g., lawyer) on this 100-point scale. Also similar to the district at the time, the sample included 29% children of ethnic-minority heritage. The participants in the PCLS study had slightly lower competence and lower adversity scores than those who did not volunteer for this intensive study, which is typical of research volunteers for such studies. Their diversity is probably attributable to the considerable effort that was made to recruit a diverse sample, assess parents at their convenience at home, gain the support of the schools in sending out letters about the study, and employ the clinical skills of the recruiters and interviewers who visited multiple times with families.

Perhaps the most notable descriptive quality of this cohort was how normative they were on standardized assessments. For example, the mean score on the Peabody Individual Achievement Test (Dunn & Markwardt, 1970), which is standardized to have a mean score of 100, was 97. On this and numerous other measures over the years, this group of children and parents showed a "bell-curve" distribution around a normative mean with a considerable range. The normalcy and diversity of the sample undoubtedly was helpful for detecting meaningful covariation in the data. High-risk samples tend to have a more restricted range of scores, which can limit the power to detect important relations among indices of competence, adversity, and other attributes of the child, family, or environment that may be functioning as mediators or moderators in adaptive processes.

Also noteworthy are the complications deriving from the fact that the PCLS was not originally designed as a longitudinal study. The children of the PCLS were originally 8 to 12 years old, in third to sixth grades. They also were recruited in two waves (1977/1978 and 1978/1979 school years). Inevitably, during follow-up assessments, we waited for some cohort members to return from the military or get out of prison to complete assessments. Over time, the age range spanned 5 to 6 years. This created interesting issues for assessments and also some unique opportunities.

The participants in the PCLS have been remarkably involved over time, even though follow-ups were spaced years apart, including both the parents or guardians and the young people. For the 20-year follow-up, 90% of the original children chose to participate, along with a very high proportion of their parents. Their steadfastness has made it possible to study nearly 200 lives through time, which affords a much different perspective on resilience and the development of competence than any one-time snapshot could provide, no matter how finely detailed the single image may be.

Methods and Methodological Contributions

Describing all the measures of this study is beyond the scope of this chapter. Generally, we followed a multiple-method, multiple-informant approach. Like other early investigators, we often had to devote considerable time and effort to developing measures and methods because so little had been done to study resilience in a community population. Measures of competence and adversity suited to a community study often needed to be adapted, and the strategies for studying resilience were not well established. We forged ahead, learning from colleagues struggling with the same issues, hoping others would benefit from some of the groundwork we were forced to do. Some highlights follow.

Competence in Age-Salient Developmental Tasks

Competence for the PCLS was defined as follows: *a pattern of effective performance in the environment, evaluated from the perspective of salient developmental tasks in the context of late twentieth century U.S. society* (Masten et al., 1995). Our conceptual approach to competence was strongly influenced by developmental theory, as well as the decades of clinical research by Garmezy and colleagues on competence in relation to mental illness. The risk consortium included developmental scientists like Arnold Sameroff, who was a leading developmental theorist as well as a risk researcher. Garmezy also spent time learning from the scientists a block down the street at the Institute of Child Development, as did his students. One of those influential faculty was Professor Alan Sroufe.

The PCLS was strongly influenced by an organizational perspective on competence in development, particularly as articulated by Sroufe (1979) and a number of the students he mentored (Cicchetti & Schneider-Rosen, 1986; Ford, 1985; Sroufe, 1979; Sroufe, Egeland, Carlson, & Collins, 2005; Waters & Sroufe, 1983). This approach emphasized the coherence of behavior across development, organized around salient developmental issues. Fundamental in this perspective was the idea that successful engagement of changing developmental issues would establish the developmental tools needed to meet the challenges of the next era. Competence referred to how well one was developing the capacities to meet these successive challenges.

Our approach to competence represented a merger of two deeply rooted traditions concerned with adaptation and its measurement, one in clinical sciences centered around understanding mental illness or health, and the other in developmental sciences centered around differences across individuals and within individuals over time in adaptation to the environment (see Masten, Burt, et al., 2006). It is not a coincidence that our project emerged at the same time and in the same context as developmental psychopathology, which represents the convergence and integration of sciences, disciplines, and theories concerned with adaptation in development (Cicchetti, 1984, 2006; Masten, 2006a). One of the core principles of developmental psychopathology is the idea that psychopathology must be understood in relation to normative adaptation and development.

For each of the major assessments of the PCLS, we aimed to measure competence in developmentally appropriate ways, defined in terms of effective functioning in age-salient developmental tasks. At the outset of the study, when the children were around 8 to 12 years of age, we focused on assessments of academic achievement, getting along with peers, and rule-abiding versus rule-breaking conduct as the observable manifestations of competence in developmentally important tasks. We also assessed these domains of function in the two primary contexts of adaptation for this age, which were home and school, although we also gathered information about activities outside of home and school. Informants included parents, peers, teachers, and the individual children themselves.

We recognized that competence develops over time and that the expectations within particular developmental task domains change as children grow older and more capable. Developmental tasks themselves develop and change over time (see McCormick et al., 2011). Thus, while the domain of peer competence remains important as children become adolescents, the nature of expected behavior changes and the measures of peer competence also need to change. Social competence in adolescents required evidence that there were deeper, reciprocated friendships. A new aspect of social competence also is beginning to emerge in the form of romantic relationships. Similarly, while academic performance remains important, the academic demands of secondary school are greater than elementary school. A new domain of work competence also is emerging in the second decade of life for most young people in the United States. By the time of the 20-year follow-up when the participants were around 30 years old on average, competence in romantic relationships and work were viewed as salient developmental tasks, while the importance of school success had waned. A newly emerging domain of competence we included for this assessment was civic engagement (Obradović & Masten, 2007).

Competence as a parent was an interesting task to consider in our assessments because the timing of parenting is less predictable than tasks imposed or expected by societies with a particular timetable, such as going to school. On the other hand, once this task is undertaken, we expect parents to care adequately for children in their custody.

Major methods for assessing competence varied over time, but they included parent and child interviews, teacher ratings, and peer assessments, as well as administrative data from school records. We also augmented these methods with ratings by employers, friends, and romantic partners for some assessments. We often were faced with measures that needed to be adapted to include more positive items. This was the case for the Revised Class Play method of peer assessment, which was based on a method developed by Lambert and Bower (1961) and successfully used by Garmezy's research group in preliminary studies of competence. In 1977, we expanded the measure to include more positive items for the initial study of competence and stress that spawned the PCLS. It has proven to be a robust strategy for assessing social behavior from the perspective of peers, widely used by other investigators as well as our group. It can be used to assess broadband competence with peers or more specific, narrowband dimensions of social function (Gest, Sesma, Masten, & Tellegen, 2006). We published a series of papers on the psychometric properties of this instrument over the years (Masten et al., 1985; Morison & Masten, 1991; Gest et al., 2006). Jennifer Roberts

Riley (2004) also did a thorough analysis of the factor structure of this instrument in the context of gender and school grade in a dissertation study using all the available school data over multiple administrations ($N = 612$), to illustrate the value of factor analysis in developmental research.

Other competence data at Time 1 came from parent and child interviews and ratings based on these interviews, the Devereux Elementary School Behavior Rating Scales (Spivack & Swift, 1967), and the Peabody Individual Achievement Test (Dunn & Markwardt, 1970). The interviews provided a wealth of data on family history and life events, as well as child behavior. Over the years, students interested in specific research questions were able to generate studies addressing their hypotheses years after the study data were collected because of the comprehensiveness of the assessments of child function at this and later assessments. Highlights can be found subsequently in this chapter.

The assessments at Time 1 and Time 3 (10 years later) were more extensive than the assessments at Times 2 and 4, each of which was conducted primarily by mail or telephone. It is extraordinarily expensive in time and funding to assess everyone in person in longitudinal studies of this kind. The more extensive assessments included interviews of the target individual about multiple domains of his or her life (school and work, friends, activities, family relationships, etc.) and if possible a parent or guardian, as well as many direct assessments (e.g., measures of intellectual function, humor) and questionnaires (on personality, life events, health and behavior problems, etc.). In order to facilitate assessments by mail, we developed a status questionnaire method of assessment for Time 2 (used again at Times 3 and 4) that also has proven useful to other investigators. The Status Questionnaire included straightforward questions about effective functioning in age-salient domains of competence, as well as questions about sociodemographic changes and subjective well-being. It was intended to capture broad indicators of how well life was going in key domains. Versions for self, parent, friend, and romantic partner were developed. A set of judges' rating scales were devised to go with these questionnaires when we found that participants conveyed information "beyond the checkbox" on these kinds of questionnaires. Trained raters could independently rate the information on these instruments with high reliability, providing consistent scores and useful data reduction (Burt, Obradović, Long, & Masten, 2008; Masten, Desjardins, McCormick, Kuo, & Long, 2010; Masten et al., 1995, 1999, 2005; Obradović, Bush, & Boyce, 2011). We have used judges' ratings, as well as the direct responses of informants, as competence indicators in various studies based on these data.

One of the most intriguing assessments of competence undertaken during the PCLS was inspired by a young anthropologist, Eric Durbrow, who came to the Institute of Child Development as a postdoctoral student at the time that we were planning the 20-year follow-up. By this time, we were well aware that one of the central questions for the study of resilience, and the criteria for "good adaptation" in particular, was "Who decides on the criteria?" (Masten, 1999; see Chapter 12). It was apparent that different investigators defined positive adaptation in varied ways that made it difficult to summarize the literature. We thought that the developmental task approach was sensible, and likely to yield robust measures of adaptive function, which appears to be the case. But we did not know if our participants shared the same views that we did about the criteria of competence. We wanted to gain their perspective on the criteria for competence without biasing them.

Durbrow was interested in studying competence across cultures and in developing measures of competence that would make sense in a new cultural context. He worked with Auke Tellegen and myself to develop an "emic" method for ascertaining the implicit criteria of competence by which people judge whether someone is doing well in life (Durbrow, 1999; Durbrow, Peña, Masten, Sesma, & Williamson, 2001). The strategy involved a two-part process, beginning with the Criteria of Competence Interview, followed by an independent sorting process that yielded a covariance matrix that could be factor analyzed to determine the implicit dimensions of competence underlying the interview descriptions of people doing okay in life.

To study the implicit competence criteria of the PCLS, just prior to the 20-year follow-up assessments, we invited a random sample of 50 males and females from the PCLS cohort to help with this preliminary study of competence (Boelcke & Masten, 2001). Results were analyzed for 42 of the responding participants (21 males and females to balance sex). Each of these participants were told the following:

> "It would be very helpful for us to know how you can tell a person's life is going well. Think of a person your age that you know is doing well, but don't tell me who it is. Then I am going to ask you a few questions about this person."

Then the interviewee was asked the sex and age of the person they had in mind and invited to provide "three or four ways that you can tell their life is going well." Most participants had little difficulty describing first one person and then a second example of the other sex. Subsequently, each description about how they could tell the lives were going well was written on a separate card, resulting in a pile of descriptions. These were pooled and a second group of 10 individuals, about the same age and background but not participants in the PCLS, were recruited to sort these descriptions into piles of items that "go together." Sorters might put items like "has a good job" with other job-related items. This procedure, developed by Tellegen, yielded a co-occurrence matrix of items ending up in the same pile. This matrix could then be factored to ascertain the underlying dimensions of the item piles, which reflected the implicit competence criteria of the PCLS respondents.

Results were quite coherent and interesting. Their descriptions fell into three broad categories: subjective well-being (e.g., happiness), accomplishments, and financial achievements. Accomplishment factors were very similar to our developmental task domains: success at work, happily married, pursuing education, and friendship. The PCLS participants also thought that owning a home and other material goods, such as a car, were indicators of doing well in life at their age. General happiness was a pervasive feature of the interview descriptions ("she is happy") and the most salient factor in the matrix. In contrast, although we measured happiness and subjective well-being in the assessments over time, and were very interested in happiness as a concomitant or consequence of competence, we did not *define* happiness as a necessary component of effective adaptation or resilience. We just expected success in age-salient developmental tasks to be associated with happiness for multiple reasons. One key reason was related to the expected pleasure in experienced mastery or success that Robert White (1959) proposed decades earlier as part of the motivation system for adaptive competence. A second was the expected consequences of failure in these tasks, which are so highly valued by others in society and the self (see McCormick et al., 2011; Obradović, Bush, Stamperdahl, Adler, & Boyce, 2010). Happiness does appear to accompany success in developmental tasks in the PCLS, both in the mind of the participants and in our empirical findings. Moreover, competence in currently important domains forecasts *later* happiness, most likely because competence forecasts later competence in key domains that yield a sense of accomplishment and go along with enriching relationships.

Findings from the PCLS, both within and across methods, have repeatedly supported the expectation that competence is multidimensional (Masten et al., 1995; Masten & Tellegen, 2012). This broad assumption was corroborated through multiple methods over the years, including factor analysis, structural equation modeling, and other multivariate strategies. Findings from the study also have supported developmental expectations about the coherence of competence in lives through time, as well as the differential significance of specific domains for later competence and psychopathology. These findings are discussed further below.

Risk and Adversity

In addition to the work on competence measures, it was essential for this study of resilience to assess adversity as well as risk factors associated with stressful experiences, such as socioeconomic status. Extensive data were gathered on family history and resources

in interviews and questionnaires over the years, along with multiple methods for assessing adverse life experiences. We focused
on cumulative indices of risk/adversity that would be challenging
or stressful for most people, including a wide range of events and
chronic conditions that could threaten child development. These
included acutely traumatic experiences or disasters and chronic
experiences of living in a home with conflict among parents, poverty, mentally ill parents, or maltreatment. We included a variety of methods, but typically used a "cumulative" approach that
attempted to evaluate the level of adversity in a given window
of time (e.g., 12 months or many years) based on multiple risks
and adversities. As noted previously in this volume, it was evident
early in the research on risk and resilience that risk factors seldom
occurred one at a time in the lives of children. We developed a
series of structured life event questionnaires for different informants and for the participants at different ages, building on the
earlier work of Holmes and Rahe (1967) and Coddington (1972a,
1972b). We developed a contextual life events interview (Linder,
1985) that reflected the influence of interactions of Garmezy with
George Brown and his colleagues (Brown, 1974; Brown & Harris,
1978). We also developed a Lifetime Life Events Questionnaire
and a life chart and rating system to further expand and pool the
information we were gathering over the years on adversity (Gest,
Reed, & Masten, 1999).

The initial LEQ included 50 items (see Masten et al., 1988).
We adapted items from Coddington's measure and included positive items to offset the negative tone of the instrument. Parents
circled yes or no whether an event had occurred in the past 12
months in the child's life. The original adversity score was a simple tally of 30 negative and ambiguous events that had been systematically judged to be independent of the child's own behavior.
We had developed weighted scores (what Holmes and Rahe [1967]
called "life change units") for this measure but discovered that
weighting did not make any difference (weighted and unweighted
scores were correlated .98). The score based on this measure was
modestly related to lower SES and strongly related ($r = .55$) to a
composite of interviewer ratings of family stress and instability.

At Time 1, one of the 2-hour family visits was devoted primarily to a contextual life events interview about events endorsed on the LEQ measure and other adversities the family brought up. The detailed information gained from this interview was analyzed in great detail in two dissertations by Herzog (1984) and Linder (1985) and subsequently utilized to develop the Life Events Questionnaire for Adolescents (self-report and parent-report versions) for the 7-year follow-up in the PCLS (see Masten, Neemann, & Andenas, 1994). Minor changes in this instrument were made for young adult versions of the LEQ in subsequent follow-ups. An LEQ for the mothers also was developed around this time for a dissertation study on competence and resilience in the mothers (Hillman, 1987). For all these LEQs, a systematic system of scoring was developed that distinguished independent from nonindependent events, chronic from acute experiences, and the valence (negative, positive, ambiguous). This made it possible to generate different scores for different purposes.

It was particularly important to distinguish between the events related to a child's own behavior and relatively independent events happening to the child. Many life event scores are confounded with the behaviors they are intended to predict. This is not to say that confounded scores are uninteresting. We found that "dependent" life event scores in adolescence were much higher for maladaptive young people (low competence with high uncontrollable adversity) as compared with their resilient peers in the study (high competence with similarly high uncontrollable adversity), even though their independent life event scores were similar and their childhood adversity scores were quite alike. It appeared that children who entered adolescence with high adversity, few resources, and little protection became more stress prone over the years, generating controllable but indeed stressful events such as trouble with peers or trouble with the law that they were poorly equipped to handle.

There also were interesting connections between chronic and acute life event scores on these LEQs. Chronic conditions of poverty or family problems were associated with higher reports of acute events as well, suggesting that the risk for theoretically "independent" acute experiences was higher in these generally stressed families (Masten et al., 1994). Acute, uncontrollable events do not appear to be randomly distributed in the population, just as tornadoes and lightning strikes do not occur randomly across places or people. Some places and situations may pose greater vulnerability for exposure to specific acute events.

All of these LEQ instruments inquired about events that had happened within the past 12 months. As we followed the families over time, we became interested in more comprehensive assessments of adversity spanning multiple years and especially the intervals between our competence assessments. For the 10-year follow-up, we developed a Lifetime Life Events Questionnaire, along with a life chart and rating approach as strategies to pool information over longer life periods (see Gest et al., 1999). Parents were interviewed about the whole lifetime of the participant, with the aid of a structured questionnaire and a visual life chart. Subsequently, we assembled a chronological database of the adversities reported across all 19 of our measures with adversity information. Life events were classified as nonindependent or independent of the target individual's behavior and the independent events were further classified by origin into categories of physical (e.g., health related), family (e.g., parent died), or community (e.g., best friend moved away, tornado). It was then possible to generate life history charts for a specific period of a participant's life, including only the independent events. These charts were subsequently rated by independent judges on the severity of adversity exposure utilizing a 7-point psychosocial stressor rating scale that ranged from "minimal" to "catastrophic" levels of stressors (*Diagnostic and Statistical Manual of Mental Disorders* [DSM-III-R]; American Psychiatric Association, 1987). Interrater agreement and intraclass correlations for these ratings were excellent (see Gest et al., 1999). These scores provided a global index of cumulative adversity exposure prior to or between assessments of competence. These scores showed modest associations with parenting quality and family SES. Although adjacent intervals were rated independently, adversity exposure in childhood and adolescence showed strong continuity on this comprehensive score (with a correlation of about .60). This is likely because many of the most salient of the stressful experiences in participants' lives involved chronic family dysfunction, including maltreatment and domestic violence or chronic alcohol or mental health problems in a parent.

Many other investigators have utilized these instruments or adapted them for their own purposes. They also were used or adapted for other studies by the Project Competence group, including research with homeless families and war refugees. For young people or their parents living in emergency shelters, we could use the same LEQs to assess exposure of children or youth to recent life events (e.g., Masten, Miliotis, Graham-Bermann, Ramirez, & Neeman, 1993). Not surprisingly, the scores on comparable tallies of the same events were much higher in homeless families than the averages observed in the more normative samples, such as the PCLS cohort.

In our studies of Cambodian survivors of the revolution and genocide perpetrated by the Khmer Rouge, we created a Traumatic Life Events Questionnaire (TLEQ) tailored to the war experiences of young refugees who were children at the time (Hubbard, Realmuto, Northwood, & Masten, 1995; Realmuto et al., 1992). The events included on this TLEQ included some items found on other Lifetime Life Event Questionnaires we had developed for the PCLS or studies of homeless families. However, there were many items pertaining to traumatic experiences rarely experienced outside of war. These included the following experiences: saw dead bodies (reported by 78% in one of our studies and 89% in another), saw stranger killed, was tortured, was captured by enemy, and parent was taken away. Scores on the TLEQ were related to trauma symptoms reported by Khmer youth. Lifetime rates of posttraumatic stress disorder (PTSD) were very high among these survivors of the "killing fields." Such studies are limited by the retrospective nature of the assessments, of course. In this work, the survivors were assessed more than 10 years after their war experiences. It is conceivable that ongoing mental health problems (particularly chronic PTSD) related to the war or its aftermath influenced recollections of traumatic experiences, even perhaps keeping such memories all too vivid.

Promotive and Protective Factors

With the goal of uncovering clues to resilience, it was also essential to assess potential resources and protective influences that we thought could play a role in adaptation to adversity. From the outset, we hypothesized that child cognitive skills and parenting quality would play a protective function in children faced with adversity, in addition to the general role these resources or assets would be expected to play in the development of child competence (as a competence-promotive influence). Thus, we included measures of parenting behavior and the closeness of parent–child relationships as well as standardized tests of child intellectual skills in assessments over the years (see Masten et al., 1988, 1999, 2004). In addition, however, we tested many other possibilities, most often through the dissertation research of students involved in the PCLS. Numerous individual differences were studied as potential factors in competence, resilience, or vulnerability over the years, including stress reactivity and other aspects of personality (Masten et al., 2004; Shiner & Masten, 2012), a sense of humor and creative thinking (Masten, 1982, 1986), social problem-solving skills (Pellegrini, 1985), motivation to adapt (Masten et al., 2004), delay of gratification (Ferrarese, 1981), self-control and planfulness (Masten et al., 2004; Shiner & Masten, 2012), and connections to adults outside the family (Masten et al., 2004).

Models of Competence and Resilience

Testing and exploring ideas about competence in relation to adversity and the variables in child, family, or environment that might explain variations in adaptation required conceptual models and corresponding strategies of analysis, in addition to measures. Examples of our conceptual models were described earlier in this volume (see Chapter 2), and appear in many of our conceptual publications (e.g., Masten, 2001; Masten et al., 1995; Masten, Burt, et al., 2006: Masten & Tellegen, 2012) and empirical papers (Garmezy et al., 1984; Masten et al., 1988, 1999, 2004, 2005). We included a variety of variable- and person-focused strategies over the course of the study, and incorporated suitable new statistical methods as they became available.

Our methods benefited over many years from the outstanding faculty and training in methodology at the University of Minnesota at the time, as well as the renowned methodological expertise of Auke Tellegen, who was a collaborator from the inception of the PCLS (see Masten & Tellegen, 2012). Robert Cudek advised the group on structural equation modeling (SEM) when we first adopted this method for analyzing the structure and coherence of competence (Masten et al., 1995), and Professor Jeffrey Long years later would guide our analyses of developmental cascades using SEM methods (e.g., Masten et al., 2005). Above all, the PCLS benefited from an extraordinary sequence of graduate students who were instrumental in designing, implementing, and analyzing the results of the study.

Our strategies for analysis were certainly affected and also limited by the sample size and design of the study. Retention was excellent but a sample size of 205 for the longitudinal data, even with contemporary imputation techniques, limits the power and complexity of the analyses that can be attempted. We have tried to be conservative in our conclusions in keeping with the limitations of the design, counting on replication by other investigators to support or refute our findings. To date, the replication of our major findings by other investigators has been encouraging.

FINDINGS FROM THE PCLS

Detailing the findings from the PCLS is not possible within the confines of this chapter. Here we highlight key results and conclusions on the themes of competence and resilience, developmental cascades, and personality, and also comment on the importance of mentoring for the contributions of this study.

Competence

Results from this study supported the multidimensional structure of competence and the significance of competence across multiple developmental task domains for future adaptation. At the broadest level, we expected to find results consistent with the basic premise that *competence begets competence*, as many developmental theorists have proposed. Results from both variable- and person-focused analyses corroborated this fundamental assertion of developmental science. Longitudinal data consistently reflect continuity within competence domains over time—such as academic achievement, rule-abiding/rule-breaking conduct, or social competence with peers—from the level of simple correlations to complex latent variables (e.g., Masten et al., 1995, 1999, 2010). Competence in age-salient domains in one period of development also were expected and found to forecast effective function in later emerging age-salient domains. For example, social competence with peers (assessed during late childhood and early adolescence) forecasts later success in adolescence and early adulthood in romantic relationships, jobs, and parenting (Masten et al., 1995, 2010; Shaffer, Burt, Obradović, Herbers, & Masten, 2009). There are likely to be numerous ways that the capacity for social interaction is shaped and sustained through experience and transfers to new developmental tasks.

Concomitantly, we observed considerable stability over time in the identification of competent people (meeting a set of diagnostic criteria for effective function in multiple developmental task domains). If we diagnosed a group of competent children or adolescents, the probability was high that they would be doing well in adulthood when we checked in on them again (e.g., Masten et al., 2004). There were some interesting changes in classification status too, but a good deal of continuity. Moreover, the proportion of the cohort that appeared to be doing at least adequately well in life was higher after the transition to adulthood. We concluded that development favors competence overall and particularly in the transition to adulthood when there is a convergence of opportunities and maturation of function conducive to positive redirection of the life course (Masten et al., 2004; Masten, Obradović, et al., 2006).

Through the course of this study, we also learned a great deal about predictors and correlates of competence in age-salient tasks. Some of these factors were related to multiple domains while others were more specific, and most of these findings were highly consistent with results from other studies before and after our reports on these analyses. Family socioeconomic advantages, the quality of parenting, and the child's general cognitive functioning, for example, all were related to multiple domains of competence across the years of the study. These are broad resource indicators that also play an important role in resilience (discussed below). Sex, on the other hand, was related to some domains more than others. Boys, for example, generally had more conduct problems over the years than girls, as often observed in the literature on conduct, although certainly there were individual girls with antisocial behavior.

If one compared competent individuals with less competent peers, whether in childhood, adolescence, or adulthood, many positive attributes were associated with competence over the years, consistent with the notion of a "positive manifold." Competent people tended to have more positive self-concepts and higher self-esteem, a variety of positive personality traits (described further below), and better social understanding, attention regulation, planning, and creative thinking (e.g., Masten et al., 1999, 2004; Pellegrini, Masten, Garmezy, & Ferrarese, 1987; Shaffer, Coffino, Boelcke-Stennes, & Masten, 2007). They also had more external resources and social capital in the form of adult support inside and outside the family (e.g., Masten et al., 1988, 1999, 2004). It seems reasonable to assume that shared processes linking multiple system levels (genetic or epigenetic, neural, behavioral, family, peer, school, or neighborhood) in development accounted for this positive manifold.

Generally, competent individuals were less likely to face severe adversity compared to less competent peers (life event exposure also was related to competence). However, if they *were* exposed to severe adversity, competent individuals were more likely to have or mobilize the resources for positive adaptation. Competent people with high-adversity exposure (our definition of manifested resilience) had a great deal in common with similarly competent people who had low-adversity exposure.

Other major findings related to competence emerged as we tested for resilience, taking adversity into account, and again when we began to consider the potential interplay of function across competence and symptoms domains, a central consideration in developmental psychopathology (Masten, Burt, et al., 2006). These findings are highlighted in the following sections.

Resilience

Perhaps the most basic finding from this study is the observation that there were individuals exposed to extremely severe or prolonged adversity who fared well on major developmental tasks, both within and across time. The study of resilience assumes such variation, and our results corroborated the expected pattern of resilience, that there would be individuals manifesting broad competence even though they had been exposed to very high levels of adverse life experiences. Multiple methods revealed resilience, including case nominations by the interviewers, empirical cut scores classifying the sample by competence and adversity, cluster analyses, and other multivariate approaches (see Masten et al., 1999). There also were individuals who had similar competence to those showing resilience, but who had experienced much less adversity, as well as individuals sharing similar adversity histories who manifested maladaptation in multiple competence domains. These three groups—competent, resilient, and maladaptive— could be compared to test hypotheses or explore new possibilities concerning "What makes a difference?"

Notably missing from the observed patterns of adaptation in relation to adversity was the "low–low" pattern, individuals who showed poor adaptation in the context of low adversity (Masten et al., 1999). As noted in Chapter 2, this is an uncommon pattern in normative samples, especially in school-based cohorts such as the PCLS. This pattern suggests an unusually vulnerable individual (lacking normal adaptive systems) or perhaps missing information about some kind of hidden or unique adversity. In a benign rearing context, relatively free from adversity, nearly everyone appears to do quite well, with the exception of individuals who have severe liabilities.

A second major conclusion from this study was that in many ways, the individuals showing resilience resembled the individuals from low-adversity backgrounds showing similar competence. Or to put it another way, competent and resilient individuals, identified in childhood, adolescence, or early adulthood, had similar adaptive advantages, in notable contrast to their maladaptive peers. The following individual characteristics, for example, were associated with both competence and resilience: good intellectual function, positive self-worth, conscientiousness, agreeableness, and happiness. Young people showing competence and resilience also were likely to have positive relationships with at least one competent and caring parent or parent surrogate, and they also had more socioeconomic resources.

In contrast, data on individuals who manifested problems in terms of major age-salient developmental tasks indicated that these individuals overall had relatively few resources and potential protective factors, both in terms of internal resources such as cognitive skills and external resources such as capable parents looking out for them (see Masten et al., 1999, 2004). On personality measures, individuals showing maladaptive patterns in the context of adversity were more stress reactive and more easily upset, less conscientious and less agreeable than their more adaptive peers (see Shiner & Masten, 2012).

The two broadest variables that we tested as hypothesized protective influences in the PCLS were general intellectual capacity and global quality of parenting (see Garmezy et al., 1984; Masten et al., 1988, 1999, 2004). Both qualities had pervasive links to multiple domains of competence, both in low- and high-adversity conditions. Given high adversity in childhood, young people with good cognitive skills and effective parenting fared substantially better than their peers with similar adversity. Results suggested particular protective effects of cognitive skills and parenting on the development of good conduct (rule-abiding vs. rule-breaking behavior), consistent with a large literature on the importance of cognitive skills and good parenting for adjustment in this domain.

These data collectively suggested that the presence (or absence) of influences that promote or protect competence across multiple domains of expected achievement are more important for explaining adaptation in development than adversity exposure per se. Therefore, adversities that undermine, harm, or damage key promotive or protective influences may carry the greatest dangers for maladaptive outcomes in development.

Early and Late Bloomers

Competence, resilience, and, of course, development in every aspect are dynamic. Thus, we expected to observe changes over time in the adaptation of the PCLS cohort. Clearly there were "early bloomers" in the study, in that we observed numerous children at the outset of the study who were showing competence across multiple domains, including children who had endured severe adversity or hardship. As the participants grew up, we were keen to learn about their ups and downs, about the persistence and changes in competence. The early bloomers usually continued to bloom, although a few were snared at least temporarily by the hazards of adolescence, such as drug use.

However, we also observed individual cases of marked change. For example, one young man who was floundering in adolescence we found to be flourishing in early adulthood when we followed him up after 10 years. Between assessments, he had fallen in love and married a young woman from a healthy family willing to provide some stability and guidance in his life. He had found work well suited to his aptitudes, and parted ways with bad habits and company of his earlier years.

One of our published studies from the PCLS focused on such changes from the 10- to the 20-year follow-up assessments (Masten et al., 2004). In this analysis we were particularly interested in testing the role of potential promotive/protective influences that might play a part in the transition to adulthood. In particular, we studied the role of planfulness/future motivation, autonomy, adult support (outside the family), and coping skills, which the literature had suggested could be important adaptive resources in this particular period of development. Results supported the expectation that these attributes would be related to current and future competence in multiple domains. In addition, we found as expected that these adaptive qualities might account in part for

the phenomenon of late bloomers who make substantial improvements in competence as they transition to adulthood (see Masten, Obradović, et al., 2006). If we compared groups of competent,
resilient, and maladaptive individuals, both around age 20 and
again around age 30, we could see the usual pattern of similarity
on these attributes for the groups showing competence or resilience, and much lower scores for the maladaptive group. For the
small group of maladaptive youth who manifested a marked shift
to resilience by adulthood, these attributes appeared to be harbingers of change. Those maladaptive cases we would later identify as late bloomers showed evidence 10 years earlier (around
age 20 at the time of the 10-year follow-up assessments) that they
were more motivated about the future, had greater autonomy
(which they may have needed to break free of difficult families or
friends), and had more adult support outside the family (such as
a mentor). Each of their paths was unique, but the late bloomers
appeared to make positive choices to go down a new road, taking advantage of opportunities provided by jobs, military service,
or college; healthy romantic relationships; supportive mentors; or
religious affiliations. Most of the late bloomers, we also noted,
were women.

Our results for "turnaround cases" were consistent with other
reports of late bloomers from studies of resilience (Burt & Masten,
2010; Masten, Obradović, et al., 2006), such as the Kauai study
discussed in Chapter 2. Werner and Smith (1992) observed that
most of the turnaround cases were women and emphasized the
salience of "opening of opportunities" in the lives of late bloomers
in the Kauai study. A number of longitudinal studies have noted
the importance of opportunities and choices in this window of
development for turning direction. We think that the transition
years spanning late adolescence and early adulthood represent an
important opportunity window for moving toward competence.
It is a period when brain development favors improved decision
making and considerations of the future, and many communities
and cultures provide structured experiences outside the family in
the adult world, ranging from military service to apprenticeships.
Development and context converge in favor of a change for the

better. The young people in the PCLS with greater motivation to succeed in the future, more adult support, and more autonomy appeared to take advantage of this convergence to change direction.

Developmental Cascades

From the outset of this study, we were interested in the possible links among domains of adaptation. Initially, we focused on the associations within and across time among domains of competence (e.g., Masten et al., 1995). However, we also measured symptoms of psychopathology, wanting to gain knowledge about the connections between traditional competence dimensions (e.g., achievement, social competence) and traditional psychopathology dimensions (e.g., internalizing, externalizing). We expected to find that the competence domain we called "conduct" (rule-abiding vs. rule-breaking behavior) overlapped with the traditional dimension of "externalizing" symptoms, partly because there were overlapping contents in the measures of these two constructs and partly because externalizing scores assess the negative end of what is actually a broader dimension of conduct expected by adults in many societies. In other cases, we expected connections across domains because behavior in one domain was expected to "spill over" to influence function in other domains. This led to a series of publications on developmental cascades.

Developmental cascades refers to the idea that function in one area or level of a system can spread to another level or domain as a result of the dynamic interplay across levels and functional domains (see Masten & Cicchetti, 2010c). This idea has a long history in developmental science and psychopathology, both for competence and problems (see Masten, Burt, et al., 2006; McCormick et al., 2011). As noted above, we expected that competence would cascade forward in time, spreading to new domains. We also expected that problems in one domain could undermine function in another domain in many possible ways, including direct interference and indirect pathways. Developmental theories about the development of antisocial behavior had postulated for decades that disruptive or aggressive behavior could interfere with social and academic competence. Patterson and colleagues at the Oregon Social Learning Center had proposed a coercion model by which noncompliance arising in the family affected subsequent school success, leading to peer rejection and academic difficulties (Patterson, Reid, & Dishion, 1992). This dual failure at school, in turn, contributed to depressed mood as these children experienced failure in two of the major developmental tasks of childhood in the school context.

Beginning in 2005, we published a series of papers testing cascade models in the PCLS. The first of these tested the links over time among academic competence, externalizing/conduct problems, and internalizing symptoms. In each of these analyses we considered three or more domains of adaptive behavior in a longitudinal assessment framework, which made it possible to control for both continuity within domains over time and cross-sectional links among domains within time, to test rigorously for "cascade effects" where there are cross-domain predictions that cannot be attributed to continuity over time or within-time covariation. Typically, these analyses employed SEM techniques to take full advantage of the multiple methods we had used to assess each domain over time. Our goal was to test hypothesized cascade effects in comparison to more parsimonious or alternative models, and also to demonstrate methods for analyzing developmental cascades.

Our findings indicated that many of the domains of interest were already related at the outset of the study, including the major domains of peer acceptance, academic achievement, externalizing problems (vs. rule-abiding conduct), and internalizing symptoms. Over time, conduct problems appeared to undermine academic achievement and indirectly affect both future social competence and psychological well-being (Masten et al., 2005; Obradović et al., 2010). These results were congruent with coercion theory and related dual-failure models, although they also could be interpreted more positively in terms of "dual success" or positive adaptation cascading across domains.

Cascade results in other studies underscored the links between childhood competence and success in early adulthood, through multiple possible cascade pathways. Work competence in adulthood showed strong connections to academic and social competence, with childhood social competence showing particularly strong predictive significance for later work success (Masten et al., 2010). Success in romantic relationships also had earlier roots in childhood competence in multiple domains (McCormick et al., 2011). Effective parenting in early adulthood (among those who were parents by the time of the 20-year follow-up) was linked to social competence in childhood, which in turn was related to receiving good parenting in childhood (Shaffer et al., 2009). This was an intergenerational cascade analysis: The quality of parenting in one generation predicted effective parenting in the next generation, through multiple pathways, including the effects of parenting on social competence in childhood, which in turn contributed in unknown ways to parenting as an adult.

These cascade analyses represent a first step in delineating the processes by which competence or problems develop and spread in development. There is considerable interest in cascade studies, reflected in the publication of two special issues of *Development and Psychopathology* in 2010, edited by Masten and Cicchetti (2010a, 2010b). Broad cascade analyses such as ours in the PCLS provide clues to where and when the action may be happening for close future study. Replication is important, as is then unpacking these processes of change.

Cascade analyses have considerable potential to inform preventive interventions because they could help identify good timing and targets for intervention efforts, early in a cascade process ("before the horse has left the barn") or with respect to which aspect of functioning to target at different times (Masten & Cicchetti, 2010c; Masten, Burt, et al., 2006). Results of such analyses also explain why some behavior problems (or successes) in childhood have such broad predictive significance for adaptation in adulthood. Early conduct problems, for example, appear to set in motion cascades that contribute to function in numerous other domains over time. Cascading effects also may afford explanations for comorbidity of disorders and commonly co-occurring symptom patterns that are widely observed in developmental psychopathology (Angold, Costello, & Erkanli, 1999).

Personality

From the outset of the PCLS, assessments encompassed a broad array of individual differences, designed to capture a deeper understanding of the children in the study. At the time, the literature on personality in the middle years of childhood was quite limited. There was a rich and growing literature on temperament and related individual differences in early childhood (Rothbart, 2011), as well as increasing interest in downward extension of adult personality measures into adolescence, but as yet little study of personality traits in childhood. Much to the benefit of the PCLS, doctoral student Rebecca Shiner became intrigued with the structure and assessment of personality traits in the great divide between early childhood and adulthood (Shiner, 1998). For her dissertation study, Shiner derived personality dimensions from the extensive set of variables on individual differences in the children that could be gleaned from child interviews, parent interviews, and a set of ratings by teachers (Shiner, 2000). Through data reduction and exploratory factor analysis, she derived a four-factor structure of personality in the childhood data from these instruments. Scores on these traits could then be related to concurrent and later competence in age-salient tasks. Children high on *mastery motivation*, for example, were curious, creative, imaginative, persistent, confident, competitive, and striving to meet high standards, reflecting a pattern of emotional engagement. Not surprisingly, children high on this trait were doing well in school at the time, and they would also do well in the future domains of achievement, both in school and at work (Shiner, 2000; Shiner & Masten, 2008; Shiner, Masten, & Roberts, 2003; Shiner, Masten, & Tellegen, 2002).

Over the years, Shiner and colleagues found many links between personality and competence in age-salient developmental tasks. Successful children tend to show a pattern of positive traits in each assessment and also across time, as noted above. Personality traits forecast later success in particular domains, as well as changes within domains. Conscientiousness, for example, predicted positive changes in achievement over 10- and 20-year spans of time. Childhood agreeableness predicted positive changes in rule-abiding conduct from childhood to emerging adulthood 10 years later.

In her initial work, Shiner noted the resemblance of the four traits she originally derived in the PCLS data to the "Big Five" personality dimensions. More recently, under her leadership, we re-analyzed the personality scores in the PCLS to specifically capture the Big Five (Shiner & Masten, 2012). Findings corroborated the links between personality and competence within and across time. Results indicated that four of the Big Five personality traits assessed in childhood—higher openness to experience, conscientiousness, and agreeableness, and lower neuroticism—were harbingers of broad adult success in developmental tasks. Results for the latter three traits were consistent with the results of other studies of the Big Five suggesting that there may be a higher-order trait of "stability" that indexes a general capability and tendency for maintaining emotional, social, and motivational control (DeYoung, 2006). The fifth Big Five trait, extraversion, had more mixed links to adult success.

The role of personality in resilience also was examined. As so often observed in this study, person-focused results underscored the similarity of personality scores in the groups marked by competence and resilience (see Shiner & Masten, 2012). Moreover, their scores were close to the average for the cohort. It was the maladaptive young people with high lifetime adversity exposure and less success in developmental tasks, both around age 20 and age 30, who showed negative scores on personality, with low conscientiousness, low agreeableness, low openness to experience, and especially higher stress reactivity or neuroticism.

PCLS findings on personality provided evidence both of continuity and change. The longitudinal data revealed considerable continuity in personality from childhood into adolescence and even stronger continuity from adolescence into adulthood. Stability and change was particularly evident when the same instrument was used to assess personality. Tellegen's (1982) Multidimensional Personality Questionnaire (MPQ) was completed by the participants in the study during the 10- and 20-year follow-ups when they were an average of 20 and 30 years old, respectively. Although there were interesting developmental trends, there was striking rank-order stability in the scores on this measure. For example, Social Potency scores had a correlation of .72 over a span of 10 years. At the same time, overall raw scores in some dimensions increased or declined over the transition to adulthood in keeping with a general trend toward maturity: The average level of constraint (including harm avoidance), for example, increased in the cohort over this decade of life. Adolescents generally embraced more risk taking than young adults.

We also were particularly interested in the ways that personality may change over the course of development and experience in relation to success or failure in age-salient developmental tasks. Results indicated that there may well be reciprocal effects of competence on personality development. Competence problems in childhood predicted increases in negative emotionality over the course of adolescence (Shiner et al., 2002). Concomitantly, the tendency to experience negative emotions or high reactivity to stress ("neuroticism") appeared to pose vulnerability or risk for dealing with adversity. Adaptive failures exacerbated this personality tendency, appearing to increase broad negative emotionality and stress reactivity. Adversity exposure (experiences out of the child's control) also was related to higher scores on this dimension of personality (greater neuroticism), suggesting that adversity itself may have contributed to negative emotionality. The concatenation of high negative emotionality and high adversity with low protection (from parents or self-regulation) may be a dire combination in the early life course, with snowballing consequences for future competence.

It is important to keep in mind, however, that positive traits also may have cascading effects. The personality traits of agreeableness and conscientious, for example, showed pervasive links to competence in multiple domains over time. Those competence domains often showed cascade effects on other domains over time. Thus, it is quite conceivable that personality traits have indirect roles in many aspects of observed adaptation over time that remain to be explored in depth.

MENTORING

The contributions of the PCLS were not limited to concepts, methods, and findings. Perhaps the most important legacy of this project stems from the mentorship provided to a sequence of student collaborators, including this author. The PCLS was founded by a renowned mentor of both students and colleagues. Norman Garmezy had a profound influence on the study of resilience and developmental psychopathology not only because of his scholarship but also as a result of a gregarious personality and generous nature, as well as the tradition of strong mentoring he established in Project Competence. This influence is evident in the special issue honoring his legacy in *Development and Psychopathology* (Masten & Cicchetti, 2012). Many students were trained over the course of the longitudinal study by Garmezy and Tellegen, and eventually, by me along with them. These students in turn have gone on to make many contributions and train many additional students in the areas of competence, risk, and resilience, in their various roles as faculty and leaders in academic and clinical institutions. Good mentoring also has cascading consequences.

SUMMARY

This chapter chronicles the origins, methods, and major findings of the PCLS, one of the early studies focused on understanding resilience. It was founded at the University of Minnesota by Professor Norman Garmezy in collaboration with his colleague Auke Tellegen and numerous graduate students, including myself, in the late 1970s. Like other early investigators, this team had to define their concepts, develop methods and measures, tackle controversial issues, and persist with a longitudinal study through the ups and downs of funding and fashion as interest in resilience waxed or waned. The legacy of this project included the concepts and methods the team developed and also a cadre of young investigators trained by Garmezy, Tellegen, and later myself (when Garmezy passed me the baton for the PCLS), together with additional methodological collaborators Robert Cudek and Jeffrey Long.

Hallmarks of the PCLS include the central focus on competence in developmental perspective, the support of the Minneapolis Public Schools for the project, and the study of a normative cohort that varied widely in SES. The core sample included 205 young people and their families, followed for more than 20 years (so far). Retention was excellent, with 90% of the original youth participating in the 20-year follow-up. A multimethod approach was taken to the assessment of adversity, adaptation, and potential protective factors, including individual and family characteristics. As a result, many different studies were possible, and to this day, students can return to this rich data set to pose and answer new questions. Contributions of this study include measures of positive adjustment, such as the Revised Class Play and Status Questionnaire methods, and also measures of adversity, such as the LEQ.

Findings from this study support the basic premise that *competence begets competence*, in that competence in childhood forecasts later competence, both in the same general domain and also in newly emerging domains. Competence was defined in terms of age-salient developmental tasks, such as academic achievement, getting along with peers, rule-governed conduct, and later on in terms of friendship, romantic relationships, work success, and (for those with children) good parenting. Results corroborated the multi-dimensional nature of competence over time. Personality traits also were broadly associated with competence in multiple domains, with evidence suggesting that a general ability for self-control (emotional, social, motivational) played an important role in life success. Domains of competence also showed cascading effects across time, domains, and generations.

Among the young people who grew up with adversity and high risk due to stressful life experiences or the vicissitudes of poverty, resilience typically was associated with more human and social capital, particularly in the form of good cognitive skills and positive relationships with caregivers or other caring adults. Competent young people from high-adversity backgrounds had many of the same advantages as competent youth from low-risk backgrounds, suggesting that there may be basic protections for human development that promote competence in general and have protective effects in the context of adversity. Some factors appear to be especially important when adversity is high: Good cognitive skills, for example, appear to be protective, whereas a stress-reactive personality appears to be a liability.

Studying individuals through time also highlighted the varied pathways of resilience. Some children from adverse backgrounds showed striking competence throughout the study, manifesting a steady course of resilience, while others struggled during adolescence and then recovered to do well. In other words, there were early bloomers and late bloomers. The transition to adulthood years appeared to be a window of opportunity for young people who had gotten offtrack to take a more positive road, often heralded by a change of heart or surge in motivation to succeed, facilitated by opportunities and adult guides.

CHAPTER 4

OVERCOMING DISADVANTAGE AND ECONOMIC CRISIS
Homeless Children

Concerns about risks posed to child development by poverty, homelessness, and economic shocks have waxed and waned over the past century, capturing the attention of scientists as well as the public (Elder, 1999; Elder & Conger, 2000; Masten, 2012b; McLoyd, 1998; Luthar, 1999; Lundberg & Wuermli, 2012; Schorr & Schorr, 1989; Zigler & Styfco, 2010; Walker et al., 2007, 2011). Concern is surging again in the aftermath of the recent global economic crisis. In 2012, the World Bank published the volume *Children and Youth in Crisis: Protecting and Promoting Human Development in Times of Economic Shocks* (Lundberg & Wuermli, 2012). Reports on homelessness (Samuels, Shinn, & Buckner, 2010) and hunger (Fiese et al., 2011) in American children also reflect concerns about the extent and effects of poverty in the United States and related issues of housing instability and food insecurity.

There is certainly reason for alarm. A large literature documents the developmental risks across the lifespan associated with poverty, socioeconomic deprivation, homelessness, and/or hunger across many domains of function from health to educational success (Evans & Schamberg, 2009; Fiese et al., 2011; Huston, 1991;

Keating & Hertzman, 1999; Samuels et al., 2010). There is a growing literature on child development in low-income countries or the "developing world" that also addresses developmental risks associated with extreme poverty (Bornstein et al., 2012; Boyden & Bourdillon, 2012; Lundberg & Wuermli, 2012; Walker et al., 2007, 2011). Child health and well-being show SES-gradient patterns, with health or cognitive problems increasing as a function of lower SES (Brooks-Gunn, Duncan, & Britto, 1999). Both chronicity and depth of poverty show risk gradients for child development (e.g., Raver, Blair, & Willoughby, 2013). Data even in wealthy countries document the multiple and cumulative risks associated with child poverty, including less-educated parents, single-parent households, dangerous neighborhoods, poor schools or limited educational opportunities, food insecurity, and inadequate health care. The combination of risk factors for development associated with poverty or low SES suggests that multiple and complex processes likely are involved in any developmental problems associated with SES.

At the same time, data also evidence tremendous variation in the shorter- and longer-term outcomes in health and behavior problems associated with economic disadvantages and stressors. Some children (and families) appear to function or turn out much better than others with similar socioeconomic background or experiences. This variation has not gone unnoticed in the literature on poverty and child development. Books published over the years herald the interest in resilience, with titles like *Escape from Disadvantage* (Pilling, 1990), *Good Kids from Bad Neighborhoods: Successful Development in Social Context* (Elliott et al., 2006), or *The Long Struggle: Well-Functioning Working-Class Black Families* (Lewis & Looney, 1983). Investigators in these reports noted how common it was for young people from impoverished families or neighborhoods to do okay in life despite socioeconomic disadvantage. Individual, family, and community factors associated with resilience in these studies included effective functioning across varying levels of analysis, such as individual cognitive skills or persistence, skilled parenting, religious affiliations, and organized neighborhoods.

Several of the classic studies of resilience also have focused on disadvantaged children or families. The risk group identified by Werner and Smith (1982, 1992) among the children of Kauai, described earlier in this volume, was indexed by poverty as well as other risk factors. Another well-known longitudinal study of resilience by Vaillant and colleagues (e.g., DiRago & Vaillant, 2007; Felsman & Vaillant, 1987; Long & Vaillant, 1984) followed up a cohort of low-income urban youth who were part of a well-known study of delinquency (Glueck & Glueck, 1950). Investigators have examined the long-term predictors of adult success in this cohort of inner-city youth in a series of publications. The Minnesota Longitudinal Study of Risk and Adaptation also has followed a high-risk cohort of the children of low-income mothers for decades (Sroufe et al., 2005). These longitudinal studies all point to the importance of relationships across the life course (e.g., with parents, friends, or mentors) as well as individual capabilities for resilience. However, variations in the social and historical context also play a role.

One of the most influential series of studies relating human development to economic and social changes was conducted by Glen Elder, utilizing longitudinal data to analyze the impact of the Great Depression and World War II on the life course. Elder drew on data from three classic longitudinal studies initiated in the late 1920s and early 1930s by investigators at the Institute of Child Welfare at the University of California at Berkeley. Three decades after these studies began, Elder recognized the potential such data held for linking major social changes to individual lives. He formulated a "life-course theory" that placed human development into historical context (Elder, 1998). Elder's work capitalized on the differential developmental timing and variations in family impact among members of these cohorts during the economic and political upheavals that accompanied global economic depression and subsequent war. His findings are summarized in *Children of the Great Depression* (1999), where he discussed the surprising resilience observed among the young people who grew up during these turbulent years: "To an unexpected degree, these children of the Great Depression followed a trajectory of resilience into the middle years of life" (p. 320). There was a notable turning period for some of these young people in the transition to adulthood that study investigators tried to explain. Some attributed this resilience to the benefits of leaving home and finding fulfilling adult roles. With his attention to the influence of changing social conditions, Elder considered the role of educational, military, and work opportunities afforded to many individuals during and following the Depression and war, including the war mobilization itself, the GI Bill, and postwar economic prosperity. He also noted the influence of earlier marriage as a source of social support and optimism.

All of these studies highlighted in different ways the cumulative effects of adversity and risk on the lives of individuals, and also the variations in success among members of a cohort at any given time and in the patterning of lives through time. Investigators followed cohorts of children for decades, which revealed changes over the life course and clues to resilience observed in many of these individuals. These studies benefited from mixed methods, ranging from case histories and qualitative analyses to complex multivariate analyses. And, again, the congruence of the findings on resilience are notable given the diversity of adversities, samples, and approaches. Their results pointed to the importance of relationships and opportunities in the lives of young people, as well as individual and development differences in stress reactivity, motivation, problem solving, or self-regulation. Developmental timing as well as historical timing played a role in resilience processes observed by these investigators. In early childhood, the quality of caregiving was crucial, whereas friends and mentors played important roles later in development. For children growing up in extreme poverty, access to high-quality child care and education was important. Later in adolescence, investigators often noted the role of opening opportunities in work, higher education, or military service, particularly in the situation of young people whose lives changed in a dramatically better direction during the transition to adulthood.

CHILDREN IN HOMELESS FAMILIES

In my own research, I have observed the risks of economic crisis through the lens of homelessness in children. I was drawn into this work in 1988, around the time that national awareness of homeless families rather suddenly emerged. It was spurred by press attention and influential reports on homeless families, such as Kozol's account of homeless families in New York City, initially appearing in *The New Yorker* and subsequently published in the book *Rachel and Her Children* (1988). I was an assistant professor in child psychology at the time, but also volunteering as a clinical psychologist for a clinic that served disadvantaged children in the community, operated by the Amherst H. Wilder Foundation. Foundation leaders were interested in knowing more about the needs of homeless families and I was asked to look into the literature and the situation in the Twin Cities, to help guide their service efforts. I discovered that virtually nothing was known about the well-being or needs of homeless children, even though their numbers were rapidly increasing in the Twin Cities and many other communities across the United States. During this process, I visited one of the largest shelters in the upper Midwest, which was located in downtown Minneapolis and operated by the nonprofit agency People Serving People. Originally housing destitute and homeless adults, this organization had responded to a rapidly rising tide of family homelessness in our metropolitan area. I also met school officials in the Twin Cities who were struggling with the challenges of educating highly mobile children who were moving in and out of shelters. Shelters and school districts needed data to guide their efforts, but little information was available about children or their parents.

With discretionary research funding provided by an early career award from the University of Minnesota, a cadre of graduate students, and community collaborators, I began a program in 1989 of community-based, collaborative research on risk and resilience in homeless children. Our goals were modest because most of us engaged in research or services concerning homelessness in families at the time expected that this problem, which had emerged so quickly, would soon subside. Homelessness in families and children, however, continued to increase for a decade. It leveled off briefly in Minnesota, and then surged here and nationwide as the crisis of the Great Recession unfolded.

One of the most important responses to the national issue of homeless children was the McKinney–Vento Homeless Assistance Act initially passed in 1987, and later reauthorized as part of No Child Left Behind (see Samuels et al., 2010). This law affirmed the rights of homeless children to a free and appropriate education. Federal action also provided funding to states to assist in meeting legislative reporting requirements while serving the needs of these children. This funding in Minnesota allowed school districts that had high numbers of homeless children to designate or hire a liaison to facilitate the education of such mobile children. Reporting requirements of this law also motivated districts to identify children who had rights under McKinney–Vento. By the 2003/2004 school year, the Minneapolis Public Schools (MPS) had developed a reliable record-keeping system, and the liaison for homeless students, Elizabeth Hinz, was advocating for research to document and address their needs. We teamed up to begin a program of research, training, and, increasingly, intervention, that expanded to include researchers, teachers, administrators, and service providers from schools, shelters, and the University of Minnesota.

Our recent research program includes longitudinal analyses of large district-level data sets, aimed at understanding the "big picture," as well as more intensive, short-term investigations of smaller samples of children and parents staying in shelters aimed at understanding or promoting resilience. Findings underscore the dire risks associated with homelessness, particularly in regard to academic success, and also the striking variability of risks and outcomes among homeless families and their children. Results have convinced us that the goal of "closing the achievement gap" related to poverty and ethnicity or race will require attention to homelessness and mobility. At the same time, the protective factors implicated in our research with homeless children (which seem very familiar), suggest that there are malleable targets for intervention to protect child development and achievement in the context of homelessness. Reducing economic burden and toxic stress exposure is vitally important, but additional strategies are needed, given the intransigence of the poverty and homelessness we currently face in the United States. In the following sections, I highlight findings from this research, including initial studies and our most recent work, and then discuss the implications for intervention and policy.

Homeless Children on a Risk Continuum: Early Findings

Our early findings from a small series of studies (1989–1996) documented high levels of risk for academic, behavioral, and emotional problems among homeless young people (Masten et al., 1993, 1997; Masten & Sesma, 1999; Miliotis, Sesma, & Masten, 1999). In our first study of families with children ages 8–17, we compared a sample of homeless families with very similar families participating in a community food program but who were not currently homeless. Homeless families closely resembled the community comparison families in terms of sociodemographic risk factors, such as a single-parent household and low maternal education. However, families in shelters had experienced more recent negative life events and parents, not surprisingly, reported more distress (Masten et al., 1993). Homeless families appeared to be higher on a continuum of risk than low-income but housed families.

At the same time, we observed widely varying risk among families staying in an emergency shelter. If we tallied up well-established risk factors for child development (e.g., single-parent household, parent did not finish high school, child exposed to maltreatment), cumulative risk scores varied dramatically among families staying in shelter, and child function was generally related to the level of family risk. Figure 4.1 shows a risk gradient for behavior problems based on a simple tally of risk factors for child development in a sample of 98 children ages 8–10, based on parental reports of risk factors and behavior problems

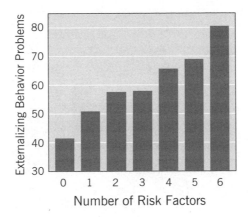

FIGURE 4.1. Example of a risk gradient showing the relation of behavioral problems to number of risk factors in a sample of 98, 8- to 10-year-old children who were staying in an emergency shelter for homeless families. Average score on the Child Behavior Checklist (Achenbach, 1991) externalizing scale (parent report) was computed for each level of risk. The risk score was a simple sum of the following risk factors: low maternal education (less than high school), single parent, a parent had died, parents had divorced, history of foster care, maltreatment history, and witnessing violence. From Masten and Sesma (1999, p. 3). Reprinted with permission from the Center for Urban and Regional Affairs at the University of Minnesota.

(Masten & Sesma, 1999). We also observed that "risk predicts risk" in the sense that a higher count on one set of risk factors also predicted risk on other indicators. Figure 4.2 illustrates how the score on a standard food insecurity measure, a widely used index of risk related to hunger, was related to the same composite risk score. Children higher on this cumulative risk index also reported higher scores on food insecurity, which is another well validated index of risk for child development. These data show a steep risk gradient for hunger in relation to cumulative risk scores. Such data illustrate the widely observed tendency for risk factors to pile up in the lives of some children, particularly among the most disadvantaged (Obradović et al., 2012).

Nonetheless, it was clear by observation in shelters, as well as in our data, that even among families with very high risk levels, there was variation in the competence and well-being of the

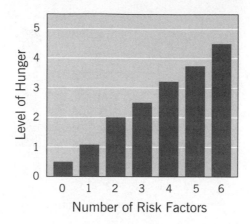

FIGURE 4.2. A risk gradient showing that average scores on a hunger index (assessed by a standard food insecurity measure) rise as the level of risk rises in a sample of 8- to 10-year-old homeless children who were staying in a homeless shelter (see Figure 4.1). From Masten and Sesma (1999, p. 3). Reprinted with permission from the Center for Urban and Regional Affairs at the University of Minnesota.

children. Effective parenting was related to better child achievement and behavior. Parent involvement predicted better school achievement for these homeless children (Miliotis et al., 1999). Higher-achieving children also had better cognitive skills. These findings hinted that typical protective factors might play a role in the adaptation of homeless children.

Longitudinal Data on the Achievement Gap with Evidence of Academic Resilience

Our collaborative research entered a new phase when reliable district-level data became available for analysis. Investigators from the office of Research, Evaluation, and Assessment (REA) in the MPS teamed up with a group of us (faculty and students) from the University of Minnesota to analyze the data on achievement, attendance, and other behavior available in administrative records that could be deidentified for secondary analysis. Our team included Professor Jeffrey Long, who was an expert in longitudinal analysis of growth and change, as well as the talented statisticians in the REA office (David Heistad and Alex Chan), Ms. Hinz, and a remarkable group of graduate students. Systematic efforts to comply with the McKinney–Vento legislation led this district to begin keeping increasingly systematic records of children who were identified as HHM in any given school year, typically when they entered a shelter. In addition, this district had chosen to administer nationally standardized achievement tests (Computer Adaptive Levels Tests by the Northwest Evaluation Association or equivalent) designed to assess growth and change over time within individuals as well as group. This combination of data made it possible for our team to analyze the levels and growth in reading and math achievement in students flagged as HHM compared with other groups of students on nationally standardized tests, using longitudinal data. We did not realize it at the time, but the quantity and quality of the data available for these analyses were unusual.

Our analyses of achievement patterns over time in the MPS district data afford a rare longitudinal perspective on risks to achievement for students identified as low income and HHM (Cutuli et al., 2013; Herbers et al., 2012; Obradović et al., 2009). Group differences on the level of achievement over time are large and stable, showing persistent achievement gaps. At the same time, the individual differences are striking and these differences illustrate the tremendous variability of achievement among students in a risk category. Data on individual differences highlight academic resilience as well as achievement disparities, underscoring the differing needs of students from the same risk category.

Results of growth curve analysis (utilizing linear mixed modeling) from one of these district-level analyses are shown in Figures 4.3 and 4.4 (Cutuli et al., 2013). In these analyses, all of the achievement test data from 5 school years (2004/2005 through 2009/2010) were pooled for all participating third to eighth graders with any test data (an accelerated longitudinal design), including 26,474 students. We focused on these grades because the same/equivalent tests were administered each fall across these grades. Four risk groups were formed for analysis, based on income and

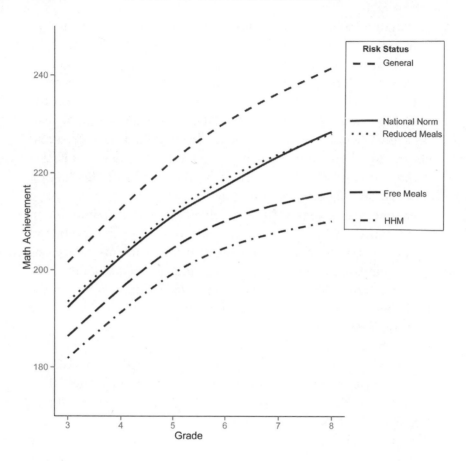

FIGURE 4.3. A longitudinal risk gradient for math achievement, showing scores over time on a standardized test for 26,474 students tested in an urban school district from 2005/2006 through 2009/2010 divided into four groups: homeless or highly mobile at any time during 6 years preceding the 2009/2010 school year (HHM; 13.8% of the students), students eligible for free lunch at any time but not identified as HHM (Free Meals, 57.2%), students eligible for reduced-fee lunch but not free lunch or HHM (Reduced Meals, 3.7%), and other students (General, 25.3%). The national average on the test is shown as a solid line. From Cutuli et al. (2013). Copyright 2012 by the authors and the Society for Research in Child Development, Inc. Reprinted with permission from Wiley-Blackwell.

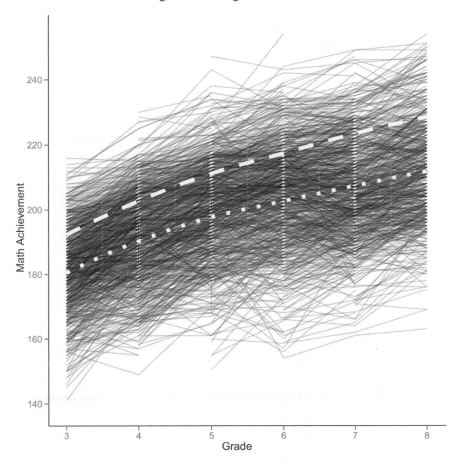

FIGURE 4.4. Individual math achievement trajectories for the homeless/ highly mobile (HHM) subgroup of 3,644 students tested in an urban school district from 2005/2006 through 2009/2010 (see Figure 4.3 for a plot of the *average* score of this group). The national average on the test is shown as a dashed white line and the dotted line indicates 1 standard deviation below the national average. Lines represent the scores of the same person over time. From Cutuli et al. (2013). Copyright 2012 by the authors and the Society for Research in Child Development, Inc. Reprinted with permission from Wiley-Blackwell.

homeless status in the district administrative data spanning 6 years preceding the 2009/2010 school year (beginning in 2003/2004). The order of presumed risk from highest to lowest was as follows: HHM (identified at any time including the school years 2003/2004 through 2008/2009), free lunch (at any time but not in the HHM group), reduced-fee lunch (but not HHM or free lunch), and general students (everyone else). Status as HHM in a given school year was defined by these conditions: living in a shelter, motel, vehicle, or campground; on the street; in an abandoned building, trailer, or other inadequate accommodation; or doubled-up with friends or relatives because housing could not be found or afforded. HHM students were identified by staff at schools, shelters, or at the district placement center. The other groups were identified according to district records of eligibility for the National School Lunch Program: free meals (income less than 130% of the poverty line), reduced-fee lunch (185% of the poverty line), and not identified as eligible or did not apply.

The proportion of students identified as HHM at any time during the study period was notable. Close to 14% of all the students in third to eighth grade over a 6-year period ending in 2009/2010 were identified as HHM at some time by the district. Moreover, almost 75% of the students in these grades in the MPS fell into one of the three low-income groups over time, a finding consistent with demographics in most large urban public school districts (Fantuzzo & Perlman, 2007).

Figure 4.3 shows the average achievement on the math test over time for each of the four groups plus the national norm on this test for comparison. The expected risk gradient was found, controlling for age, gender, ethnicity, attendance, special education placement, and English language learner status. Results for reading were similar. HHM students had significantly lower achievement than students who qualified for free lunch, who were lower than those in the reduced-fee lunch group, who were lower in turn than the relatively advantaged students in the general group. Average achievement of the HHM group (12th percentile reading, 18th math in third grade) and free-lunch groups (21st percentile reading, 31st math in third grade) were markedly low compared with the national average (50th percentile), while the reduced-fee lunch group tracked the normative level quite closely (46th percentile reading, 54th math in third grade), and the more advantaged students were above average on their scores (75th percentile reading, 79th math in third grade). These achievement gaps were present at the earliest test point and persisted (reading) or worsened (math). Attendance also was lower for the HHM group than other groups, although this and other differences on the control variables do not account for the magnitude of the gaps among groups.

In this study (Cutuli et al., 2013), we also were able to examine whether the rate of change in achievement (an index of learning rate) was slower the year after identification as HHM compared with non-HHM years. This was indeed the case for math, where growth was significantly slower in the year following identification as HHM. The rate of gains in reading did not vary significantly by HHM-identification timing. Math learning may be more acutely affected by residential mobility or the stress related to it than reading achievement, whereas both domains reflect the chronic risk associated with HHM status, regardless of timing.

The data shown in Figure 4.3 depict a longitudinal risk gradient for achievement, with HHM students showing the highest risk. However, these average scores for group obscure the individual trajectories of achievement within each group. To illustrate the marked individual differences within group, Figure 4.4 shows individual plots of achievement for the HHM group. The individual variability is now visually apparent, with many students testing in the average range or better on this test. Indeed, we found that 45% of the students in the HHM group scored consistently within or above the "average range" on this test over time.

We have consistently found these patterns of risk and resilience in district data. Our findings corroborate a continuum-of-risk model, in which HHM children have similar but greater risk than other socioeconomically disadvantaged children (Masten et al., 1993; Samuels et al., 2010). Additionally, there appear to be chronic and acute manifestations of academic risk associated with HHM status.

Individual differences among students in the higher-risk groups beg the question of what might account for the differences. For those who want to mitigate risk or promote school success, these differences hold potential keys to intervention. Data available in school records provide some clues, such as attendance, which is lower among HHM students. However, the scope of the individual differences far exceeds the potential explanatory power of the routine variables that schools monitor in administrative data. Thus, our search for resilience and vulnerability factors led us to pursue more detailed studies with families in shelters, with a particular focus on malleable influences that would be amenable to intervention.

IN SEARCH OF TARGETS FOR CHANGE: PREVENTING HARM AND PROMOTING RESILIENCE

Interventions to shift the odds of better lives for children from homeless families could focus on a range of system levels, from housing policy and economic supports to strategies targeting schools, teachers, parents, or individual children. Intervention could be directed at preventing homelessness or mitigating the associated risks before, during, or after it occurs. Federal and state policymakers and welfare agencies concerned with homeless families have traditionally focused on supports or policies related to housing, food, educational access, health care, child care, and employment (see Samuels et al., 2010). The Department of Housing and Urban Development (HUD), for example, has been conducting a large-scale experiment testing alternative housing strategies as an intervention for homeless families. The earned income tax credit might be a target for change among economists (Duncan, 2012). Educators, including early childhood educators and psychologists, have focused on direct interventions to facilitate success in age-salient developmental tasks, such as training or enrichment or tutoring to promote school readiness and success, while others have focused on preventing emotional and behavioral problems or treating symptoms of stress and trauma, often by helping parents with parenting and emotional support of children.

As a team of developmental, clinical, and educational psychologists; social workers; and early childhood teachers, our attention has been directed at understanding vulnerability and protective processes that potentially might be targets of intervention for families that already have experienced homelessness or are at considerable risk for homelessness, as well as strategies that can be implemented readily in shelters, schools, and other contexts where these children and parents are located. We were particularly interested in systems that show promise for change through intervention. We recognized early on in our work that although HHM families were similar in many ways to other low-income families, their mobility itself posed special challenges. Many evidenced-based interventions require a level of time and commitment that is impossible or impractical for many homeless families.

Our research in recent years has focused on stress, parenting, and executive function (EF) systems as promising targets for change that span multiple levels of analysis in the individual and the family. As noted above, our early work suggested that effective parenting skills and child cognitive skills, and particularly their cognitive control skills, were related to resilience in HHM children, as is often apparently the case in other children contending with adversity. We learned that parents were generally interested in the academic success of their children, and that within the constraints of a very difficult time in their lives, parents supported efforts to promote school readiness and achievement in their children. We have focused on the school context, because of the promising evidence that teachers and curriculum influence key systems we have targeted for change, such as EF skills.

In a series of basic studies, we focused on clarifying the roles of stress, parenting, and cognitive skills with respect to the competence and adaptability of children staying in shelters with their parents. At the same time, we were determined to move forward on developing interventions directly related to our models of malleable change, to test whether we were on the right track in regard to protective factors that matter for child development in homeless and similar families. Two related domains of child and family function strongly implicated in studies of risk and resilience as predictors of success in school that consistently relate to stress and adversity exposure and also show considerable promise in regard to change through interventions are EF skills and parenting.

Executive Function Skills

As individuals develop, they acquire the skills to direct their capabilities toward achieving their goals. We often refer to these self-control skills in terms of self-regulation. Some of these functions occur automatically, out of conscious awareness, while others require voluntary effort. Voluntary management of one's own mental and physical capabilities to meet a goal often are referred to as "cognitive control processes" or EF. EF capabilities depend on integrative neurocognitive processes that develop over time, and most notably on prefrontal processes in the brain (Carlson, Zelazo, & Faja, 2013).

EF encompasses a variety of skills essential to success in everyday life and over the longer term. These include paying attention, switching attention from one thing to another, suppressing an impulse or automatic response in order to make a preferred or novel response that is more adaptive, keeping multiple rules in mind, inhibiting short-term impulses for long-term gains, making yourself do something boring, and so on. Scientists often group these skills into three major categories: working memory, cognitive flexibility, and effortful or inhibitory control (Miyake et al., 2000; Zelazo & Carlson, 2012). These skills are fundamental for adaptive behavior and learning in novel situations, and play a central role in adaptation to changing experiences.

EF skills develop and change over the life course in conjunction with brain development and experiences (Zelazo & Bauer, 2013). There is a rapidly expanding body of science on neural systems related to these skills and their development in both typically developing and atypical populations (Best & Miller, 2010; Blair & Raver, 2012; Carlson et al., 2013; Zelazo & Carlson, 2012). These skills improve rapidly in preschool-age children and appear to be a good indicator of school readiness (Blair, 2002; Diamond & Lee, 2011). In addition, there is growing evidence that EF skills can be improved through intervention or training (Diamond & Lee, 2011; McDermott, Westerlund, Zeanah, Nelson, & Fox, 2012; Raver et al., 2011; Riggs, Jahromi, Razza, Dillworth-Bart, & Mueller, 2006; Zelazo & Carlson, 2012).

The resilience literature has long implicated self-regulation skills as important for positive outcomes in adverse environments

(Masten & Coatsworth, 1998). In addition, our own observations at shelters, where many of our team have volunteered and conducted research for more than two decades, influenced the decision to focus on EF skills. There appeared to be dramatic variation in the self-control skills of children in activities, in school, and in their interactions with parents. Parents also varied in their observable capabilities for staying calm in a crisis, managing the family, and planning in the midst of all the ongoing stresses and chaos accompanying homelessness.

In 2006, when we began pilot studies for our new work on malleable protective factors, one of our talented doctoral students, Jelena Obradović, decided to focus on EF skills in homeless children for her dissertation study. We did not really know at the time if it would be feasible to bring EF measures typically administered in controlled laboratory settings at universities into a homeless shelter environment, though we knew that it would be very difficult to assess homeless families at the university. So we proceeded to develop methods for field assessment. Obradović decided on a battery of well-established (in labs) tasks to try to capture EF skills broadly in the children. We focused on children who were about to enter kindergarten or first grade, to study how EF was related to teacher ratings of their behavior and academic success at school.

Obradović's (2010) study was very successful, although the sample size was modest. We learned that many of the measures worked well, were appealing to children, had expected patterns of associations, and also predicted how the children did in school from a teacher's perspective. EF skills were related as expected to age and parenting quality, and performance on more traditional "IQ" test measures. Yet even with all of these controlled, EF still had unique significance as a forecaster of school adjustment across multiple domains. For homeless children staying in an emergency shelter, EF tasks seemed to be a good indicator of how well children would do in kindergarten or first grade. We found, and continue to find in subsequent studies, that parents are generally enthusiastic about participating in research on school success. This initial study of EF was encouraging and we therefore continued research to refine and develop EF assessments for children, and build evidence of their significance for school readiness and potential as a target for intervention. We also learned that EF skills were related (negatively) to a widely used index of biological stress reactivity. Higher levels of the stress hormone cortisol (assayed from saliva samples) were related to worse EF performance (Cutuli, 2011).

Data from subsequent studies based on more recent data collection has essentially corroborated and expanded these initial findings. A larger study was implemented (during 2008–2010) in the years immediately after the Great Recession began with families from three shelters. Again, a battery of EF tasks was administered, along with several traditional IQ measures (Masten, Herbers, et al., 2012). We expected these measures to be related since performance on any kind of cognitive test requires a child to follow instructions and pay attention. Yet we hypothesized that EF skills would also have "added value" as a predictor of school adjustment, over and above any shared component of basic skills with IQ measures. Results supported these expectations. EF composite scores had a unique role in predicting school adjustment in comparison to IQ scores, as well as a shared component. EF scores were broad predictors of school function, including academic achievement, getting along with peers, relationships with the teacher, prosocial behavior, and externalizing problems.

Data from the same families also corroborated the finding that EF skills are related to levels of the stress hormone cortisol. Children with higher cortisol (adjusted for time of day) had worse performance on EF tasks (Cutuli, 2011). These data are consistent with a growing body of evidence that adverse life experiences, biologically mediated by dysregulation of the stress-regulation system, can undermine EF performance in the short term and EF development in the long term (Blair & Raver, 2012; Evans & Schamberg, 2009; Shonkoff, 2011). These processes are discussed further in Chapter 7.

Parent–Child Relationships and Parenting

In our recent research on potentially malleable protective factors for resilience in homeless and similar children, we also focused on

parenting. Effective parenting and high-quality parent–child relationships are implicated in virtually every study of resilience in children (Luthar, 2006; Masten, 2007), including the limited research
on homeless families (Miller, 2011; Miliotis et al., 1999; Herbers et
al., 2011). Moreover, there is considerable evidence now, including
"gold-standard" randomized trials, that parenting practices and the
parent–child relationship qualities are malleable through intervention and that improvements in the parenting system predict better
child outcomes (Belsky & de Haan, 2011; Patterson et al., 2010;
Sandler, Schoenfelder, Wolchik, & MacKinnon, 2011).

The wide variation in parenting behavior is easily observed in
a shelter context. We had informally observed for many years that
some parents appeared to be struggling with the complex tasks
of caring for their children during an episode of homelessness,
while others appeared to be managing well. Well-behaved children often seemed to be part of families where at least one parent
was navigating this inherently difficult situation effectively. Our
early research supported these observations through interview-
based assessments of parenting, as noted above (Miliotis et al.,
1999). In our most recent work, we have expanded our methods
for assessing the qualities of the parent–child relationship. These
include both brief and easy to code methods, along with more
time-consuming observational methods.

The "five-minute speech sample" method is an example of a
brief measure that appears to work well with homeless families
(Narayan, Herbers, Plowman, Gewirtz, & Masten, 2012). Parents
are simply asked to talk about their child for 5 minutes, which is
taped and later coded with standardized systems for expressed
emotion (e.g., negative, harsh, or critical; positive or warm; Caspi
et al., 2004; Magaña-Amato, 1993). Scores on this brief measure
(based on systematic and reliable coding systems) were related
to considerably more labor-intensive assessments of observed
parent–child interaction, as well as teacher ratings of classroom
behavior. Parents who talked about a child in more positive and
less negative ways also showed more effective and positive parenting behavior in structured interactions with the child, as coded by
independent observers.

In order to ascertain the utility of different methods for coding observed parenting for HHM families, we have compared three different coding systems, each highly reliable, for observational coding of structured parent–child interactions. Observational coding is often viewed as the "gold-standard" approach to assessment of parenting or parent–child interaction. In one study, we adopted a set of structured parent–child interaction tasks that were originally developed by investigators at the Oregon Social Learning Center (OSLC) for assessing parent–child interaction for their basic and intervention research on parenting and later adapted for use with low-income families (Gewirtz, Forgatch, & Wieling, 2008). In a sequence of structured tasks, parent and child were directed to play a game, discuss a family issue, solve a problem, clean up toys, or play a variety of games (Herbers, 2011). This session of approximately 45 minutes was video recorded for later coding. Three separate coding approaches were completed by different coders. Each method showed excellent interrater reliability. The three methods included (1) global clinical judgments, (2) the most recent version of the OSLC rating scales (Forgatch, Plowman, Gewirtz, & Stubbs, 2010), and (3) microsocial coding for a state space grid (SSG) analysis (Herbers, 2011). Parenting scores based on each of these three methods were strongly interrelated and basically equivalent indicators of a broad, underlying dimension of parenting quality (Plowman, Narayan, Masten, Desjardins, & Herbers, 2012).

Observable parenting skills in this session were associated with child outcomes at school and also with the child's EF skills. Analyses indicated that EF skills mediated in part the link between specific aspects of parenting and child behavior at school as reported by teachers. These findings were congruent with our hypothesis that one way good parenting "goes to school" is through its role in the development of effective self-regulation skills in the child.

Parenting, of course, is not a one-way process, but an ongoing transactional process between parent and child (Sroufe et al., 2005). EF task performance by the child measured immediately before the parent–child interaction session predicted child "on-task" behavior observed and assessed by microsocial coding of the child for the SSG analyses. Parents respond differently to on-task behavior than they do to distracted, negative, or otherwise off-task behavior in their interactions with children. Over time, these dyadic processes would be expected to cascade and reinforce positive or negative trends in the development of EF skills and the quality of the parent–child relationship.

Observing these interactions, it also became clear to us that parents varied widely in their own EF and that their self-regulation capabilities were playing a central role in family resilience. In our subsequent research we have begun to assess the EF of parents, and the risk and protective factors that may influence how well parents manage stress and maintain good self-regulation in self and family members.

In the situation of homelessness or family life in a temporary shelter, conditions are quite taxing for any family. Ongoing economic strain, chaos, fatigue, and realistic worries or stress could take a toll on EF in the parent as well as the child, with corrosive effects on parent–child interaction. Yet some families manage to maintain routines, effective parenting, and good self-regulation of children and parents. Good EF in this context—by parent or child—probably indicates that there are potent protective processes operating to support EF, although there also may be variation in the sensitivity or susceptibility of individual parents or children to the challenges posed to EF in this context. Understanding these processes may be crucial for interventions designed to support positive family and child function during periods of economic crisis and concomitant family turbulence.

STRESS: THE ELEPHANT IN THE ROOM

In our efforts to promote resilience among HHM children and similar families, we do not want to ignore the proverbial elephant in the room, which is the inherently stressful nature of the situation for parents and their children. As I discuss in Chapter 11, there are multiple ways to intervene in the interplay of adversity and individuals in the promotion of resilience. These strategies include preventing exposure or mitigating its impact.

We suspect that stress plays a central role in the processes by which poverty or homelessness affect child development, some direct and others indirect. Families that end up homeless often have experienced a sequence of highly stressful events and experiences prior to any specific episode of homelessness. Homelessness itself imposes an additional series of very stressful experiences on a family. Overwhelming stress can overload physical and mental capacities for adaptation in the parents as well as children. We know that chronically high stress is bad for parenting as well as the health and development of children. We concur with Shonkoff's (2011) argument that it is essential to prevent or reduce exposure or mitigate stress effects for children in addition to whatever actions are taken to increase resources or protective factors. Preventing or reducing stress through intervention is itself a protective action, and one of the fundamental strategies for changing the odds of resilience (see Chapter 11).

In focus groups and our parent education groups, homeless parents often talk about the enormous stress they experience in their everyday lives and their concerns about the toll stress is taking on their children, as well as their own health and well-being. Leading scientists in multiple disciplines share their concerns about the long-term consequences of stress on individual development and the health of subsequent generations (Blair & Raver, 2012; Evans & Schamberg, 2009; Hackman, Farah, & Meaney, 2010; McEwen & Gianaros, 2011; Shonkoff, 2011; Walker et al., 2011). Evidence points to multiple strategies by which the stress on families or children might be reduced (Yoshikawa, Aber, & Beardslee, 2012).

It is notoriously challenging, however, to implement most of the best-validated evidenced-based interventions with residentially unstable families. Residential stability as well as adequate safety, nutrition, and health care may be a prerequisite for long-term stress reduction in families. Coordinated efforts that span private and public sectors, as well as local, state, and national governmental and nongovernmental agencies may be required. Meanwhile, parents, as well as local agencies and schools, are asking for assistance for currently HHM students.

IMPLICATIONS FROM FINDINGS ON RISK AND RESILIENCE IN HOMELESS CHILDREN IN THE UNITED STATES

Our findings on the "big picture" in the district data on achievement, attendance, and other administrative data have major implications. HHM status is surprisingly common when one considers the cumulative data. HHM status also is associated with higher risk than poverty alone, as indexed by federal eligibility criteria for reduced-price or free school meals. This risk appears to be largely chronic in nature and persistent, although there also was evidence of acute effects on math achievement during the year following HHM identification. *These findings strongly suggest that the goal of closing the achievement gaps observed for children in poverty or with minority status in the United States is going to require explicit attention to HHM students.* Moreover, the strategies that work with stable children may prove inappropriate or insufficient for mobile children. Mobility itself poses challenges for interventions or policies aimed at addressing the issues of HHM families.

The risks and issues posed by residential mobility for learning and education have been summarized in a report from a workshop organized by the Board on Children, Youth, and Families published in 2010 by the National Research Council and Institute of Medicine. A White Paper commissioned by HUD raises similar concerns, with a sharper focus on homelessness in children (Samuels et al., 2010). It is unlikely that there is "one solution" for the complex and intertwined issues of poverty, homelessness, and school mobility in children.

While the risks and problems observed in homeless families show many similarities with other disadvantaged families, our research, together with the larger body of studies, also suggests familiar protective factors. These include adaptive capacities embedded in individuals, parent–child relationships, and families, as well as communities and cultures.

Our findings have consistently supported the idea that EF skills, or self-regulation more broadly defined, are associated with resilience or maladaptation in children experiencing

homelessness. Our findings align well with the few other studies on self-regulation in similar populations (e.g., Buckner, Mezzacappa, & Beardslee, 2009). Such data do not necessarily indicate that EF skills have a causal role in resilience. However, this
possibility motivated us to pursue intervention strategies that
might provide better evidence about the role of EF in this context.

Over the past few years, we began developing intervention
strategies to test the possibility that fostering EF skills could promote success in these high-risk children, particularly in regard to
school readiness and adjustment (Casey et al., 2014). This work
is collaborative, including university experts on EF (Stepha-
nie Carlson and Philip Zelazo), family interventions (Abigail
Gewirtz), and early childhood education (Barbara Murphy and
Marie Lister), as well as community partners with extensive experience in education and services for homeless and disadvantaged
children. We are currently developing an intervention for HHM
children designed to build EF skills during a developmental window of opportunity in preschool. EF skills develop rapidly in the
preschool years, and they appear to have considerable plasticity
during this developmental period (Carlson et al., 2013; Zelazo &
Carlson, 2012). Moreover, there is growing evidence that these
skills can be improved through explicit training and preschool
curricula focused on their development (Blair & Raver, 2012; Diamond & Lee, 2011).

Our project is designed to boost EF training in early childhood settings with HHM students. Given the mobility of these
students, we are attempting to improve EF skills in a short time
frame (within a month). Our intervention has three related components, all designed to motivate and help children practice EF
skills: preschool curriculum activities, parent education, and
individual training. Our theory of change is focused on activities
that encourage reflective thinking and practice EF skills. Teachers
learn how to increase EF skill building through classroom management strategies and specific activities. Parents learn that EF
skills matter for school readiness, how family routines can facilitate EF skills, and how to include fun EF practice in everyday life.
At family fun nights, parents and children practice games that tax
a child's emerging skills to concentrate and remember rules or

cards that have been played (e.g., Memory, Go Fish!), switch rules with flexibility (e.g., Blink; sorting by color and then by shape), stop or go as called for (e.g., Red Light, Green Light; "freeze dancing," where children freeze position when the music stops), and so on. They discover books that use humor and imagination to encourage flexible or reflective thinking and concentration (e.g., *Don't Be Silly Mrs. Millie*, *Spilt Milk*, "I Spy" books), and how to turn any early reading activity into an EF practice session by asking more questions about what comes next, what the characters are thinking, or a different ending. For children who need more intensive practice, we have focused on EF games and training exercises with a tutor or "EF coach." Our goal is to test whether a combination of EF-training components can improve children's EF skills and also the EF-teaching skills of parents and teachers with beneficial effects on school readiness of the children. Early results suggest that each of the components can be implemented with high-risk children and their parents, including in shelter settings. Families, as well as teachers, have responded with interest and enthusiasm to the evolving intervention, but it remains to be seen whether this kind of intervention will have any lasting effect on EF or school outcomes, especially in a context of extremely high ongoing stress exposure.

Preventing or mitigating stress may turn out to be an essential prerequisite of any intervention with children or parents experiencing homelessness. We are just beginning to consider intervention strategies suited to short-term programs for parents and children that target stress reduction, beyond the family fun nights built into our EF-training programs. Many options are available, ranging from mindfulness or meditation to exercise and music, although these strategies may have only temporary effects while long-term stress-reducing solutions are implemented, including stable housing and income supports.

SUMMARY

Homelessness in American children is a broad indicator of high cumulative risk to development that is strongly linked with the risks of deep or chronic poverty to health, education, and development. Homelessness appears to indicate an even higher level of academic risk compared with free school lunch eligibility, congruent with general evidence on the effects of mobility on achievement. Yet there is considerable variation among children who fall into this category, both with respect to the level of risk or adversity in their lives and also in how well the individual child or other members of the family are functioning. Many children who move into or out of homelessness do surprisingly well in school, for example, and their resilience provides clues to promotive or protective influences. Some of these children may simply have more resources and fewer risks than other children experiencing homelessness. Others may be actively protected by an effective parent or teacher, while others may be less susceptible biologically to the potential stress of adverse experiences. Stress, parenting, and self-regulation processes and their development appear to be promising directions for future research aimed at promoting adaptation and protecting development in the context of economic crisis.

The broad literature on adversity and resilience among children growing up in poverty underscores familiar conclusions about risk and protective processes. Risks often accumulate in the lives of children and families, and this burden often takes a cumulative toll on development. Yet there is impressive evidence that outcomes vary among children exposed to similar risks related to poverty and mobility. Dose matters, and so does the developmental timing of exposures to adversity or deprivation, but resources and protective factors also matter. Children with more effective parents and other stable, caring relationships fare better, as do children with better cognitive and self-regulation skills and opportunities to attend good early childhood programs and schools. Successful interventions appear to effectively address exposure and stress, as well as resources and protections, supporting the systems that protect children and child development, including parenting, family, education, child care, health care, and other community systems. The literature on resilience in war and disaster, discussed in the next chapter, also echoes these themes.

CHAPTER 5

MASS TRAUMA
AND EXTREME ADVERSITIES

Resilience in War, Terrorism, and Disaster

S ince the beginning of this century, millions of children have been affected by disasters, war, terrorism, and severe political violence across the globe. Children worldwide were exposed to the terror of the September 11, 2001, attack on the World Trade Center, both directly through loss of family members or proximity to Ground Zero, and indirectly through media exposure, effects on their caregivers or classmates, or the disruptions of everyday life. Three years later, on September 1, 2004, another terror attack horrified the world, when armed separatists occupied a school in the Russian town of Beslan. Over the course of 50 hours, more than 1,100 hostages, including close to 800 children, were held captive without food or water, were wired with explosives, and witnessed the murder of other hostages. After 3 days and a series of explosions, Russian forces stormed the school, ending the siege. The death toll was 334, including 186 children. Later the same year, during the holiday season in late December, a massive megathrust earthquake in Indonesia triggered major tsunami waves in the Indian Ocean that took over 200,000 lives, killing many children outright and leaving countless others without parents or homes. Hurricane Katrina arrived in the Gulf of

Mexico the following year, leaving a huge area of destruction in its wake. In 2008, thousands of Chinese children died in the Sichuan earthquake, many of them students killed by collapsing school buildings. In 2011, a triple catastrophe occurred after the Tōhuko earthquake off the coast of Japan triggered a tsunami that not only destroyed a large coastal region but also caused the meltdown of the Fukushima Daiichi nuclear power plant, with still-unfolding consequences for children in this and future generations.

During this same period of time, chronic wars and conflict zones around the globe generated trauma and misery for millions of children who have suffered consequences in the form of injury or illness, exposure to extreme violence, kidnapping as child soldiers, starvation, and the loss of parents, friends, homes, and nationalities. Most of these ongoing conflicts occur in low-income countries where children already suffer from inadequate nutrition and health care (Reed, Razel, Jones, Panter-Brick, & Stein, 2012).

Concerns about children exposed in large numbers to such extreme adversities have played a central role in resilience research throughout its history. A literature on children in war was sparked by the plight of children in World War II, threatened by bombings, starvation, execution, abandonment, bereavement, and persecution. Anna Freud and her colleague Dorothy Burlingham published the influential volume *War and Children* in 1943 summarizing their observations and clinical experiences. They described the signs of "traumatic shock" they observed among children but also noted the profound importance of maternal care in child responses. Children in the care of mothers and mother surrogates showed fewer signs of such trauma. During the London Blitz, accounts of how children fared during this massive and rapid evacuation also noted the traumatizing consequences of separating children from their parents; some children returned to London despite the dangers from bombing because they were faring so poorly (Garmezy, 1983). This observation on the buffering effects of proximity to caregivers for children exposed to terrifying adversities is one of the most robust findings reported in the literature on children in mass disasters, including war and natural disasters.

After the war ended, Freud played a key role in interventions for orphaned child survivors rescued from concentration camps. In another influential work, published in 1951, Freud and Dann described their experiences supervising the treatment of a group of six young children sent to England after liberation of the Terezin concentration camp. They described numerous behavioral and emotional problems among this group of children when they arrived, but also the strong attachment bonds among them. These children, and many others from Terezin, showed dramatic improvements over time. Yet, during the same period, many also showed evidence of lingering effects, often described as "scarring" or "sensitization" effects. This mixed picture of resilience and lingering consequences of extreme adversities has been observed in both the anecdotal and empirical literature on children in war and disaster (Masten & Narayan, 2012; Masten, Narayan, Silverman, & Osofsky, 2015).

Two of the most powerful images of child survivors of war capture this mixture of terror, resilience, and scarring. Both are photographs of Kim Phuc, the "girl in the picture." On June 8, 1972, Nick Ut took one of the most famous photographs ever captured of children in war. The photo featured 9-year-old Kim Phuc, badly burned by Napalm, fleeing in terror down the road with other villagers. This Pulitzer Prize-winning photograph appeared on the front page of newspapers around the world the next day and it has been reprinted many times, bringing the horrific pain and suffering of children in war to global attention. Kim Phuc survived and eventually settled in Canada, where another evocative photograph was taken of her by Joe McNally in 1995 for *Life* magazine. This photograph shows her holding her sleeping baby on her shoulder, seen from the back with her badly scarred skin exposed. Only the external scarring shows in a photograph; we are left to consider the internal scars. These two images tell a powerful story of resilience and recovery but also the terrible cost of war for children. Kim Phuc's story was told by Denise Chong (2001) in the book, *The Girl in the Picture*.

There are many accounts of children surviving war and political violence. The story of a young Cambodian girl, Thida Butt

Mam, is recounted in the biography *To Destroy You Is No Loss* by JoAn Criddle (1998), quoted in Chapter 2. This book was named for the motto of the Khmer Rouge. A more recent example is provided by the chilling, brutally honest, and moving autobiography of Ishmael Beah (2007), *A Long Way Gone: Memoirs of a Boy Soldier*. Born in Sierra Leone, he recounts how he became a boy soldier, the dehumanizing atrocities he experienced, his liberation, and his rehabilitation. In his autobiography, Beah expresses his appreciation for the professors at Oberlin College who encouraged him to begin his book while he was a student and facilitated its publication.

These single-case accounts suggest that for some young people there may be solace or something therapeutic about "telling the story" of terror and recovery. Perhaps these narratives, and other artistic expressions about similar experiences in art or music, provide a means for victims to gain a greater sense of control and meaning in their lives.

Child survivors of natural disasters face calamities that are not of human design, but they also encounter terror, devastation, loss, starvation, horrible injuries, and many other traumatic situations. It is therefore not surprising to find striking similarities in the research on disasters and war, both with respect to risks and protective processes (Masten & Narayan, 2012; Masten, et al., 2015).

Concerns about the effects of disasters on children also played a key role in the history of research on resilience. Historically, two of the best-documented disasters in terms of their effects on children, both in the short term and over the long term, are the Buffalo Creek dam disaster and an Australian bushfire.

The dam disaster, not entirely "natural," occurred in 1972 in a mining community when a dam above Buffalo Creek, West Virginia, burst and flooded the town below. This small community was devastated, with 125 deaths, many more injuries, and lingering consequences (Erikson, 1976; Gleser, Green, & Winget, 1981; Korol, Kramer, Grace, & Green, 2002). A subsequent lawsuit resulted in extensive documentation of the observed effects on the survivors. Although this context raised numerous issues of bias, the accounts have been influential because of their comprehensiveness and the scarcity of other data available on the consequences of mass trauma on families. In addition, there was a follow-up study 17 years after the disaster, which was even more rare (Green et al., 1994; Korol et al., 2002).

Lawsuit notwithstanding, conclusions based on survivors of the Buffalo Creek disaster have been widely replicated (Masten & Narayan, 2012; Masten et al., 2015). Dose effects were observed, with young people exposed to greater death and devastation showing more symptoms. Anxiety and trauma symptoms, such as fearfulness, nightmares, or jumpiness, were particularly salient, and anxiety symptoms forecasted more lasting effects. Girls generally were rated higher on anxiety symptoms, whereas boys were rated higher on aggressive–disruptive behavior, or "belligerence." Older age at the time of the disaster was related to more overall symptoms, and particularly to greater anxiety. Adults had more symptoms than adolescents who generally had more symptoms than younger children, although young children exhibited more specific fears and regressions in recent developmental achievements, such as toilet training. Child problems after the disaster also were related to general family function and how well parents were adjusting in terms of irritability, violence, gloomy mood, and less supportiveness.

Seventeen years later, most of the survivors had recovered, although as a group they had higher current (7%) and lifetime (32%) rates of PTSD than a comparison sample (4 and 6%, respectively; Green et al., 1994). By this time, dose effects had largely dissipated, although major losses (family and friends) had lingering significance. These findings suggest that over time, resilience and recovery were typical, even for a disaster of this magnitude in a community.

The Australian bushfire of 1983 provides a second example of influential disaster research, with results that also have been widely replicated. McFarlane and colleagues conducted a large study about 2 years postfire (McFarlane, 1987; McFarlane, Policansky, & Irwin, 1987) and a follow-up study 20 years later (McFarlane & Van Hooff, 2009). Over 800 children attending primary schools in the fire-exposed region were compared with a group of 725 children from a neighboring region not directly affected by the fire. The fire-exposed children had more symptoms than the comparison group in 1985 at the time of the initial study, consistent with "dose" effects (in this case contrasting high levels of direct exposure with lower levels of more indirect exposure). However, one of the most notable results of this study was the finding that separation from mothers and maternal symptoms were more important predictors of child well-being than dose itself, underscoring again the protective effect of proximity to attachment figures in terrifying situations. In the follow-up study, there were some differences between the high- and low-dose groups, but again the differences were few and small in magnitude. Fire victims reported higher rates of PTSD symptoms, such as intrusion symptoms (memories, images, or thoughts) or hyperarousal, related to the fire. On the whole, however, this study also suggests that resilience is normative.

Reviews of the early literature on the extreme stressors of childhood drew conclusions that have held up well over the years (Eth & Pynoos, 1985; Garmezy, 1983; Garmezy & Rutter, 1985; Rutter, 1983). Early reviewers concluded that dose matters, and that trauma exposure can have lasting effects, although usually the effects are short term. They observed that threats and loss of loved ones had greater effects than material losses, and that parents or surrogate caregivers played key roles in the responses of children. How well the parents were functioning themselves, the support they could muster for their children, and their simple proximity all mattered. Community supports also played a role. The early reviewers noted dramatic individual differences in apparent vulnerability and response to what appeared to be very similar experiences. These observations continue to be prominent in subsequent reviews of the recent literature (Masten & Narayan, 2012; Masten et al., 2015; American Psychological Association, 2010; Furr, Comer, Edmunds, & Kendall, 2010). At the same time, considerably more evidence has accumulated, from higher-quality studies, and with a stronger focus on unpacking the processes that may account for both risk and resilience in disaster. Selected evidence from recent research is highlighted below, with a focus on dose effects, individual differences, the protective roles of community or culture, and effective interventions. In the chapter conclusion, implications of these findings for disaster preparedness are discussed.

DOSE EFFECTS: CUMULATIVE RISK IN THE CONTEXT OF MASS TRAUMA

Evidence continues to mount that there is generally higher risk for symptoms, suffering, and other consequences of mass trauma when children are exposed with greater frequency or intensity and there is a piling up of severely threatening or traumatic experiences (Dimitry, 2012; Furr et al., 2010; Masten & Osofsky, 2010; Masten et al., 2015; Norris, Friedman, & Watson, 2002; Norris, Friedman, Watson, et al., 2000; Pine, Costello, & Masten, 2005; Qouta, Punamäki, & El Sarraj, 2008). A variety of severity indicators show dose gradients of this kind. In disasters with clear paths of destruction, literal distance from areas of greatest devastation can serve as a proxy for exposure. In situations without a single epicenter or path of destruction, assessments of severity and number of traumatic experiences often are utilized to index the degree of exposure, tallying exposure to specific adverse experiences such as rape, loss of loved ones, torture, or witnessing death. Psychological proximity also shows dose effects, where the closeness of relationships and identification with victims of a catastrophe or perceived danger to self and loved ones is associated with greater effects on survivors. Emotional proximity can have more effects than physical proximity (Dimitry, 2012; Masten et al., 2015).

Increasingly, efforts are made to assess dose in ways that account for multiple parameters of traumatic exposures. Shortly after 9/11, research showed dose effects on school children in New York related to personal exposure (e.g., injury, witnessing), family death or injury, and media exposure (Hoven et al., 2005). Researchers also consider the context of ongoing or new adversities that may precede or follow a specific disaster or acute traumatic exposure.

Combined effects of this kind can be viewed as dose effects or as evidence of sensitization to trauma triggered by earlier exposures (Masten et al., 2015). A study of the 2004 tsunami in Sri Lanka found that children with greater direct exposure to the devastation and children from war-ravaged areas of the country were more affected by this disaster than children with less direct exposure or children from more peaceful areas (Catani et al., 2010). Childhood abuse experiences appeared to have a sensitizing effect for adolescents in the Second Lebanon War in Israel, with abused youth showing higher rates of PTSD (Schiff et al., 2012). After war or displacement due to political conflicts, recovery does not go as well for youth who experience ongoing or new abuse, rejection by the community, or other adversities (Reed et al., 2012).

Studies of dose effects often pack together many aspects of exposure to gain a general understanding of risk. However, there is also value in "unpacking" risk to understand which experiences may have specific or more extreme effects. In their meta-analysis of posttraumatic stress (PTS) studies, Furr et al. (2010) were able to demonstrate that greater effects were observed in disasters where there was greater loss of life, when children had greater physical proximity to the disaster, when children reported greater perceived threat, and when there was loss of a loved one or friend. Based on their study of Bosnian adolescents exposed to war and political conflict, Layne and colleagues (2010) identified particular experiences that appeared to be more potent risk factors, including exposure to life threat and traumatic death. Their observations align with broader studies of trauma on events that pose high risk for posttraumatic symptoms or disorder among youth and adults. Similarly, in their study of child soldiers, Betancourt et al. (2010) described the experiences of rape and killing others as "toxic" experiences associated with distinctive and long-lasting effects.

There is growing interest in dose–response patterns, and particularly in the possibility that this relation is not always linear. It is conceivable that there are response ceilings, where response stops rising as a function of rising exposure, resulting in a kind of asymptote effect. This could happen at levels of exposure so high that everyone has passed the threshold for a full reaction. Beyond this level, dose effects wane and other factors may become salient, including individual and situational differences in resources, protective systems, or recovery context. In a recent study of child soldiers in Uganda, where young people were exposed to extreme, prolonged, and horrific atrocities, severity of exposure during captivity did not relate to adaptation during rehabilitation (Klasen et al., 2010). Instead it was experiences and support characterizing the recovery context that related to how well the former child soldiers were faring.

Another nonlinear possibility is that individuals do well up to a threshold and once they pass this threshold, dose is strongly related to response. In this scenario, response is not related to dose until the threshold is past. This could be described as a depletion or exhaustion model, in which children have a limited capacity for handling traumatic exposures. When this capacity is surpassed by the demands of adjusting to repeated or prolonged trauma exposure, disturbances emerge.

In their summary of research on Palestinian children in Gaza, Qouta and colleagues (2008) describe yet another nonlinear pattern. They observed that adaptive behavior declined as adversity exposure rose at lower exposure levels, but then when exposure became extreme, responses changed, as if youth were inspired to rally in response to very extreme political violence.

Time may not "heal all wounds" but dose effects often diminish with time. As noted above, long-term follow-ups of major disaster suggest that recovery is normative, although there often are lingering effects for some individuals. The meta-analysis by Furr and colleagues (2010) indicated that there was greater PTS for assessments conducted within a year after the disaster than after a year had passed. A study of mental health following 9/11 in adolescents (Gershoff, Aber, Ware, & Kotler, 2010) found only small dose effects 15 months after this trauma; it is conceivable that effects of the trauma experience were already declining by the time of this assessment. There are additional "timing" issues related to the developmental timing of the exposures, discussed in the next section.

The meta-analysis by Furr et al. (2010) also indicated that children self-reported more PTS than their parents reported about them. This finding has important implications for assessment and intervention following mass trauma. Parents and other adults may underestimate the exposure dose or trauma response of children. On the other hand, young people may also attempt to protect their parents by withholding information about trauma exposure and their symptoms. In either case, the end result would be underestimating the needs of children, with children and youth not seeking or receiving the support they need to adequately address the consequences of trauma.

Media Exposure

Since World War II, there have been massive changes in the role and nature of media in the lives of adults and children. Vivid and visual coverage of disasters and political violence continues to expand, with a 24-hour news cycle, widespread access to the Internet, viral spreading of recorded events through websites for posting video recordings by individuals, and the spread of social media and mobile devices that enable individuals to share experiences with millions worldwide. Although research has lagged behind technological advances, it is clear that exposure through media can be extensive during and following a crisis and that there are dose effects related to media exposure (Comer & Kendall, 2007).

Media-based exposure effects, to date typically referring to television exposure, have been reported after the Challenger space shuttle explosion (Terr et al., 1999), after the Oklahoma City bombing (Pfefferbaum et al., 2001, 2003); and after 9/11 (Lengua, Long, Smith, & Meltzoff, 2005; Otto et al., 2007; Phillips, Prince, & Schiebelhut, 2004; Saylor, Cowart, Lipovsky, Jackson, & Finch, 2003; Schuster et al., 2001). Data from these studies are consistent with dose effects but complicated by variations in the nature of media access and use, developmental and age variations in the viewers studied, parental monitoring of use, and assessment strategies. In a study of Boston families after 9/11 (Otto et al., 2007), media exposure was related to PTS in younger children. There is considerable concern that younger viewers do not understand that events are being replayed rather than happening again (Franks, 2011). Older viewers, on the other hand, could have greater exposure because they have more unmonitored access to media and have a better understanding of the full scope of what they are seeing and its possible long-term significance (Comer & Kendall, 2007; Comer, Furr, Beidas, Weiner, & Kendall, 2008).

More research is clearly needed on the media with respect to exposure dose, as well as the potential roles of media in communication, preparation, and intervention about terror and disaster. Media exposure has the potential to be monitored and moderated by parents, teachers, producers and broadcasters, individuals, and societies, in ways that direct exposure to disaster cannot be controlled. Evidence of dose effects has prompted clinical experts and educators to recommend caution with respect to exposing children, and especially young or anxious children, to media coverage of disasters, war, and terror (Bonanno, Brewin, Kaniasty, & Greca, 2010; Comer & Kendall, 2007; Lengua et al., 2005; Masten et al., 2015; Masten & Obradović, 2008; Pine et al., 2005).

Determinants of Dose

Dose matters, so it is important to consider the determinants of exposure dose. Variations in individual sensitivity to the same experiences, what might be viewed as "subjective dose," are discussed in the next section. However, it is also the case that objective exposures vary in their randomness: There are places, historical times, families, jobs, sociodemographic addresses, and situations where the likelihood of traumatic exposures to natural and human-made disasters is much greater. The risk of exposure to war atrocities is much higher in some regions of the world, just as the risk of hurricanes or earthquakes is higher in some areas. For children, two of the most widely observed determinants of exposure in mass trauma situations are age and sex.

In disasters and war, older children often have higher exposure, probably for multiple reasons (Masten & Osofsky, 2010;

Masten et al., 2015). They understand more about what is happening, they have more freedom of movement, greater media exposure, and they are called on to help or get involved more than young children. Older children are more likely to be recruited or forced into war as child soldiers and more likely to be raped in the course of war. In their national survey study of exposure to violence and disaster, Becker-Blease, Turner, and Finkelhor (2010) analyzed data from a Developmental Victimization Survey of 1,000 adolescents (ages 10–17), and 1,030 caregivers of children (ages 2–9). Age was associated with reports of higher exposure to disasters (including terror attacks), both within each age group and across the two groups.

Sex has a complex relation to exposure. Males and females may experience different events, be more or less likely to report them when they happen, or interpret them differently, and they also may experience different treatment or stigma as a result of similar experiences (American Psychological Association, 2010; Masten & Osofky, 2010; Masten et al., 2015). Betancourt et al. (2010), for example, found that female former child soldiers reported more rape experiences than males, which also carried greater stigma for females in the recovery community. In their report on studies of Palestinians living in Gaza, Qouta and colleagues (2008) noted that parents were more protective of girls, whereas they encouraged boys to participate actively in the conflict, which would convey very different exposure risks for males and females.

Exposure Processes

There are many exposure pathways by which disaster or war experiences could affect child function and development. These include direct injuries and starvation; radiation poisoning and contaminated water; and the psychological stresses of witnessing death, torture, or destruction; experiencing threats of death or injury; and loss of caregivers, siblings, friends, or pets. Indirect pathways include the effects of severe trauma on parents and other loved ones and the impact of destroyed communities, school, or opportunities on the life course. Even before a child is conceived, trauma could affect the future parents in ways that will later affect their children. At the time of a disaster, children are very adept at reading the emotional state of their parents as a source of information about what is happening and safety, a phenomenon called "social referencing" in the developmental literature (Walden & Ogan, 1988). A terrified parent can be terrifying to a child, regardless of whether the child understands the situation that is terrifying the parent. Additionally, disasters and wars often dislocate and impoverish families, disrupting all familiar routines, and may require migration to new cultures.

Processes by which exposure influences individuals, directly or indirectly, is a topic of global research interest. As noted in Chapter 2 and discussed further in Chapter 7, there is growing interest in the processes by which severe adversity exposure alters the organism and its development, perhaps by altering stress regulation or immune function, and inducing epigenetic change. Timing of exposures appears to play a significant role in these processes, as do individual differences in susceptibility.

INDIVIDUAL DIFFERENCES IN RESPONSE

Early accounts of children in war and disaster noted the marked variations in responses by individual children (Garmezy, 1983; Masten, 2011; Masten & Osofky, 2010; Masten et al., 2015; Rutter, 1983). It was not simple curiosity that inspired closer examination of these differences, but rather a search for understanding potential protective processes that might inform efforts to help children before, during, and following mass trauma.

The puzzle of individual response differences to highly similar experiences was a thorny one. It was often unclear whether observed differences arose before or after exposure, since there rarely was data on how children were faring before the disaster. In addition, it was difficult to ascertain whether reported differences reflected different objective exposures, different subjective experiences or reactivity to the same objective dose, or reporter bias among the observers. Nonetheless, consistencies among the studies of individual differences suggested clues to uncovering processes that might be helpful for intervention.

Sex Differences

Sex differences provide a case in point. Differences are often observed but it is difficult to sort out the role of preexisting differences, different exposures, and differential interpretations by victims or their communities based on sex, including stigma (American Psychological Association, 2010; Bonanno et al., 2010; Masten et al., 2015). After disasters and violent mass-trauma experiences, females often—though not always—are found to show more symptoms of distress, depressed mood, or anxiety (Barber & Schluterman, 2009; Furr et al., 2010; Masten et al., 2015; Reed et al., 2012). However, girls who have not been exposed to extreme trauma also usually report more internalizing symptoms than boys of the same age, particularly in adolescence and beyond (Crick & Zahn-Waxler, 2003). If there were a general increase in these symptoms related to traumatic experiences, one would expect girls to have more symptoms than boys. Numerous reports, including results of the PTS meta-analysis by Furr et al. (2010), indicate greater distress and PTS among girls. Following an industrial disaster in France, for example, Godeau et al. (2005) reported more symptoms consistent with PTSD among younger and older adolescent girls compared with boys the same age. Similarly, two studies of symptoms post-Katrina found more symptoms of trauma and depressed mood among girls than boys (Kronenberg et al., 2010; Vigil, Geary, Granger, & Flinn, 2010). The study by Vigil et al. (2010) was unusual in having a socioeconomically matched low-exposure comparison group. It is interesting to note that there was an interaction effect for sex by depressed mood in this study indicating that hurricane-exposed adolescent girls had higher levels of depression symptoms compared with nonexposed girls, whereas the two groups of boys did not differ on depression symptoms.

Evidence generally continues to indicate sex differences in the expression of aggressive or externalizing behavior following disasters or mass-trauma exposures, with males showing more aggressive behavior (Barber, 2009a, 2009b; Dimitry, 2012; Dubow et al., 2012; Masten & Narayan, 2012; Masten et al., 2015). Once again, however, it is important to keep in mind that males generally show more aggressive behavior, particularly physical aggression, on diverse measures of externalizing behavior (Crick & Zahn-Waxler, 2003). Thus if there was a general increase in aggressive behavior, boys would be expected to have more elevated scores than girls. Moreover, cultural expectations and social roles may encourage greater aggression or violence in males (Belsky, 2012). Male youth are often engaged more directly in political conflicts, recruited and trained to fight, and expected in many cultures to take responsive actions in war or violence that involve aggressive behavior (Dimitry, 2012; Qouta et al., 2008).

There is growing evidence, as well, that sex differences may be quite complex (Masten et al., 2015). In a study of symptoms following terrorist attacks in Israel, girls had more symptoms of PTSD and fear, but the *severity* of symptoms among boys was greater (Laufer & Solomon, 2009). After a wildfire disaster, girls reported more perceived threat but not more PTSD (McDermott, Lee, Judd, & Gibbon, 2005). Research after Hurricane Charley found that girls showed more PTS during the first year, but not in the second year (La Greca, Silverman, Lai, & Jaccard, 2010). Moreover, studies of stress measured at a biological level, such as studies of the stress hormone cortisol, find complex relations to sex (Delahanty & Nugent, 2006).

Developmental Timing

Developmental timing of exposure is another important but complex aspect of individual differences research on mass-trauma exposure. Developmental theory suggests several major ways that developmental timing of disasters and other severe traumatic experiences could matter (American Psychological Association, 2010; Franks, 2011; Masten et al., 1990, 2015; Masten & Osofky, 2010). First, the nature of exposures, both objective and subjective, vary by age. As noted above, younger children are less likely to experience some traumatic events, such as kidnapping to become a child soldier, and also may be buffered by their cognitive immaturity from full apprehension of the scope and implications of a disaster. Infants do not have close friends to lose, reducing risk of traumatic loss of friends, but they are also highly dependent on care and thus extremely vulnerable to loss of care in a disaster. Young children may misinterpret replayed media coverage as new events, increasing exposure.

Second, there may be varying sensitive periods in development when the developing human organism is more or less vulnerable to the consequences of extreme trauma, just as radiation exposure has differential impacts on human health and development depending on the timing of exposures (Fushiki, 2013). There is great interest and concern about the possibility that traumatic stress has biological programming effects, such that early exposure, including fetal exposure, may alter important adaptive systems, including functions of the immune system, autonomic system, or hypothalamic–pituitary–adrenal (HPA) axis (Essex et al., 2011; Fox, Levitt, & Nelson, 2010; Hochberg et al., 2011; Meaney, 2010; Miller, Chen, & Cole, 2009; Phillips, 2007; Shonkoff, et al., 2009; Shonkoff, 2011). Recent delineation of epigenetic processes offer plausible explanations of how traumatic experiences could "get under the skin" to affect long-term health (Hertzman & Boyce, 2010; Hochberg et al., 2011; Meaney, 2010; Rutter, 2012a).

During development, key regulatory systems emerge, organize, and change. Recent perspectives on the effects of severe trauma, either to the pregnant mother or a child, suggest that these regulatory systems, such as the HPA axis, could be altered by extreme adversity, and that these alterations could have lasting effects on health and well-being. Yehuda and colleagues have suggested that fetal programming as a result of trauma could increase the risk for PTSD across the lifespan (Yehuda et al., 2007; Yehuda, Bell, Bierer, & Schmiedler, 2008; Yehuda & Bierer, 2009). Children of pregnant mothers exposed to the 9/11 terror attack who developed PTSD had lower salivary cortisol than children of mothers who did not develop PTSD. This effect was greater for mothers with more severe exposure and also for timing later in gestation. Yehuda's team also has found that children of Holocaust survivors with PTSD have lower cortisol levels than children of survivors without PTSD and nonexposed parents. These studies suggest that there could be intergenerational transmission of trauma effects through epigenetic programming, in addition to the possible behavioral pathways mediated by disturbances in parenting (perhaps due to chronic PTSD) that stem from extreme trauma experiences.

Longitudinal data related to the nuclear disaster at Chernobyl also suggest that fetal exposure to stress may alter biological development in lasting ways through programming effects (Huizink et al., 2008). When the explosion occurred in April 1986, there was widespread fear among residents of Finland due to potential radiation exposure. It also was well known already that pregnant women and their unborn children were vulnerable to radiation exposure. Thus, Chernobyl propagated an intense and extensive fear vector throughout the country as well as a modest objectively measurable and variable exposure to radiation. As part of a large, longitudinal study, twins born in Finland over a number of years have been followed in the "FinnTwin12" study. In this study, investigators compared individuals in gestation during Chernobyl with a cohort in gestation a year later. They sampled saliva in these two cohorts of twins at age 14, comparing levels of two hormones that have shown programming effects related to prenatal stress (cortisol and testosterone). Results indicated that there were higher levels of the stress hormone cortisol for both sexes and also higher testosterone levels for adolescent girls for children who were in utero during Chernobyl, particularly with exposure during the second trimester. The interpretation is that prenatal stress (mothers fearful of radiation effects on their unborn children) altered fetal development in the Chernobyl-exposed sample, with greater effects during a sensitive developmental window. Radiation exposure was not viewed as a likely explanation of the differences because exposures levels were low in Finland and not related to adverse outcomes.

Developmental timing also has been implicated for protective processes as well as vulnerabilities, raising the interesting question of inoculation versus sensitization effects of early exposure to trauma (Masten & Narayan, 2012; Rutter, 2013). There is growing recognition that some level of challenge may be needed to organize, calibrate, or "tune" adaptive systems, including the immune system and stress-response system. Some exposure prepares the organism for effective responses to challenges, analogous to vaccinations. Thus the relation of dose to healthy development shows a familiar, nonlinear inverted U form: Neither no exposure nor extremely high exposure to stress is optimal for development. Early descriptions of "steeling effects" of manageable exposures to adversity in the literature on resilience reflect this idea (Rutter, 1987; see Masten, 2012a). The "hygiene hypothesis," linking the rising prevalence of asthma, allergies, and related immune dysfunctions in modern, wealthy societies to the decreasing exposure of children to microorganisms, offers an analogous example for another key regulatory system (Okada, Kuhn, Feillet, & Bach, 2010; see Chapter 7).

The unifying theory for these contrasting effects of sensitization versus inoculation is the idea of plasticity and experience-driven programming of the developing organism that enhances adaptation to the "anticipated" environment (Hochberg et al., 2011). In these models, evolution favored organisms that developed adaptively, altering regulatory systems in keeping with signals of environmental conditions. However, extreme exposures (either very low stress or very high stress) could cause problems, especially if the prevailing conditions during sensitive developmental windows differ markedly from the subsequent environment. Theoretically, for example, it could be adaptive for the HPA system in conditions of extreme early adversity to down regulate cortisol production to protect the developing brain. Chronically high levels of cortisol can have toxic effects on neurobehavioral development; thus it could be adaptive to down regulate the responsiveness of this system in a chronically stressful environment (Gunnar & Quevedo, 2007; Lupien et al., 2011). However, the cost of this adaptation may be considerable if the environment changes to more normative conditions that favor a flexible and responsive HPA system.

In addition to the effects of extreme stress, such programming effects on regulatory systems have been proposed in relation to the nutritional environment during early development both in animal and human models (Schulz, 2010). One of the most powerful studies of such effects stems from research on the consequences of the human-caused famine during the German occupation of the Netherlands in the winter and spring of 1944. This tragic "natural experiment" revealed the importance of timing for lifelong health consequences of malnutrition. Fetal exposure to this nutritional disaster during the first trimester was associated with later obesity and related health problems. The heightened risk for obesity, presumably related to changes in metabolic systems, can be viewed as an adaptive mechanism gone awry; the fetus was programmed for an environment of scarcity but grew up in a context of plentiful food.

Child Characteristics

At the level of individual child differences, several major attributes have been implicated as important for adaptation in studies of mass trauma, including general intelligence or problem-solving skills, cognitive control, agency or self-efficacy, and personality traits such as negative emotionality. These characteristics have been widely implicated in the broader literature on risk and resilience as well, discussed throughout this volume.

Cognitive capabilities may be a double-edged sword. Greater comprehension of the situation could increase exposure dose, whereas problem-solving skills could enhance survival in a novel and challenging context. For example, good language-learning skills could be crucial to adaptation of refugees who start life anew in new language environments. Language fluency is associated with greater success in school (e.g., Hubbard, 1997), as well as fewer PTSD symptoms (Halcón et al., 2004) in studies of war refugees. Studies of youth in Palestine suggest that cognitive capabilities are protective (Qouta et al., 2008). Yet, in a study of 5- to

8-year-olds following Hurricane Katrina, Sprung (2008) found that children who have more advanced cognitive development (theory-of-mind skills) had more intrusive thoughts (a trauma symptom). However, those same children were more receptive to learning strategies for coping with trauma symptoms.

Self-regulation skills, and particularly the top-down cognitive control of attention, emotion, and behavior, also have shown specific effects in studies of mass trauma, though research is somewhat limited. In a rare study with predisaster data, Kithakye, Morris, Terranova, and Myers (2010) found that self-regulation skills in preschoolers measured prior to an outbreak of political violence in Kenya generally predicted better postconflict outcomes in the children, both less aggression and more prosocial behavior, controlling for preconflict behavior. Better self-control also appeared to moderate the effects of exposure severity on prosocial behavior. A study of sixth graders after Hurricane Katrina suggested that cognitive control skills moderated the risk of PTSD symptoms, consistent with a protective effect (Terranova, Boxer, & Morris, 2009).

Self-efficacy, perceived agency or competence, higher self-esteem, and confidence in one's own abilities to cope and be effective also have been studied as potential promotive or protective factors in mass-trauma research. These cognitive attributions and beliefs are theoretically associated with a powerful intrinsic motivation system that drives learning and adaptation in human development and many other species (Bandura, 1982, 1997; White, 1959), discussed further in Chapter 6. People with a greater sense of effectiveness, agency, control, and self-confidence are more likely to take action and persist in the face of adversity. Betancourt et al. (2010) found that child soldiers in recovery who had survived rape had greater confidence than other child soldiers, which the authors attributed to their reflections on enduring prolonged hardships during the years of captivity. In a study of 9/11-exposed adolescents, higher self-esteem was associated with less PTS (Lengua et al., 2005). After Hurricane Floyd, competence beliefs were related to posttraumatic growth among children ages 6–15 (Cryder, Kilmer, Tedeschi, & Calhoun, 2006). Barber (2008) has reported positive effects of activism for Palestinian youth participating in the *Intifada*.

Hope and a sense that life has meaning may be close relatives of perceived effectiveness and agency. Resilient people identified across diverse adversities, including disasters, often identify hope and meaning as protective influences in their lives. The passage about Thida Butt Mam quoted in Chapter 2 recounts a dramatic shift in perceived agency and hope, accompanied by renewed motivation to survive the killing fields of the Khmer Rouge. Spiritual beliefs and religious faith, also commonly reported in resilience case reports, may afford similar protections (Crawford, Wright, & Masten, 2006). The empirical literature remains quite limited in this area. However, Klasen et al. (2010), in their study of Ugandan former child soldiers, report that youth with better mental health also reported more spiritual support.

Individual differences in personality also have the potential to exacerbate or ameliorate stress. The broader literature on risk for mental health suggests that negative emotionality and stress reactivity are good candidates for vulnerability factors, as is the tendency to ruminate on negative experiences (Klein, Kotov, & Bufferd, 2011). Here again, research on disaster is limited, in part because of the scarcity of predisaster information on personality. In one small study of adolescents exposed to Katrina, prehurricane-assessed negative emotionality predicted postdisaster symptoms of depressed mood, anxiety, and traumatic stress (Weems et al., 2007). On the other hand, another Katrina study suggested that the tendency to ruminate predicted posttraumatic growth (Kilmer & Gil-Rivas, 2010). These investigators speculated that ruminative style may have facilitated the reconstruction of meaning, processing of trauma, or reintegration of identity following the disaster.

It seems quite possible that the same personality trait could be protective in one situation but problematic in another, or protective in regard to one aspect of outcome and harmful with respect to another (Masten et al., 1990). Much more nuanced studies are needed to understand the role of personality in adaptation during or following mass-trauma situations.

Family Characteristics

From the beginnings of research on children in mass-trauma situations, investigators were focused on the significance of family separations and family function for child adaptation. As noted above, it was clear that loss of parents and separation from caregivers played a vital role in child well-being, and also that parent function moderated child response to severe trauma exposures. Recent studies continue to corroborate these influences. Strong family relationships predicted resilience in Palestinian children exposed to political violence (Qouta et al., 2008). The quality of the parent–child relationship moderated the effect of tsunami exposure on PTSD symptoms and depression in Sri Lankan adolescents (Wickrama & Kaspar, 2007). Family acceptance was associated with all of the adaptive recovery indicators in child soldiers (Betancourt et al., 2010). After 9/11, preschool children with parents who had more mental health symptoms were not doing as well (Chemtob et al., 2010).

Nonetheless, the question of overinvolvement of parents in disasters has been raised as a potential threat to resilience, presumably through effects on self-efficacy or agency. In a study of PTSD in adolescents following a flood disaster, Bokszczanin (2008) found that highly involved parents had adolescents with more PTSD risk. Of course, it is difficult to distinguish the direction of effect in most studies. Still, it is an interesting and important question to consider nonlinear effects of parent behaviors on child adaptation, especially in relation to the question of too little or too much scaffolding or protection.

Community and Culture

Mass trauma affects entire communities and the recovery of families and individual children, whose everyday lives are embedded and entwined in community context and function. Thus, is it important to consider the role of community and cultural-level influences on families and their children (Betancourt & Khan, 2008; Norris, Stevens, Pfefferbaum, Wyche, & Pfefferbaum,

2008). The devastation (analogous to dose) and response (dysfunction, adaptation, recovery, etc.) of communities would be expected to play a role in the resilience of families and individuals living in those communities. Resilience across these levels of individuals, families, and communities involves interdependent and interactive processes. If a community is completely destroyed (e.g., washed away in a tsunami), people must resettle at least temporarily and the capacity for resilience afforded by the community resources and functional integrity may be unavailable or gravely affected for a time. Yet communities are not simply material and geographical in their nature; the relationships and cultural belief systems shared in community groups can play a sustaining role in the midst of physical destruction.

Norris and colleagues (2008) have provided a conceptual framework for understanding and promoting community resilience for disaster that is highly analogous to the framework that I have advocated for understanding individual resilience. Community resilience is defined in terms of a set of networked adaptive capacities, facilitated by resources in the domains of economic development, information/communication, social capital (relationships, sense of community), and what they term community competence (collective know-how and effectiveness). Communities can be prepared to respond with flexible organization, effective communication, physical distribution of essential physical resources (such as water and medical care), and actions to support social cohesion.

In the aftermath of disasters, some of the most important functions for children afforded by communities, beyond emergency supplies, safety, and medical care, are restoring community routines and structures central to the lives of children, including child care, school, and safe places to play. Virtually every overview of how children fare in disasters and war, whether based on anecdotal reports, research, experts' experience, or a combination, notes the importance of restoring community functions and structures of this kind for children and families (e.g., American Psychological Association, 2010; Betancourt & Khan, 2008; Masten & Obradović, 2008; Masten et al., 2015; Osofsky, Osofsky,

& Harris, 2007). In addition to providing individual care, respite, peer interaction, learning, and opportunities to be active and experience agency, the restoration of community-level routines and structures appears to be highly symbolic of recovery and a sense of normalcy. Thus, they provide a sense of hope and efficacy across an affected population. Prompt resumption of schooling was one of the most highly endorsed postdisaster practices in a Delphi consensus study based on surveying experts from leading humanitarian agencies that intervene in many crises worldwide (Ager, Stark, Akesson, & Boothby, 2010).

Research on the individual impact of community-based protective factors is limited to date. However, some individual studies are consistent with the key role of community resilience for children. Staying in school was associated with better recovery in former child soldiers from Sierra Leone (Betancourt et al., 2010). The same study found that community acceptance was a key factor associated with better adjustment during rehabilitation of these severely traumatized youth. Community support was a core theme in a small case study of resilience in Columbian child soldiers (Cortes & Buchanan, 2007). Community acceptance and forgiveness may be particularly important for child victims of war who have engaged during captivity or forced service in behaviors forbidden in their own cultures or horrific atrocities (Boothby, Crawford, & Halperin, 2006).

INTERVENTION

The research described above has implications for what might be done to prepare for better response to disaster or facilitate recovery. To date, however, there remains a concerning lack of research on interventions for children who face such catastrophic adversities given the scope of ongoing and anticipated exposures to mass-trauma experiences worldwide (Masten & Narayan, 2012). When Peltonen and Punamäki (2010) searched the literature for a meta-analysis of intervention studies in situations of terrorism or armed conflict, they only found four studies that met their critieria for the review. This is perhaps understandable given that it is extraordinarily difficult to conduct research in the context of disaster, as well as terrorism or war (American Psychological Association, 2010; Bonanno et al., 2010; Hobfoll et al., 2007; Jordans, Tol, Komproe, & De Jong, 2009; Tol et al., 2010). On the other hand, given the huge numbers of children worldwide who are exposed to mass trauma, the likelihood of continued exposure in the future, and the scope of humanitarian efforts to intervene and help in these situations, intervention research would seem to be a clear global priority.

There are a small but growing number of studies that meet the gold-standard design feature of randomized assignment to intervention or control/comparison group (a randomized control trial [RCT]). One of the earliest examples in the literature is a study by Dybdahl (2001), conducted a year following the end of the war that accompanied the breakup of the former Yugoslavian countries. The intervention focused on Bosnian mothers of young children (5 or 6 years old) who had been exposed to severe war atrocities, in an effort to protect and improve the quality of parent–child interaction. Families were randomized to two groups. One received only medical care, while the other group received medical care plus an intervention focused on warm and supportive interactions of mothers with children during group treatment meetings spanning 5 months. Mothers and children in the intervention focused on parenting had better mental health outcomes and the children also had greater weight gain.

In a later study in Bosnia, Layne and colleagues (2008) also conducted an RCT study, focused on reducing symptoms in war-exposed adolescents through a school-based program. Classrooms received (by random assignment) a program of psychoeducation and skills training or a more intensive intervention that added a manualized group treatment for trauma and grief (17 sessions). Both groups improved over time, but the youth with the added trauma and grief intervention showed greater improvement in maladaptive traumatic grief.

Intervention trials with former child soldiers also have shown efficacy as well (Betancourt, McBain, Newnham, & Brennan,

2013). Ertl, Pfeiffer, Schauer, Elbert, and Neuner (2011), for example, found that narrative exposure therapy (NET) was successful with young people 12 to 25 years old in Uganda in a randomized treatment trial. NET is a brief intervention that combines autobiographical narrative or testimonial therapy with trauma exposure therapy for PTSD (Neuner et al., 2008).

Additional studies support the use of NET with children, sometimes called "KidNET." KidNET typically involves 4 to 10 sessions during which children gradually construct a story about their trauma experiences, often involving drawings or symbolic supports (e.g., a rope "timeline" with stones of different sizes placed for difficult times and flowers representing positive experiences). The goal is to construct a narrative and habituate (desensitize) to the emotions aroused by recalling what happened, gaining a sense of control while reducing avoidance and fear. A study in Germany found this approach to be efficacious in reducing PTSD symptoms among refugee children (Ruf et al., 2010). KidNET also has shown promising results in another RCT for children in Sri Lanka exposed to the 2004 tsunami in the midst of an ongoing civil war (Catani et al., 2009).

In another intervention study done in Sri Lanka, Berger and Gelkopf (2009) assigned groups of 9- to 25-year-old students to treatment or waitlist control conditions, where the treatment consisted of 12 sessions of "ERASE-Stress Sri Lanka." ERASE stands for enhancing resiliency among students experiencing stress. The treatment included psychoeducation, training in coping skills, and experiential group activities, carefully adapted to cultural traditions in Sri Lanka. On multiple measures of PTSD and symptoms, as well as hope, the treatment group showed more improvements than the controls.

There also is interest in preparing children for disaster, either for potential attacks in violence-prone regions of the world (Ayalon, 1983; Wolmer, Hamiel, & Laor, 2011) or for disaster response in regions prone to natural disasters. Some of these efforts are conceptualized as stress inoculation, in which children practice responding to low doses of the potential threat. Prospective studies of their effectiveness are extremely rare. However, circumstances resulted in one such study in Israel, after a school district implemented a stress inoculation training program in some schools in a high-risk area for armed conflict. Subsequently, there was a 3-week-long conflict ("Operation Cast Lead") with frightening rocket attacks and high trauma exposure. It was later possible to compare the mental health of students (fourth and fifth graders) from six schools who received the intervention with the symptoms of students from six schools who had not received the training (Wolmer et al., 2011). Results suggested that stress inoculation training had preventive effects on PTS and other symptoms.

Consensus Guidelines for Intervention

There are two kinds of consensus on how to intervene to protect children in the event of disasters and mass violence (Masten & Narayan, 2012; Masten et al., 2015). One kind is based on systematic efforts to reach a consensus. For example, Ager et al. (2010) conducted a Delphi study, which is a qualitative research strategy, to glean the wisdom of leaders from leading humanitarian agencies that respond to many emergencies around the world. Another group of experts (Hobfoll et al., 2007) reached a consensus by discussion, yielding five broad intervention principles for mass-trauma situations: promote a sense of safety, promote calming, promote a sense of self- and collective efficacy, promote connectedness, and promote hope. These broad recommendations align well with the idea of protecting, supporting, or restoring the most fundamental adaptive systems believed to generate the capacity for resilience, summarized in the next chapter.

The second kind of consensus is based on reviewing research and recommendations stemming from empirical studies, to ascertain consistent themes. There are many similar recommendations about children stemming from reviews of this literature published since 9/11 (American Psychological Association, 2010; Bonanno et al., 2010; Jordans et al., 2009; La Greca & Silverman, 2009; Masten et al., 2015; Masten & Osofky, 2010; Norris, Friedman, & Watson, 2002; Norris, Friedman, Watson, et al., 2002b; Norris et al., 2008; Peltonen & Punamäki, 2010; Pine et al., 2005). First and foremost, it is recommended that the special needs of children and families with children be considered in emergency planning. Amazingly, this is not always the case. Other core recommendations frequently made in these reviews are the following: keep families together whenever possible and plan for reuniting separated families, train emergency responders on the needs of children, recognize that parents and teachers also are "first responders," and make it a priority to restore normal routines and places so that children can go to school and play. There also is a consensus that some time should be allowed for natural recovery to unfold once emergency needs, safety, and basic community supports are restored for families. Then screening for children who may have additional needs is usually recommended, although there is not a consensus on the best timing for such screening.

There also is a consensus on "cautions" for intervention in mass trauma with families (Masten & Narayan, 2012). Developmental sensitivity and cultural attunement are important. There are concerns about intervening at the wrong time, too intrusively, or with strategies that have little basis in research. Bonanno et al. (2010) have recently questioned the value of immediate intervention after disasters, beyond the provision of basic tangible necessities and information, and efforts to facilitate keeping natural social units together. There is little evidence that intrusive prophylactic efforts in the field immediately after disaster, such as "critical incident debriefing" or grief counseling, have positive effects, and these strategies may disrupt naturally occurring recovery processes or undermine the perceived efficacy of individuals or communities (Bonanno et al., 2010; La Greca & Silverman, 2009).

SUMMARY

Clearly, more systematic research is needed to inform preparation and response efforts in the context of mass catastrophes, which will certainly continue to occur. Nonetheless, there is a substantial body of work to guide those who cannot wait for future research.

And, once again, there appears to be remarkable consistency in the conclusions and recommendations emerging from this work. Dose and developmental timing matter, as do individual differences in sex, personality, and cognitive tools. Context matters, in terms of family, friends, community, culture, and the conditions for recovery. Some conditions are so terrible for children that resilience can only be observed after adversity abates and some semblance of normal nurture and life are restored. When major protective systems are destroyed—parents are killed, the brain is injured or deprived of essential nutrients and learning opportunities, friends are lost, the fabric of community is torn, faith and hope are extinguished by atrocities—children do not function or develop well. If these major protective systems are sustained or restored, many children show recovery, especially over the long term, although there can be lifelong or intergenerational consequences of prolonged or extreme trauma exposure. Beyond immediate survival needs, it is essential in the aftermath of disaster or war to protect or restore the adaptive systems that protect and promote child development. The next section of this book is focused on these fundamental adaptive systems in the child, relationships, community, and culture.

PART III

ADAPTIVE SYSTEMS IN RESILIENCE

CHAPTER 6

THE SHORT LIST AND IMPLICATED PROTECTIVE SYSTEMS

After five decades, there is a wide-ranging body of research on resilience in development in young people that encompasses many different kinds of stressful life experiences, individuals, families, communities, and cultures. This body of work, like all rapidly emerging scientific fields of inquiry, could be and has been criticized in many respects (Masten, 1999, 2012a, 2013b; Luthar, 2003, 2006, Luthar et al., 2000; Rutter, 2012b; Ungar, 2012). These criticisms and controversies, discussed further in Chapter 12, are probably essential for progress in the science of resilience. Moreover, there is considerable substance at the heart of these criticisms. There has been a confusing array of definitions, situations, samples, measures, methods, and findings that make it very challenging to reach a consensus on concepts or to evaluate the evidence.

Nonetheless, despite all the controversies and confusion, there has been a striking degree of consistency across the diverse body of research on resilience in children and youth. Years ago, I and others who were keeping track of this literature began to notice that findings converged around an increasingly familiar list of attributes in the function and lives of young people who manifest resilience. Early reviewers highlighted commonly observed correlates of manifested resilience (Garmezy, 1985; Rutter, 1979, 1987) and this continues to be the case (Luthar, 2006; Masten,

2001, 2007; Wright et al., 2013). Twenty years or more ago, I began to think and speak about these recurring correlates of psychosocial resilience as the "short list," and I pondered the meaning of this recurring list of resilience factors. My essay on resilience as "ordinary magic" in *American Psychologist* (Masten, 2001) was a succinct effort to address this question.

Table 6.1 illustrates a contemporary short list. The list has not changed all that much in 20 years, although the research literature

TABLE 6.1. The "Short List" of Widely Reported Factors Associated with Resilience in Young People and Implicated Adaptive Systems

Resilience factors	Adaptive systems
Effective caregiving and parenting quality	Attachment; family
Close relationships with other capable adults	Attachment; social networks
Close friends and romantic partners	Attachment; peer and family systems
Intelligence and problem-solving skills	Learning and thinking systems of the CNS
Self-control; emotion regulation; planfulness	Self-regulation systems of the CNS
Motivation to succeed	Mastery motivation and related reward systems
Self-efficacy	Mastery motivation
Faith, hope, belief life has meaning	Spiritual and cultural belief systems
Effective schools	Education systems
Effective neighborhoods; collective efficacy	Communities

Note. CNS, central nervous system.

grows by leaps and bounds. Occasionally, a change in the short list seems warranted, and that would be expected, given research progress. However, these changes seem surprisingly minor given the scope of the growing literature.

In more informal ways, the short list has been corroborated by many different audiences of students and colleagues at lectures and workshops over the years. I invite members of the audience to think about a child or adult whom they know well who has shown resilience (by whatever criteria they hold to be important). Then they are asked to consider what seemed to make a difference in this person's life, or what made it possible for this individual to overcome serious adversity. Pooled responses typically result in a list of attributes that bears an impressive resemblance to the list in Table 6.1. Sometimes unusual talents or resources or more specific aspects of broad items on the short list are mentioned, but most of the time, a familiar list of "what made a difference" keeps coming up.

WHAT DOES THE "SHORT LIST" MEAN?

Resilience in young people is associated with a set of attributes of child, context, or their relationships that turn out to be well-established general predictors of positive development. The short list, in other words, looks like the factors associated with good development in general, and I have argued that this recurrent list suggests that there are fundamental adaptive systems that protect human development under many different circumstances (Masten, 2001, 2007). These fundamental systems are the product of biological and cultural evolution, shared in basic respects across many contemporary societies because different individual people and cultures around the world share many of the same biological and social functions, potentials, limitations, resources, vulnerabilities, and adaptive challenges.

My speculations about the meaning of the items on the short list are also indicated in Table 6.1, in terms of implicated adaptive systems. There is extensive theory and science on each of these potential adaptive systems, which have been studied at multiple levels of analysis in multiple disciplines. A full discussion is well beyond the scope of this book. In this chapter, my aim is to highlight briefly how these systems may function to promote resilience in young people, with a particular focus on the most widely implicated factors and the systems strongly linked to those protective factors. In the following chapters of this section, I expand on the neurobiology related to these protective systems and the role of important contexts in child development implicated by the resilience literature to date, including families, schools, and cultures.

The short list reflects the focus of initial waves of resilience science by developmental investigators, and particularly the work of social scientists. Recent work on the neurobiology of resilience is likely to lead to additions or refinements of the short list and hypotheses about the adaptive systems it signifies (see Chapter 7). The short list also reflects the shortcomings of resilience literature to date, which are noted in the following discussion and throughout this volume.

ATTACHMENT AND CLOSE RELATIONSHIPS

The central significance of close relationships for resilience has been noted in virtually every review on resilience in development over the past half-century. In young children, the role of caregivers is paramount, including primary caregivers supplemented by extended family and other individuals in caregiving roles. As the contexts for development expand to school and neighborhood, relationships with other people can become important as well, including teachers or ministers or coaches or mentors. Friends and romantic partners eventually become important potential protective relationships.

In developmental theory, a powerful and universal biological system is implicated by the ubiquity of relationships in competence and resilience: the *attachment system*. Attachment theory was initially described by John Bowlby (1982) in his masterpiece on attachment and loss and later elaborated by many developmental theorists (e.g., Ainsworth, 1989; Bretherton & Munholland, 1999; Cassidy & Shaver, 2008; Sroufe, 1979; Sroufe, Carlson, Levy, & Egeland, 1999; Thompson, 2000). Many of Bowlby's ideas about the attachment system emerged from his clinical observations as a child therapist observing the reaction of young children to separations and reunions, and the many children in World War II who were traumatized by separation or loss of caregivers. Bowlby viewed attachment as a protective system that evolved biologically to protect vulnerable young animals from predators and other dangers. He and other attachment theorists proposed that during the latter part of the first year, human infants form a special bond with the primary caregiver (and other caregivers to a lesser degree) that serves the functions of safety, emotional security, and learning. This organized relationship is typically bidirectional, reflecting an organized pattern of behavior between the caregiver and the infant. Once the attachment system organizes in a caregiver–child dyad, then a threat perceived by either party can activate the system and trigger attachment behaviors. A frightened child will cry and/or seek contact/proximity to the caregiver for comfort. Similarly, the attached caregiver perceiving a threat will seek proximity to the child and attempt to soothe or comfort the child. In contrast, when the world is perceived as safe, a child will venture out to explore and the caregiver will allow the exploration without anxiety. The presence of an attachment figure provides a "secure base" for exploration and learning.

The attachment system is associated with strong motivation and emotions. Separation in the presence of a threat can trigger enormous anxiety or panic, and reunion often brings joy and relief. This phenomenon can be observed in everyday life at playgrounds or shopping centers when, for example, a toddler playing happily nearby a parent responds to a big dog or a loud siren with fear, running back to the parent. A child who wanders off from the parent may suddenly panic when he or she realizes the parent is not there or that he or she is clinging to the wrong pair of jeans. The parent who suddenly realizes a toddler is out of sight may also panic. Both parent and child may show relief or joy at reunion (although parents may also express some anger as well). Attachment behaviors, theorists assume, were naturally selected to bring vulnerable individuals and their protectors into proximity with each other when danger was perceived by either party.

Attachment plays a lifelong role in human adaptation. Moreover, the proclivity of humans and other species that show attachment (many social mammals) to bond is so fundamental that they may show such bonds across species, with objects (like blankets and stuffed animals), with their homes, and in the case of humans, with spiritual figures and other nonphysical characters (such as avatars). As children grow older, they form attachment relationships with other adults in nurturing roles, such as teachers. They form attachments with peers, initially with friends and later with romantic partners. Eventually, they form attachment bonds with their own children. Over the course of development, the balance in attachment relationships shifts. Initially, the infant is in the protected role and the parent is the protector. Peer relationships are more balanced, with friends and romantic partners protecting each other.

Developmental theorists also have argued that responsive and sensitive caregiving contributes to high-quality, secure attachment relationships between caregiver and child that are then carried forward into future relationships (Sroufe, 2005; Thompson, 2000). Sensitive caregivers also provide external regulatory capacity for the developing child until the child is mature enough to regulate his or her own biological functions, emotion, arousal, stress, and behavior. This "coregulation" of child function by parent is believed to play a key role in the development of self-regulation, another set of adaptive skills discussed below.

The protective functions of parents, however, extend well beyond comfort and coregulation. Parents play central roles in the development of other adaptive systems in their children, including cognitive development and related problem-solving skills, as well as mastery motivation. They also serve as cultural conduits, transmitting cultural practices that may foster resilience. They actively seek help for their children as needed, anticipate dangers, and try to prepare their children to deal with expected challenges.

As a result of their multifaceted functions, it is not surprising to find that an effective parent or someone in this role has proven to be the most important and pervasive influence on resilience in children. Concomitantly, one of the greatest threats to child development is an ineffective or abusive parent in this vital role. Nonetheless, even in the situation of maltreatment, at least one good relationship with a caring parent or other caregiver has been associated with resilience (e.g., Alink, Cicchetti, Kim, & Rogosch, 2009; Collishaw et al., 2007; Egeland, Carlson, & Sroufe, 1993; McGloin & Widom, 2001).

Some of the most effective interventions testing resilience theory have focused on bolstering the quality of attachment and caregiving in the lives of children exposed to high levels of adversity. The case of Sara (see Chapter 2) provides a single-case example of intervention to promote resilience by providing effective caregiving in a loving and stable family. Even more compelling is the growing gold-standard evidence based on experiments with randomized control designs. Successful intervention experiments to improve the quality of parenting in a parent–child dyad or to provide higher-quality foster care have demonstrated the power of targeting the attachment system. Examples are discussed in Chapter 11.

Observations of risk and resilience in war and disaster, highlighted in Chapter 5, also affirm the central role of attachment across the lifespan in varying forms. Immediately after 9/11, telecommunications and the Internet were flooded with the efforts of humans of many ages across the world seeking contact with one another. The urge to seek contact with attachment figures (bidirectional) is striking in such life-threatening situations. In war and disaster, it is important to consider the overwhelming nature of the biological attachment response in training first responders and responding to dangers for children. Those who plan for such emergencies now recognize that separating children from parents should be avoided if possible. And if the primary caregivers are lost to death or unavoidable separations, it is crucial to provide children with a capable, caring, and consistent adult in this role as soon as feasible for as long as needed.

INTELLIGENCE, INGENUITY, AND PROBLEM-SOLVING CAPABILITIES

Individual differences in measurable capabilities for thinking and problem solving in the service of learning and adapting to the environment have been linked to better outcomes in many domains of function for a century. These differences, broadly described as *intelligence*, and their measurement in the form of intelligence tests that assess IQ, are associated with competence in developmental tasks and most particularly with academic or work achievement (Masten, Burt, et al., 2006). This is not surprising since they were developed in large part for this purpose. Moreover, intelligence often is defined in terms of the mental activities or processes associated with adaptation to the environment. At the very outset of intelligence testing, Alfred Binet regarded intelligence as a collection of abilities involving judgment, common sense, initiative, and adaptive behavior (Masten, Burt, et al., 2006; Sattler, 1988). David Wechsler, who developed one of the most successful IQ tests of the past century, defined intelligence broadly as "the aggregate or global capacity of the individual to act purposefully, to think rationally and to deal effectively with the environment" (1958, p. 14). The tests designed on the models put forward by Binet and Simon over a century ago, and Wechsler half a century ago, are still dominant in global assessment of individual differences in cognition. These tests focused on measuring a variety of cognitive skills applied to brief but integrative problem-solving tasks (requiring a combination of attention, memory, motor skills, language, and other skills), rather than more basic faculties such as reaction time. These tests of higher cognitive reasoning included two broad kinds of thinking that have come to be called fluid reasoning (applying cognitive skills to novel or abstract problems, such as assembling some blocks into a pattern, presumed to require less explicit information or knowledge) and crystallized intelligence (requiring specific knowledge acquired through learning, such as vocabulary). Intelligent behaviors, such as those assessed on IQ tasks, depend on brain development and learning through experience, with myriad influences from nutrition, parenting, education, and the interplay of individual genes with experience.

Many studies of resilience as well as competence in human development have observed that intelligence scores are associated with better function, both in low- and high-stress conditions (Luthar, 2006; Masten & Coatsworth, 1998; Masten, Burt, et al., 2006). IQ is clearly a marker of good odds for adaptive success in modern societies or a promotive influence on success under a variety of conditions. However, there is also evidence that IQ has a *protective* influence particularly when adversity is very high (Masten et al., 1999; Masten & Obradović, 2006). In the PCLS, IQ scores were generally associated with competence, but even more so for those with extremely high lifetime adversity exposure. Numerous other longitudinal studies of resilience have implicated IQ as protective (Lösel & Farrington, 2012; Werner & Smith, 1992, 2001). Individual cases of resilience also implicate general intellectual abilities. Some doors opened to Dr. Maddaus (see Chapter 2) because of his intellectual talents, once he decided to apply his intelligence to education rather than delinquent activities.

Resilience does not appear to require extraordinary intelligence. Protection may be afforded by average or better thinking skills that can be applied to problem solving in novel and challenging situations. These capabilities likely reflect a human brain "in good working order" combined with knowledge to understand what is going on, what to expect, and what to do or how to get assistance from others who do know. These capabilities will develop as the brain develops and learns, and decline as cognitive function declines, but they also will depend on connections to other intelligence resources, both human and electronic. Stress, illness, sleep deprivation, starvation, and many other conditions associated with adversity exposure could degrade these capabilities.

It is also important to consider the possibility that intelligence can be a double-edged sword in adaptive function, because awareness and knowledge also can increase exposure dose and influence morale. As noted in the chapter on war and disaster, sometimes a *lack of understanding* is protective. Intelligence also may bring existential *angst* or worries that can increase the risk of anxiety or depression. Nonetheless, it seems evident that human resilience often depends on our unique capacity for ingenuity in the face of challenge and our well-developed capacity for sharing information about adaptation across people, space, and time through language, learning, and technology.

Also important to remember is that the strategic application of intelligence may require motivation, self-regulation, and knowledge derived from a history of effective parenting, teaching, and other opportunities. As a result, the adaptive functions of human information processing systems and intelligence, broadly construed as a complex, cognitive adaptive system, is rather difficult to separate from other related adaptive systems, such as attachment, self-regulation, and mastery motivation systems, all of which may play a role in shaping the development of the others. The human brain develops and functions as an integrated network of interacting systems.

The development of intelligence is influenced by interactions with many other systems, including family, education, and community. Cognitive development is promoted and protected by good nutrition and health care, secure attachment, access to good education, and safe neighborhoods, while it is undermined by toxins in the environment or toxic stress in the home or community (Shonkoff, 2011; Shonkoff & Phillips, 2000). Poverty, discrimination, and war all can threaten brain development and cognitive development in many ways that can influence the development and application of intellectual skills.

SELF-REGULATION AND SELF-DIRECTION

Self-regulation skills, including self-management of attention, arousal, emotions, and actions, also appear to play a central role in human adaptation, development, and resilience. Extensive research links such skills to good adaptation over the lifespan (Carlson et al., 2013; Masten & Coatsworth, 1998; Zelazo & Carlson, 2012; Reich et al., 2010). Early in development, caregivers coregulate many of the adaptive systems of their infants and toddlers, soothing them when they are upset, stimulating them to laugh and learn, monitoring their behavior closely, setting limits, teaching them rules of society and enforcing them, and so forth. As children develop, we expect them to gain control of their own attention, arousal, emotions, or impulses, and take responsibility for their own actions. Parents plan for young children, but we expect older children and adults to plan for themselves and take action to implement those plans. Developmentally appropriate self-regulation skills are associated with both concurrent adjustment (competence in developmental task domains and fewer mental health problems) and future adjustment (Carlson et al., 2013; Masten & Coatsworth, 1998; Rothbart, 2011).

When conditions arouse high levels of negative emotion (fear, anxiety, anger) and/or physiological alarm or stress, it is not surprising to find that the capacity to keep adaptive control and take adaptive action to manage the self in relation to the environment would be associated with better outcomes. Similarly, individuals who may be more reactive to adversity, in terms of arousal or emotion, especially may need effective internal and external sources of self-regulation to retain or recover good function.

Self-regulation capacity includes an array of skills and adaptive systems that develop and fluctuate over the life course. Theory and research on self-regulation dates back a century to concepts like the *ego* and ego control (Masten, Burt, et al., 2006). Recent theory and research has focused on *executive function* (EF), a suite of cognitive control processes that depend on neural networks associated with prefrontal brain development (Best & Miller, 2010; Blair & Raver, 2012; Carlson et al., 2013; Diamond & Lee, 2011; Zelazo & Carlson, 2012). As noted in Chapter 4, multiple functions are included under the broad umbrella of EF, including working memory, inhibitory control, and cognitive flexibility. These skills develop rapidly in the preschool years and continue to improve into early adulthood (Zelazo & Bauer, 2013; Zelazo & Carlson, 2012). Many advantages and disadvantages can influence EF development; the neural networks associated with EF may be especially sensitive to the risks associated with poverty, adversity, trauma, toxins, and neglect, and this may be particularly true in early development (Blair & Raver, 2012; Shonkoff, 2011). At the same time, some children in high-risk contexts develop good EF skills.

EF skills appear to be a key protective influence for high-risk children, enabling them to succeed in a context of severe adversity or poverty (Blair & Raver, 2012; Sapienza & Masten, 2011). Buckner and colleagues (Buckner, Mezzacappa, & Beardslee, 2003; Buckner et al., 2009) found that more successful youth from low-income families (many of whom were formerly homeless) had better self-regulation skills based on interviewer ratings. In our work with HHM children, described in Chapter 4, EF skills are associated with better school adjustment (Masten, Herbers, et al., 2012; Obradović, 2010). Moreover, better EF skills in these young homeless children were related to better observed parenting and lower stress hormones.

Prevention science also provides compelling evidence that EF skills are central to better adjustment and responsive to intervention. Preschool programs that target EF skill development have promising effects on school readiness, particularly among high-risk children (Diamond & Lee, 2011; Raver et al., 2011).

Long-term longitudinal evidence also underscores the significance of early emerging evidence of self-regulation skills for later competence and adjustment (Duckworth, 2011; Zelazo & Carlson, 2012). Recent data from a highly regarded and large cohort study of individuals from New Zealand showed that childhood measures of self-control (assessed by multiple methods over time before age 10) predicted better adult outcomes at age 32 in multiple domains, including health, substance abuse, criminality, and SES, over and above IQ and social class of origin (Moffitt et al., 2011). In another classic study of self-control, children who resisted the temptation to eat a marshmallow now in order to wait for a larger reward 15 minutes later showed greater competence and fewer problems in adolescence and early adulthood (Ayduk et al., 2000; Mischel et al., 2011).

Caregivers and other socializing agents, including extended family and teachers, play critical roles in the early development of self-regulation. In attachment theory, effective caregivers shape the development of self-regulation through their sensitivity, responsiveness, monitoring, and coregulation efforts. Parents can tailor their parenting to individual differences in the child, helping sensitive or reactive children toward better self-regulation through different strategies than they might use with children who have a different personality (Kochanska & Knaack, 2003).

Development of self-regulation skills accelerates during the preschool years, but continues for a much longer time, well into early adulthood. The most advanced EF skills, such as self-reflection, evaluating one's own life, and planning for the future, may require that the neural systems supporting self-control are quite mature, which happens fairly late in brain development. The phenomenon of "late bloomers" in resilience may reflect this late surge of capacity for self-reflection and planning, combined with the opportunities that societies may offer for finding a new path in the transition to adulthood. Thus, while the preschool years offer an important window of opportunity for the development of self-control skills, there may be later windows for redirecting the life course that are tied to later-emerging cognitive capabilities and opportunities.

MASTERY MOTIVATION, AGENCY, AND RELATED REWARD SYSTEMS

From an early age, children often show delight or satisfaction in making things happen in the world. They throw things off the high chair as infants, laughing. New walkers toddle across the room, beaming with joy. Older children may try over and over to hit a ball or solve a puzzle. In the seminal essay "Motivation Reconsidered: The Concept of Competence," Robert White (1959) argued that humans and other animals were motivated to master the environment through a motivation system that evolved through natural selection. Based on a brilliant integration of research on behavior in children and animals, White argued that there is a biological predisposition to engage with the environment in ways that promote learning and adaptation. He termed the motivation *effectance* and the experienced feelings of satisfaction associated with perceived accomplishment related to this motivation system *efficacy*. Experiencing pleasure in mastery functioned to reward efforts to achieve successful interactions with the environment. In this theory, children make an effort to explore the environment and try things out because they experience intrinsic pleasure in doing so, and not just to eat or please their parents. This system evolved because it favored learning to function successfully in the environment, which favored survival. Humans, more than any other species (to our knowledge), develop the greatest capacity to orchestrate their own lives, and mastery motivation appears to play a central role in this process.

The idea and function of a motivation system for agency in adaptation and pleasure in perceived effectiveness has been elaborated by other highly influential theorists in developmental science. Susan Harter elaborated on the development of mastery motivation and perceived competence, and also developed a widely used measurement strategy for assessing perceived competence in multiple domains of competence, differentiating social, cognitive, and physical competence (Harter, 1978, 2012). Harter linked White's ideas to the growing developmental literature on perceived success and failure, locus of control, and intrinsic versus extrinsic motivation. Ryan and Deci (2000) elaborated on the role of intrinsic motivation in the development of competence. In all of these related ideas, investigators proposed that the striving for competence is motivated by needs to have effects on the environment that are internal in origin though shaped by experience.

Albert Bandura proposed a somewhat different account for the striving for mastery in his social cognitive theory, elaborated in his book *Self-Efficacy* (1997). Bandura proposed that the striving for competence was motivated by "the various benefits of competent action," shaped by learning opportunities and efficacy beliefs that develop over time (p. 15). In Bandura's theory, agency and related efforts to exert control in one's life are motivated by anticipated benefits rather than an intrinsic or inborn drive for mastery. These beliefs emerge and develop through experience.

Bandura argued that self, self-efficacy beliefs, and a sense of agency are all socially and cognitively constructed through interactions with the environment. Self-efficacy beliefs in Bandura's theory can be highly differentiated in regard to specific kinds of competencies. Bandura recommended designing self-efficacy scales that were multidimensional, with specific items (How certain are you that . . . you can stick to a diet during the holidays? How certain are you that you can solve algebra problems?).

Other people, and particularly responsive caregivers and teachers, play an important role in promoting the development of agency and self-efficacy beliefs by providing many opportunities for young children to experience effects on the environment, which promotes a sense of agency. Children with efficacy experience gain a sense of control and agency, and are more likely to try to overcome challenges. Thus, self-efficacy beliefs would be expected to promote resilience. On the other hand, if children have little experience in making things happen, they begin to feel powerless, will not be motivated to try, and would be less likely to persist in the face of challenges. Thus, self-efficacy arises from the experience of overcoming manageable challenges and a robust sense of self-efficacy in turn fosters persistence in the face of adversity, which is more likely to lead to success than giving up.

Although these ideas on mastery motivation vary in theories about origins and specificity, and also in strategies for measurement, there is consistency among these various concepts in proposing that there is a powerful motivational system involved in learning and striving for adaptation and competence. This motivation system develops early in children and continues to develop and change over the life course. These investigators also agree that parents and teachers are central contributors in shaping the development of mastery motivation or self-efficacy beliefs, with opportunities for mastery experiences playing an important role in these processes.

One of the most effective strategies is to provide opportunities for mastery experiences wherein a child can achieve new skills and confidence in his or her skills through graduated steps well-suited to the child's capabilities. Perceived agency—"I did it myself"—in the course of overcoming a challenge is often accompanied by positive emotion, which rewards the effort involved in meeting the challenge. At the same time, there also is something profoundly social about the development of mastery motivation in human children. This system emerges in the context of social interaction in the family, with peers, and with teachers, and the joy in mastery appears to be enhanced in the context of positive attachment relationships. It is much more fun to fling the Cheerios off the high chair or toddle across the room with a responsive parent looking on.

This motivational system is a powerful engine for learning and efforts to take action in adversity. Unfortunately, circumstances may shut down this system or extinguish the motivation to adapt. Grossly neglected children, bereft of simulation and opportunities to play and experience mastery, often become apathetic or depressed (Zeanah, Smyke, & Settles, 2006). Children chronically tormented by bullying or abuse may become hopeless and despondent. Teenagers who see no opportunities to experience mastery due to discrimination or lack of opportunities may turn to contexts and activities disapproved by society where their needs for experiencing competence and pleasure in mastery can be met. Mental or physical illnesses, such as major depression, also can take a toll on this system.

One of the greatest challenges in clinical practice with children is working with a child who has experienced overwhelming adversity, lost a sense of agency, and given up on trying to cope. Competence motivation or self-efficacy beliefs may fall victim to chronic exposures to trauma or the chaos of multiple foster care placements and other forms of chronic stress and inadequate caregiving. Rekindling the mastery motivation system may be vital to resilience in such situations.

In turnaround cases of resilience, where late bloomers change direction dramatically, mastery motivation appears to be one of the "leading indicators" of change. In Project Competence and other studies of resilience, as well as anecdotal case reports, one of the early reported signs of change is a surge in desire or motivation to change (Masten, Obradović, et al., 2006). The power of the drive for mastery in resilience was underscored by Hauser, Allen, and Golden (2006) in *Out of the Woods: Tales of Resilient Teens*. These authors highlighted the role of "agency and the quest for mastery" in detailed case narratives illustrating resilience in a group of young people who were hospitalized for psychiatric treatment as adolescents but managed to find their way "out of the woods" by adulthood. These young people were part of a larger study of young adults hospitalized as adolescents for serious emotional and behavioral problems, assessed by interviewers blind to their psychiatric history. Nine of these young adults who were thriving as adults were compared with a sample of peers who were not doing well, and in this book, the authors present four of the resilient cases in detail to illustrate what they learned from intensive narrative analysis. Three protective qualities stood out in the resilient group: personal agency, an inclination to reflect, and an interest in relationships. The authors describe the striving and persistence of these resilient young people as they moved their lives forward, in striking contrast to their peers who gave up, blamed others, and floundered. The choices and behavior of the resilient group, especially as they struggled to change direction or seize control of their lives, were not always fruitful, wise, or traditional—the teens who later would show resilience were often rebellious as well as feisty—but they were highly motivated to drive their own lives and keep on trying to get it right.

Desistance from delinquency also is associated with active choice and pride in making the change. When Laub and Sampson (2003) interviewed in late life the individuals in the classic study of delinquency by Sheldon and Eleanor Glueck (1950), they were struck by the role of agency in the lives of the men who desisted from a life of crime and their satisfaction in what they had accomplished.

It also is telling that this urge to change often is accompanied or followed shortly by future-oriented goals and the appearance of a mentoring adult who facilitates the opportunities for change. Hauser et al. (2006) emphasized in their account that the teens headed for resilience seemed to actively seek relationships. It is probably not just luck that draws the partners in effective mentoring or other kinds of positive relationships together. There may well be complex interplay among the processes of motivation, relationships, opportunities, and goal formation that converge for positive change in late bloomers (Masten, Obradović, et al., 2006). Another signal of change that often accompanies turnarounds in direction is a new or renewed sense of hope and meaning.

FAITH, HOPE, AND BELIEF THAT LIFE HAS MEANING

In numerous case reports and studies, resilience is associated with hope, optimism, faith, and belief that life has meaning. As noted in earlier chapters, classic works on resilience repeatedly have noted that those who overcame adversity had a more positive outlook on life. Some late bloomers report transformative epiphanies when they experienced a surge of hope or belief that life could be meaningful; Thida Butt Mam and Michael Maddaus, described previously, both report transformative experiences of this kind. In *Man's Search for Meaning*, Viktor Frankl (2006) recounted the power of perceived meaning in the midst of overwhelming suffering in his harrowing account of life in a concentration camp.

In her autobiography, Elizabeth Smart describes the feeling of being broken and her despair after her initial rape by her kidnapper, Brian David Mitchell. She reports the ray of hope she felt when she realized her family would always accept and love her no matter what happened. Throughout her story, Elizabeth describes how her faith, as well as the love of her family, kept her going, and also how she managed to manipulate her captor into returning from California to the Salt Lake City area, where she was recognized and rescued (Smart & Stewart, 2013).

Human capacity for *meaning making* in the midst of suffering or seemingly overwhelming adversity suggests that systems of belief, personal or shared, may be important for resilience, particularly in situations of great suffering with loss of control. These belief systems may also sustain the mastery motivation system, protecting self-efficacy and mastery motivation from extinction in the face of lost control. When we have asked parents in emergency shelters what has helped them get through the experience, many respond by saying "my faith" or "God." Faith and spiritual support is widely reported in studies of resilience as a protective factor (Crawford et al., 2006).

On the other hand, terrible life experiences can shatter deeply held systems of belief that the world is safe, there is a benevolent God, or life has meaning (Janoff-Bulman, 1992). Traumatic experiences that involve betrayal of trust appear to be particularly difficult to overcome in this regard, including sexual abuse by a parent or religious leader (Janoff-Bulman & Frantz, 1997; Wright, Crawford, & Sebastian, 2007). Children who suffer great pain or betrayal at the hands of trusted adults may have difficulty recovering trust in future relationships or religion.

Religions and cultures of the world impart complex, organized systems of belief and also rituals and practices that are important for resilience in communities as well as individuals. These functions and practices are described further in Chapter 10.

WHAT ABOUT TEMPERAMENT AND PERSONALITY?

From the beginning of systematic research on resilience in children, there was interest in the possibility that individual differences in temperament or personality might play a role in adaptive behavior. Consequently, numerous studies of competence and resilience included temperament or personality trait measures. Early reviewers (e.g., Garmezy, 1983; Masten et al., 1990) noted that an appealing, agreeable, or easy-going personality or temperament was often (though not always) associated with resilience, whereas stress reactivity or negative emotionality (neuroticism) appeared to convey vulnerability in highly adverse circumstances. Resilient children also were described as more cooperative, having a positive outlook on life, high self-confidence or self-efficacy, an internal locus of control, and/or more emotional stability. Many of these personality characteristics have been linked to competence under low adversity as well (promotive functions). In Project Competence, the competent and resilient groups differed from the maladaptive group on three traits associated with a broad "meta-trait" of stability: low neuroticism, high conscientiousness, and high agreeableness (see Chapter 3; Shiner & Masten, 2012).

The most consistent evidence of *protective effects* for personality appear to be for the role of conscientiousness and effortful control (or constraint) for school or work success in the context of high risk or adversity (Shiner & Masten, 2012; Lengua & Wachs, 2012). These personality traits overlap conceptually with the capacity for self-regulation and EF discussed above. There also is evidence that agreeableness has protective effects on social competence in adversity (Shiner & Masten, 2012).

There also is *mixed evidence* on personality, raising the possibility that the same trait may serve varying functions in different situations or for different outcomes of interest. This issue surfaced early in the resilience literature, when Rutter (1989) and others pointed out that "easy" temperament in infants, often construed as a protective factor, was not always associated with resilience in non-Western contexts. In a provocative field study of Masai children studied longitudinally in the context of a severe drought in 1974, it was expected that easy babies would fare better, but it was those with a "difficult" temperament (more reactive, more difficult to soothe, etc.) who were more likely to survive (deVries, 1984). Moreover, aspects of personality viewed as problematic in American middle-class households, such as intensity and assertiveness, and therefore labeled as "difficult" in research on such samples, were admired as desirable traits in the Masai culture.

The trait cluster related to inhibition, shyness, and fearfulness also presents a mixed picture in the literature on competence and resilience (Masten et al., 1995). Inhibited personality or shyness may be more desirable in Asian cultures than it appears to be in American schools, particularly for boys. This personality disposition may also function differently for the outcome of delinquency or risk-taking behavior (where evidence suggests a promotive or protective effect) than it does for other outcomes, such as anxiety or social problems (where it may confer vulnerability).

Recent interest in individual differences in sensitivity to context raises somewhat different issues in regard to the functional role of traits. This work highlights the role of the context in defining whether an enduring individual difference is viewed as favorable or unfavorable. In a context fraught with peril and adversity, high sensitivity poses a vulnerability, whereas in a benign or enriched environment, the same proclivity would have a positive or enhancing function. Thus, it is the *function* of the trait that matters, considered in a particular context. The trait itself is not inherently a vulnerability or protective factor; the function arises in the interplay of individual and context. Furthermore, evidence is growing that personality traits (including sensitivity to context) can be shaped by adversity itself. Sensitivity to experience is discussed further in Chapter 7.

RESILIENCE IS *NOT* A TRAIT

Various scholars over the years have suggested that there is a trait of "resiliency," although there is little evidence to support this view (see Chapter 12; Masten, 2012a, 2013b). Such a trait would be akin to the idea of a healthy immune system that conveys resistance to disease and also responds to infections by mounting a suitable antibody response. At best, the notion of a general resiliency trait appears to be a convenient fiction to describe many different attributes and processes, often correlated, that are helpful to individuals in various situations calling for adaptive behavior. Some of the protective processes involved in resilience are not in the individual at all, but in their relationships and connections to external resources. For those attributes that are enduring individual differences associated with resilience, there does not appear to be evidence of a singular "master trait" of resiliency, but rather a multiplicity of characteristics often associated with better adaptation. At worst, the idea of a resiliency trait carries the risk for "blaming the victim" who does not show resilience (which could occur for many reasons having little to do with the individual's attributes) as somehow deficient. This issue is discussed further in Chapter 12, along with other perennial controversies in resilience research.

WHAT ABOUT HUMOR?

The idea of humor as a coping strategy or antidote to stress probably dates back thousands of years ("A merry heart doeth good like a medicine . . ."; Proverbs 17:22). A century ago, Freud (1928) viewed humor in its highest form as a "triumph of the ego," a defense mechanism revealing human capacity for liberating the self or asserting a sense of control, even in objectively terrible or uncontrollable situations (e.g., joking on the way to the gallows). Many anecdotal accounts of resilience implicate some role for humor as protective. In research, however, the role of humor in resilience has been difficult to investigate because of its complexity.

Humor is multifaceted, including the elements of appreciation (both cognitive and affective, thinking that a joke or cartoon is funny vs. expressed mirth), comprehension, creativity (generating humor), and biological changes in arousal. Humor can enact in a few moments the "pleasure in mastery" experience, combining a cognitive challenge or surprise (usually some form of incongruity) and some kind of resolution (sudden insight as one "gets" the humor) that engenders amusement and laughter. Laughing can reduce social tension or spur relaxation. Shared humor can be viewed as a form of play that serves to smooth interaction and boost attachment. Reputation for "a good sense of humor" is one of the items strongly associated with popularity in classroom assessments of peer reputation (Masten et al., 1985).

Humor develops and changes over the life course, as children acquire cognitive skills, share jokes, and gain life experiences (McGhee, 1989; McGhee & Chapman, 1980). Laughter and smiling often accompany playful social interaction. Appreciation shows a cognitive congruency pattern, in that children often prefer humor that is challenging but not incomprehensible (too difficult to understand). Jokes that children find funny at one age may seem "stupid" or silly later in development. Adolescent humor, compared with toddler humor, reflects the cognitive capabilities as well as the issues and experiences of adolescents.

Humor is associated with multiple aspects of personality, as well as a variety of cognitive skills, intelligence, social competence, and academic competence. In Project Competence, we found that multiple aspects of humor were related to multiple aspects of success over the course of the study (e.g., Masten, 1986). Humor was also related to IQ scores, social problem-solving skills, personality, and creative thinking. Peers viewed children who expressed more mirth, understood humor, and could generate it as leaders with good ideas for things to do, as more popular, outgoing, and happy. Teachers viewed such children as more engaged, attentive, cooperative, response, and productive.

Humor, however, also can be used to demean and bully others, or express hostility (Lefcourt, 2002). Children may laugh along with the "class clown" but not want to socialize with him or her and teachers rarely appreciate this kind of humor. Like many human capabilities, humor can be used as a destructive or maladaptive tool, as well as a resource or coping strategy. Laughter can occur in contexts of anger, fear, or anxiety as well as joy and fun. These complexities have complicated the study of humor in resilience.

Humor may be associated with coping and resilience because of its integrative nature, reflecting many of the systems already discussed that could facilitate adaptation (Kuiper, 2012). Understanding, appreciating, and generating humor all appear to require high-level integration of cognitive and emotional processes, and humor often involves arousal modulation, reframing, or cognitive control. Thus, humor may index capacity for integrated thought or action or reflective thinking and self-regulation, as well as aspects of personality associated with adaptation, such as agreeableness. Joking about a dire situation may facilitate distancing or reflection, which in turn could facilitate adaptation. Laughter also has physiological effects that can lower arousal and stress, and perhaps also improve immune function (Lefcourt, 2002; McGhee, 2010; Southwick, Vythilingam, & Charney, 2005).

˙Given the prominent role of humor in human life, the research on humor remains surprisingly limited. To date, the functions of humor (or component processes) in resilience are not well studied or understood, although humor in part appears to encompass multiple processes related to cognitive capabilities, mastery motivation, positive reframing or reflection, and self-regulation capabilities discussed above.

ADAPTIVE SUBSYSTEMS WITHIN THE INDIVIDUAL

The processes that lead to resilience clearly involve many systems *within* the individual as well as many systems *outside* the individual. The adaptive systems above were described from a behavioral and social perspective, but of course all these behaviors and social relationships are shaped and influenced by many lower-level systems within the organism and many other systems outside the organism in constant interplay. This is the nature of complex, living systems like human individuals. Adaptive function of the individual is interdependent with many other systems at different levels of function that are continually interacting. Intelligent behavior develops in conjunction with brain development and neural function, which depends on the adaptive function of a cardiovascular system, immune systems, and many other internal systems of the human organism. Human biology coevolved with microorganisms on which we also depend for healthy function, generally referred to as the microbiome. Current estimates indicate that only about a tenth of the cells in our body are human; the Human Microbiome Project is an effort that was launched to understand the intertwined nature and role of the microbiota in human function and development (Turnbaugh et al., 2007).

Efforts to explore the role of internal systems in resilience, such as neurobiological, microbiotic, and neuroimmunological, have progressed with advancing tools and knowledge over the past decade (Cicchetti, 2010, 2013; Feder, Nestler, & Charney, 2009; Sapienza & Masten, 2011; Russo, Murrough, Han, Charney,

& Nestler, 2012), but this domain of work remains in its infancy. In Chapter 7, some of the more promising current directions of this research are highlighted. This work comprises a major portion of the fourth wave of resilience science.

THE INDIVIDUAL IN CONTEXT: MICROSYSTEMS AND MACROSYSTEMS THAT SUPPORT RESILIENCE

The individual also develops in continual interaction with the environment, including the family system, sociocultural systems, and the physical environment (Bronfenbrenner & Morris, 1998; Lerner, 2006). The genotype of the individual may not change much at all (barring mutagenic exposures) but the *active* genotype appears to be highly and variably responsive to experience. As a result, the interaction of the organism at many levels (including molecular, neural, and behavioral) is altered by interaction with all aspects of the environment, and these changes can be highly dependent on timing of exposure.

The contexts of development also shape resilience in many direct and indirect ways. The adaptive systems described above are influenced by the experiences of different children in the contexts of interactions with family, friends, schools, communities, and culture, in addition to the physical interactions related to nutrition, water or air quality, microbes, toxins, or disease-causing organisms. Increasingly, children are exposed to an extensive set of interactions on social media and information coming through the Internet or mass media. The role of these microsystems and macrosystems in the lives and adaptation of young people also are receiving more attention in resilience science (see Southwick, Litz, Charney, & Friedman, 2011). These systems contribute in many ways to the development of the adaptive systems described above, but they also afford resources and protections for the resilience of whole communities or societies at higher levels of analysis. A full discussion of the emerging science of resilience in all the systems that touch the lives of children is well beyond the scope of this volume. In Chapters 8–10, I discuss the systems most proximal to child development, where there has been considerable research pertinent to resilience in recent years: family (Chapter 8), school (Chapter 9), and culture, including religion (Chapter 10).

Burgeoning theory and research on the resilience of communities and societies, as well as the social ecology of resilience, has been reviewed by Norris and her colleagues (Norris et al., 2008; Norris, Sherrieb, & Pfefferbaum, 2011), and also by Ungar and colleagues at the Resilience Centre at Dalhousie University (see Ungar, 2011, 2012). Research on resilience in the broader ecosystems linking physical with social ecology have been examined for decades by a leading group of ecologists studying resilience, including Holling, who launched the study of resilience in ecology, and his students and colleagues (Holling, 1973; Gunderson, Allen, & Holling, 2010). These scientists founded the Resilience Alliance, which maintains an informative website and publishes the open-access journal *Ecology and Society*.

ADAPTIVE SYSTEMS GONE AWRY: A CAUTIONARY NOTE

Much of the resilience observed in young people appears to be due to the fundamental adaptive systems described in this and subsequent chapters. However, it is important to keep in mind that these powerful systems can be misdirected or subverted in ways that lead to maladaptive outcomes or outcomes not desired by parents, self, or society that are harmful to individuals or groups. Reward systems that normally foster learning, agency, or healthy activities can be "hijacked" at a neural/biochemical level by addiction (Dackis & O'Brien, 2005). Gang leaders or pimps can recruit young people seeking the security of a surrogate family or attachment relationships and opportunities to experience self-efficacy, using their influence and rewards to encourage behaviors not approved by mainstream society or parents. Similarly, religions or religious leaders who provide comfort and support in times of need to their members also can perpetrate atrocities against nonbelievers or abuse their own young members. Sometimes resilience is threatened by the breakdown or unavailability of powerful systems, but at other times these same systems are co-opted for purposes or goals that would be widely condemned as maladaptive or harmful to young people. This issue is discussed further in Chapter 12.

SUMMARY

Many studies of resilience in human development over decades of research implicate a short list of promotive or protective factors often associated with good or better adaptation in conditions of high risk or adversity. This suggests that there are fundamental adaptive systems that protect human development or promote resilience under widely varying circumstances. These powerful systems afford the capacity for close relationships, self-regulation, problem solving, learning, motivation to adapt, persistence, keeping faith or hope and making meaning of life, and keeping a sense of perspective. Families, schools, communities, and cultures all play a role in nourishing, sustaining, or facilitating the development, stability, and recovery of these systems.

Each of these systems is connected to a large body of research, past and ongoing. I have argued that the short list and implicated systems offer "hot spots" for continued research, in that they implicate "where the action is" and call for deeper understanding and interdisciplinary research to integrate knowledge across levels of analysis (Masten, 2007). Each of these systems operates in constant interaction with many other systems of human life, both within the organism and in interaction with the environment. Either a life-threatening infection for an individual or a natural disaster for a large region offers devastating evidence of the inherent interdependence of systems in human resilience.

CHAPTER 7

THE NEUROBIOLOGY
OF RESILIENCE

From the outset, resilience investigators were interested in the neurobiological and genetic processes that might account for resilience as well as vulnerability (see Masten, 2007). Moreover, early models of resilience drew on powerful metaphors from medicine and neurology, such as the protective effects of vaccination. This is not surprising because many of the early investigators who became intrigued with resilience were clinical psychologists, psychiatrists, pediatricians, and similar clinical professionals. In addition, many of them were engaged in studies of developmental risk based on premature birth, low birth weight, having a biological parent or twin with schizophrenia suggesting genetic vulnerability, or neurological anomalies. At the time, however, the tools for directly measuring risk or resilience processes in children at a genetic, neural, or other biological level were limited. As a result, early waves of research on resilience tended to focus on behavior and psychosocial processes that could be more readily observed and assessed.

In the meantime, tremendous technological advances were rapidly changing the potential for studying the human genome and epigenetic processes, brain structure and function, stress and related systems, and many other processes in human adaptation at the level of systems within the human organism as it developed. These advances reawakened the long-standing interest in

174

the neurobiological processes that might be involved in resilience, and served to energize what was described above as the fourth wave of resilience research.

In this chapter, I begin by briefly reviewing key biological ideas and findings that shaped early concepts and models in resilience science. Then I describe examples of currently emerging research on the neurobiology of resilience. These include research on the neurobiological processes related to adaptive systems initially studied at a behavioral or social level, genetic studies, research on stress response systems and differential sensitivity to experience, and studies of neurobiological programming and plasticity. Although this work is relatively new, efforts to integrate neurobiological processes are rapidly transforming resilience science.

EARLY BIOLOGICAL MODELS OF PROTECTIVE EFFECTS

Medicine and medical research provided several key models of protective processes that influenced concepts and models in early resilience science. One of the most powerful concepts stemmed from the idea of *vaccination* to stimulate the body to make protective antibodies to a dangerous pathogen. In 1796, a country doctor in England, Edward Jenner, performed the first vaccination on a child to prevent smallpox using material drawn from cowpox lesions in a dairymaid (Stern & Markel, 2005). Jenner had figured out that exposure to cowpox conferred protection for one of the most dangerous diseases in human history. Over the ensuing two centuries, vaccines would be developed for many of the most destructive diseases in the world, including rabies and polio. Stimulating the immune system to respond protectively, and with great specificity in making antibodies, offered a powerful metaphor for promoting resilience through successful engagement with milder but still challenging forms of adversity. The ideas of *steeling effects* and *stress inoculation training* continue to be important concepts in resilience science.

A contemporary but related idea stems from the "hygiene hypothesis" concerning the modern rise in asthma, which asserts in effect that modern lives are "too clean" (Guerra & Martinez, 2008). In this case, exposure to microorganisms at the right time mobilizes the immune system to down regulate its reactivity to a potential biological stressor, serving to calibrate the immune system (Okada et al., 2010). Evidence on the genetics of asthma suggests that early exposure to microbes on farms among children with genetic sensitivity confers protection from asthma, whereas later exposure in individuals with the same genetic sensitivity would trigger asthma (Guerra & Martinez, 2008). In other words, there appears to be a developmental window of opportunity during which exposure to a particular environment programs the organism for adaptation in that environment, in this case conferring protection for the sensitive farm children. Growing up on a farm is protective for respiratory allergy (von Mutius & Radon, 2008). Recent research on other developmental programming effects in stress reactivity, discussed below, builds on this model.

Developmental timing also was implicated by early neurological studies of brain plasticity in relation to injury (see discussion by Cicchetti & Curtis, 2006). The classic example in this case was the observation that injury to the language centers of the brain after they were fully developed was more devastating to language function than injury to the same brain regions earlier in development. When injury came early in the processes of hemispheric specialization of the brain for language, then the other hemisphere developed capability for language. If the injury came late in development, language capabilities were much more impaired. The interpretation of these data focused on the greater plasticity, or capacity for change and reorganization, of the brain in early development. In more recent research, discussed subsequently in this chapter, some of the assumptions about plasticity and irrevocable sensitive periods in development are being brought into question, as scientists begin to unlock the nature of neural plasticity itself.

Another important idea in resilience theory stems from the observation that the same genetic factor could confer risk or vulnerability in regard to one problem and protection for a different problem. The classic example, invoked by Rutter (1987, 2006) and others, was the gene for sickle-cell anemia, an autosomal recessive disorder. When two sickle-cell alleles are present, the child develops this life-threatening disease. Given the grave risk associated with the disease, epidemiologists were initially puzzled by the observation that this risk factor continued to be so prevalent in some regions of the world, particularly sub-Saharan Africa. Then they realized that in the heterozygous form, with only one of these alleles instead of two, the sickle-cell trait provided protection from malaria, which was rampant in regions where the gene was more prevalent. The heterozygote state (one sickle-cell allele) in certain regions (with high risk for malaria) was more advantageous (more likely to survive malaria, while not developing sickle-cell disease) than the homozygous state (either zero or two sickle-cell alleles). This situation provides an example of "balanced polymorphism," where the heterozygous individual has a survival advantage. The protective effect of the sickle-cell allele under certain conditions explained why this risky gene showed high prevalence in specific regions, despite the dangers of the disease. This medical example provided a powerful reminder that what matters is the protective effect in a given context with respect to a particular outcome. The same trait could be protective under one set of circumstances and dangerous in another, or protective for one problem and conducive to another. In other words, the same attribute could have a protective function in regard to one context or outcome and confer vulnerability with respect to another problem or in a different context.

A final example of a protective effect drawn from the medical literature illustrates another point made by early reviewers in resilience science. Just as inoculations are not pleasant, functional protective factors may not be experienced as positive. The *ALDH2*2* allele has a protective effect with respect to alcohol abuse (see Irons, Iacono, Oetting, & McGue, 2012). Individuals with this gene variant, more common among those of Chinese, Japanese, or Korean ancestry, have an adverse reaction to alcohol, due to the way the liver metabolizes alcohol, resulting in symptoms like facial flushing, nausea, or rapid heartbeat. Given these reactions, the unpleasantness of the drinking experience could have a protective effect with respect to risk for alcohol abuse. Recent studies also suggest that this liver-mediated protective effect is influenced by development and context. The protective effect appears to increase over the course of adolescence and early adulthood and also is influenced by parental drinking behavior (Irons et al., 2012).

NEUROBIOLOGICAL PROCESSES UNDERLYING ADAPTIVE SYSTEMS

Resilience literature on major adaptive systems, such as attachment and problem solving, was initially focused on observable, behavioral, and social levels of analysis. In the meantime, research on the biology of these systems was progressing and gaining momentum as methods and knowledge accumulated on the neurobiological processes involved in normal and abnormal functioning of these adaptive systems. Application of this burgeoning literature to the goal of understanding and potentially promoting resilience is under way, although still limited at this time. In this section, I briefly highlight examples of this growing edge of resilience science for specific adaptive systems implicated by the short list described in the previous chapter.

The Neurobiology of Attachment

As noted in Chapter 6, attachment was conceptualized as a naturally selected biological system by Bowlby (1982) and many other scientists who have expanded theory and empirical evidence on this adaptive system. Animal models played a key role in the research on attachment from an early point in the history of this science, with many mammals serving as illuminating models of the development and biological underpinnings of attachment behaviors, as well as models of depression and other problems related to disrupted attachment, maltreatment, or deprivation

(Bowlby, 1977; Šešo-Šimić, Sedmak, Hof, & Šimić, 2010; Stevens, Leckman, Coplan, & Suomi, 2009). The work of Harry Harlow, Stephen Suomi, and their collaborators on attachment and stress responses and attachment in primates has played a major role in delineating risk and protective processes related to attachment and deprivation of caregiving (Kobak, 2012; Stevens et al., 2009; Suomi, 1999, 2006). Research on maternal licking behavior and the development of rat pups has played a seminal role in recent research on gene expression, epigenetic processes, stress biology, and the protective effects of maternal care on development over the lifespan and into the next generation (Karatsoreos & McEwen, 2013; Meaney, 2010).

Research on the neurobiology of parenting in animal and human studies has clearly demonstrated that the quality of care experienced, in combination with individual differences in the biological makeup of the individual (monkey, rat, or person), has the potential to alter gene expression, with lasting effects on the organization and function of the stress response system, risks for mental and physical health, and brain development, in myriad ways. Like other crucial adaptive systems for development, this system shows powerful motivational features at a biological as well as behavioral level. Caregiving is experienced as rewarding, activating major, universal reward circuits in the human brain and other mammals projecting along the medial forebrain bundle and involving dopaminergic neurons (Šešo-Šimić et al., 2010). If this reward system is hijacked (e.g., by drug addiction) or blocked (deliberately in some animal experiments), nurturing by mothers can be profoundly affected, with potentially devastating consequences for the development of young individuals in their care.

Generally, the neurobiological systems associated with attachment have implications beyond attachment per se. Attachment relationships and "good-enough parenting" appear to play a foundational role in the neurobiology of other adaptive systems, including stress-regulation systems and EF. Groundbreaking work by Meaney and others (see Meaney, 2010) on the consequences of licking behavior in rat mothers for the development of rat pups illustrates not only a seminal example of parenting experience as a protective process but also the interplay of adaptive systems in development across multiple levels of function.

Licking and grooming by rat mothers play an important role in the development of rat pups. Pups that are reared by mothers in early life with high levels of licking and grooming behavior (high-LG) show healthier development, particularly in regard to their capacity for stress regulation. They also grow up to be better (high-LG) mothers. Even pups known to be genetically at risk for poor stress regulation, fearfulness, or low-LG behavior (bred from lines high or low in these behaviors) respond to high-LG foster mothers in cross-fostering experiments (Gross & Hen, 2004). In effect, "good parenting" in the form of high-LG of mother rats changes development of at-risk rat pups. Moreover, this protective function applied in rat infancy has enduring effects over the life course and even into the next generation. Increasing evidence indicates that the experience of high-LG (good rat mothering) alters gene expression, effectively turning genes off or on, altering the impact of the DNA on function. This work has shown that expression of the glucocorticoid receptor gene is affected by rat-mothering behavior and the expression of this gene is centrally involved in stress regulation among other functions. Rat pups genetically likely to grow up more anxious and ineffectively reactive to stress that were reared by high-LG mothers grew up with better stress response systems, showing less trait fearfulness.

Subsequent studies have shown that the consistency of maternal care plays a key role in the adaptive development of rats (Karatsoreos & McEwen, 2013). Work by Tang, Reeb-Sutherland, Romeo, and McEwen (2014) suggests that the capacity of rat mothers to regulate stress plays a mediating role in the quality of their maternal care, with lasting consequences for their offspring.

Growing evidence in primates and human research implicates the influence of good or poor parenting on genetic risk, presumably through complex gene × gene and gene × experience interactions and processes (Karatsoreos & McEwen, 2013; Meaney, 2010; Gonzalez, Jenkins, Steiner, & Fleming, 2012). Research has shifted to focus on epigenetic processes that alter gene expression, such as the "silencing" of a gene by methylation (the addition of a methyl group that turns off gene transcription). Animal models of parenting and gene expression have demonstrated that the quality of parenting can have "programming effects" or lasting influences on gene expression related to behavior. Thus, experience is rendered into the biology of the organism and carried forward into the future, probably into many aspects of behavior, including later parenting behavior.

The rat model also suggests that developmental timing of parenting experiences are important, in that high-LG by rat mothers has lasting effects when it occurs during a specific early window of development. Yet the stability of such epigenetic changes does not mean that later change, even in adulthood, is impossible. Indeed, there is growing interest in the idea of reprogramming or altering gene expression in mature animals (Meaney, 2010).

The experience of high-LG mothering for rat pups also is associated with better learning later in development, at least in low-stress environments. Meaney (2010) and others have suggested that brain plasticity may be influenced biologically by the quality of rat mothering. The relative adaptive advantage potentially conferred by specific effects of high- or low-LG parenting may depend on the nature of the context.

Compelling studies of rhesus and other macaque monkeys also demonstrate at multiple levels of analysis the promotive and protective effects of effective caregiving and the attachment bond that accompanies this care (Stevens et al., 2009; Suomi, 2006, 2011). Macaques normally form strong attachment bonds to their mothers, with both partners maintaining close proximity during early life. Then, gradually, the young monkey begins to explore the world from this secure base, which provides opportunities for play and learning. Rhesus monkeys deprived of maternal care or reared with peers during important periods of early development develop a multitude of problems, including poor social skills and dysfunctional biological stress-regulation systems. Less normal engagement with peers interferes with learning many of the skills needed for the development of competence in these primates.

Primates also vary in temperament, with some monkeys inclined to be more outgoing and bold, while others are fearful and anxious (Suomi, 2006). However, when monkeys bred for fearfulness and high-stress reactivity are cross-fostered for rearing by experienced and highly effective mothers, they develop normal competence and adaptive function.

Studies of gene by experience interactions in rhesus monkeys parallel research in other species (rats, humans) suggesting that good parenting could have a protective function for offspring that have a biological vulnerability conveyed by genetic risk or temperamental variation. Given that gene expression can be regulated or influenced by the quality of parenting, it is likely that numerous vulnerability and protective moderating influences will be uncovered in future research. Meaney (2010) has emphasized the complexity of these processes, which can easily be oversimplified by focusing too much attention on single gene × environment effects. Increasingly, this field is moving toward "gene network" × experience studies, focusing on groups of genes that are functionally related (Meaney, 2010).

The sensitivity of the infant or juvenile to the quality of the parenting also is important to keep in mind. Rhesus monkeys, like humans, appear to vary in their sensitivity to parenting experiences. Moreover, variations in sensitivity based on experience likely also are changing with development and experience. Sensitivity is discussed further below.

Another neurobehavioral area of research with implications for attachment processes has centered on the roles of oxytocin and vasopressin in social affiliation and attachment behavior (Adolphs, 2009; Carter & Porges, 2013; Porges, 2011). These hormones facilitate social engagement and appear to work together in complex ways. In "The Biochemistry of Love," Carter and Porges (2013) have suggested that the neuropeptide oxytocin plays a key role in reciprocal attachment bonds in addition to its well-known roles in birth and lactation. Moreover, they argue that oxytocin is involved in adaptation to stress in various ways, facilitating protective forms of social engagement, neurogenesis and tissue repair, and other adaptive responses. Evidence suggests that oxytocin moderates the protective effects of social support during stress exposure.

Many of these ideas have been tested in prairie voles, a well-established model for social behaviors and parenting in a species with monogamous pair bonding, but findings in human behavior also support the role of oxytocin in a wide range of social behaviors important for attachment relationships (Carter & Porges, 2013; Meyer-Lindenberg, Domes, Kirsch, & Heinrichs, 2011). Intranasal administration of oxytocin, for example, facilitates eye contact, empathy, and social cognition in human experiments. There is a rapidly expanding literature on the neuroendocrinology of attachment behaviors in mammals, including humans, that may have important implications for the neurobiology of resilience.

The Neurobiology of Adaptive Thinking and Problem Solving

Problem-solving skills and learning generally are viewed as important tools for adaptive behavior in humans and other species. Adaptive thinking depends on brain development and function, which depends on many other aspects of biological function and development (Brancucci, 2012; Gray & Thompson, 2004). Toxic stress impedes cognitive development (Shonkoff, 2011). Deprivation of essential nutrients or interactions with a stable caregiver or learning opportunities all have profoundly negative effects on the development of adaptive cognitive capacity (Gray & Thompson, 2004). For example, if the level of glucocorticoid hormones involved in the biological stress regulation remains too high for too long, brain structure and function can be affected, with many consequences for development. The hippocampus, involved in many aspects of cognition, including memory, is especially susceptible to harm from high levels of unmitigated stress (Gunnar & Herrare, 2013; Shonkoff, 2011). Thus, a young child who is unprotected from stress by an effective parent or, worse, assaulted with stress by an abusive parent is at risk of suffering cognitive consequences to learning and intellectual capacity.

Over the past several decades, advances in tools for studying the neurobiology of brain development and function, including structural and functional magnetic resonance imaging and related methods for studying functional connectivity and other aspects of the brain at work, have produced a rapidly expanding literature on the neuroscience of intelligent behavior (Brancucci, 2012). It is now possible to study what is going on at a neural level while a child or adult is solving problems, and these tools continue to improve.

What promotes the development of good problem-solving skills, especially the fluid reasoning abilities required to deal effectively with novel challenges that might be posed by adverse experiences? A long and controversial body of research has been directed at this question (Blair, 2006; Gray & Thompson, 2004). Nonetheless, it seems clear that the quality of physical and emotional care and education all play central roles. Controlled experiments to improve the quality of parenting, nutrition, and/or learning opportunities show clear evidence that brain development and neurobiological function, as well as intelligent behavior and learning, are effectively altered by strategic interventions targeting the quality of parenting, nutrition, or early education (e.g., Diamond & Lee, 2011; Fisher, Van Ryzin, & Gunnar, 2011; Fox, Almas, Degnan, Nelson, & Zeanah, 2011; Nelson et al., 2007). Natural experiments that yielded improvements in these aspects of the environment also show the effects of improved environments on the development of cognitive skills. Children adopted from Romanian orphanages marked by profound physical and emotional privation, particularly those adopted early, showed often dramatic developmental gains in cognitive function even though there appeared to be lingering negative consequences of this experience (Rutter, Sonuga-Barke, & Castle, 2010).

As delineated in Chapter 9, many cultures and communities assign to their education systems a primary role in honing the problem-solving skills of children. Increasingly, school is coming to be viewed as a "neurocognitive–developmental institution" (Baker, Salinas, & Eslinger, 2012). Concomitantly, evidence grows that exposure to schooling changes cognitive function in ways that can be measured through imaging and other neuroscience methods. At a behavioral level, the Flynn effect—the substantial rise in average performance on fluid intelligence tests observed over the course of the 20th century—may reflect the impact of a widespread increase in formal schooling in many nations (Baker et al., 2012; Blair, 2006).

EF and Self-Regulation

Research on fluid intelligence also informs the neurobiology of EF and self-regulation skills. The capabilities usually encompassed by the latter concepts depend to a considerable extent on the neurobiological processes implicated in studies of fluid intelligence and follow a similar developmental course, improving into early adulthood and then leveling off or declining with age (Blair, 2006; Brancucci, 2012; Carlson et al., 2013; Zelazo & Bauer, 2013). EF improves as brain functions involving the prefrontal cortext develop, but it also improves with educational experience, practice, and training (Zelazo & Carlson, 2012). Growing evidence links these improvements with observable changes in neural structure and function that can be assessed by various brain-imaging techniques.

Self-regulation in the context of high arousal or emotion, sometimes referred to as "hot cognition" or "hot EF," holds particular interest for understanding resilience because threats and adversities typically elicit strong emotions or high arousal levels that galvanize multiple response systems. Emotional arousal itself, such as intense fear, can be viewed as adaptive in readying the organism to fight or flee, either away from danger and/or toward the safety of the attachment figure. However, intense emotion or arousal can interfere with adaptive thinking and action at levels well past the peak of the Yerkes–Dodson performance–arousal curve.

Controlling attention, considering alternatives, making decisions, and taking suitable action in the context of a terrifying threat or an extremely appealing temptation are quite different from the "cool" processes of reflection or self-control needed for taking a test of fluid reasoning or performing on an abstract test of cognitive flexibility in the absence of threat or temptation. Tasks designed to be "hot" appear to engage different brain circuits, including orbitofrontal cortex (Zelazo & Carlson, 2012).

Adaptive behavior in high-stakes situations likely requires the coordination and management of numerous systems simultaneously. Conscious cognitive control emerges and develops in childhood and adolescence, but there still are many other biological processes outside awareness involved in stress response and adaptive behavior.

Stress Regulation

Much has been learned about the neurobiology of stress reactivity and regulation over the decades since Hans Selye first published his classic works on biological stress response systems (Gunnar & Herrare, 2013; Gunnar & Quevedo, 2007; Karatsoreos & McEwen, 2011, 2013). A "symphony" of processes is involved in stress regulation, serving to maintain homeostasis or return the organism to healthy function across many biological systems following disturbances (Joëls & Baram, 2009). The adaptive processes that help regulate homeostasis have been described as "allostasis" (Sterling & Eyer, 1988). However, allostasis in the service of maintaining essential aspects of homestasis can take a toll on the body, a kind of cumulative "wear and tear" that McEwen and colleagues have termed *allostatic load* (McEwen & Gianaros, 2011; McEwen & Stellar, 1993). Individuals vary in their capacity for minimizing or reducing allostatic load, which can be viewed as a biological form of resilience (Charney, 2004; Feder, Charney, & Collins, 2011; Karatsoreos & McEwen, 2011, 2013).

There are two major stress-regulation systems, both of which involve the adrenal gland and the central nervous system (Gunnar & Quevedo, 2007). The autonomic sympathetic adrenomedullary (SAM) system is associated with rapid preparation of the body for "fight" or "flight" through the effects of circulating epinephrine. This is a fundamentally adaptive system, which can be maladaptive if it is triggered at the wrong time or by misperceived threats. The HPA is a slower-acting system associated with production and regulation of glucocorticoids, hormones that influence gene transcription at receptor sites in cells in the human brain and body. The complex effects of the HPA system may afford protection from stressors in the short term but can have deleterious effects on brain function and development if they are prolonged, as they might be with chronic stress (McEwen & Gianaros, 2011). High levels of cortisol are not good for brain development, and the brain sometimes appears to down regulate or turn down the reactivity of this system if there continues to be too much cortisol detected for too long. Studies of prolonged trauma in the context of child maltreatment or war described previously suggest that some individuals become hyporesponsive to stress, which may serve the adaptive function of protecting neural function and development, despite the potential cost of failing to respond to actual threats. Repeated deployment or continued high activation of the HPA system can contribute to allostatic load. Thus, efficient or effective function of the HPA system may contribute to resilience (Gunnar & Quevedo, 2007; Feder et al., 2011; Karatsoreos & McEwen, 2011, 2013; McEwen & Gianaros, 2011).

The quality of early care and parenting also influences the HPA system. As noted previously, the development of the efficiency of the HPA axis in rat pups is influenced by maternal care. High-licking maternal behavior, for example, alters the methylation and thereby the expression of genes in the hippocampus that are glucocorticoid receptors involved in the HPA system. High-LG mothers have a protective effect on this system. Studies of maternal deprivation or child abuse in human children and primates also show the effects of early social experience on the development of stress-regulation systems. Separation of infant monkeys from mothers or rearing in conditions that disrupt the quality of care can produce dysfunction in the HPA system, whereas interventions to provide or restore effective care can restore or improve HPA function (Gunnar & Quevedo, 2007; Gunnar & Herrare, 2013; Stevens et al., 2009; Suomi, 2006, 2011). In human children, positive attachment relationships have been shown to buffer physiological stress responses in research on mild stressors (Gunnar & Quevedo, 2007). In addition, improved quality of care in experimental intervention studies shows positive effects on HPA function. For example, a training program to improve parenting by foster parents had positive (normalizing) effects on diurnal cortisol patterning, a signature of effective HPA function (Fisher et al., 2011).

Maltreated children generally have an elevated risk for dys-regulated HPA function, showing both high rates of flattened diurnal cortisol levels, with lower than normal levels of morning cortisol secretion, or hyperarousal (Cicchetti, 2013). Adults who were maltreated as children show other possible indications of lingering stress-related effects as well. One is shorter telomere length, which may be a sign of cellular aging related to early stress exposure and allostatic load (Tyrka et al., 2010). Telomeres are repeats of deoxyribonucleic acid (DNA) at the ends of chromosomes that appear to protect the integrity of DNA and keep it stable through replication. In this case as well, there are variations among maltreated individuals, which may indicate many other processes that influence telomere length in addition to the effects of stress hormones like cortisol. These patterns of variation in HPA function and telomeres may indirectly reflect trade-offs of stress adaptation that are protective in the short run and potentially problematic for the long run.

There is considerable interest in the idea of promoting telomere growth and/or protecting telomeres from the negative consequences of stress (Blackburn & Epel, 2012). A classic study of stress effects on telomeres in mothers (Epel et al., 2004) found that mothers caring for chronically ill children had shorter telomere length. Greater perceived stress and longer time caring for the ill child were both associated with shorter telomere length. Additional research indicates that early negative life experiences may have lasting negative effects on telomere length, while there is some evidence that efforts to boost the activity of telomerase (involved in producing telomeres) or reducing stress can improve telomere length (Blackburn & Epel, 2012).

It is also conceivable that flexible stress response is an important sign of adaptive capacity. Life brings many unexpected and varying challenges. Inflexible stress response patterns may be both inefficient and maladaptive and thus particularly problematic for development. Understanding how a flexible stress-regulation system is spared, protected, or recovered may be very important for interventions to prevent damage to this crucial adaptive system or promote adaptive function.

Active Coping to Regulate Stress

Deliberate efforts to reduce stress or negative emotions related to adversity can take many forms, but it is clear that many of these strategies alter the biological processes of stress, sometimes successfully mitigating physiological stress and allostatic load or boosting immune function (Feder et al., 2011; McEwen & Gianaros, 2011; Troy & Mauss, 2011). Strategies might include talking with a friend or a therapist, exercising, biofeedback, mindful meditation, turning on a funny television show, making jokes, or deliberately reframing the situation in a more positive light. Although adults would be expected to have a larger repertoire of strategies for self-regulation of stress or emotion and more experience in their application, children clearly develop coping capabilities from an early age, with varying levels of skill and success. Those skills continue to develop with improving self-regulatory capacity and experience. Children also can learn techniques for lowering their stress through relaxation, biofeedback, yoga, and other methods (e.g., Pop-Jordanova & Gucev, 2009). Smartphones and tablet computers are opening new horizons for portable biofeedback games designed to help children relax or focus their attention. These systems often rely on finger sensors that monitor heart rate, galvanic skin response, or similar physiological indicators of arousal or anxiety.

Research on active coping in children has focused on describing common ways of coping, understanding their development and effectiveness in different situations, and promoting coping skills for particular adversities, such as medical procedures or chronic illnesses (Compas, Jaser, Dunn, & Rodriguez, 2012; Skinner & Zimmer-Gembeck, 2007). Coping often is defined as efforts to regulate the self or the environment under stress (Compas et al., 2012). Common coping strategies described in this literature include efforts to reduce exposure, get help or support, and regulate one's own responses to the stressor. Self-regulation and seeking support are particularly important in situations of uncontrollable adversity, such as cancer or essential medical treatments. Coping includes active strategies such as problem solving and seeking support, as well as accommodating strategies such as minimizing pain, self-encouragement, or self-distraction, all of which can be adaptive for managing pain or illness or the fears, stress, and anxieties that accompany severe adversities. Passive coping strategies include avoidance or disengagement, which is generally not found to be effective as a coping strategy in the context of chronic illnesses. Intervention studies of children with serious illnesses indicate that interventions focused on active or accommodative coping strategies can reduce pain, anxiety, and depressed mood, and improve quality of life (Compas et al., 2012).

The therapy literature for children with a variety of mental health problems also indicates that interventions focused on active coping can reduce physiological symptoms of anxiety or distress. "Coping Cat," for example, is a widely used and manualized cognitive-behavioral intervention for children with anxiety that has shown efficacy for reducing anxiety symptoms in a variety of disorders (Kendall, 2006; Kendall & Hedtke, 2006). Children (and their parents) learn strategies for managing anxiety in sessions and homework assignments that facilitate active coping skills practice, planning, and controlled exposure.

The science on coping in children appears to be converging with the developmental literature on stress regulation and EF, described previously. A particular concern for resilience in the context of severe illnesses in childhood is the possibility that the illness or the treatment, such as radiation for brain tumors, can harm adaptive systems due to effects on brain development or other neurobiological systems (see Compas et al., 2012).

Reward Systems

Behavioral findings on resilience suggest that powerful reward systems play a role in motivating efforts to adapt and persist in the face of challenges. Research on self-efficacy, agency, intrinsic motivation, and humor all suggest that positive emotions or pleasure experienced in the context of exercising agency or successfully solving a problem have reinforcing effects on effort, expectations of success, perceived efficacy, and the motivation to keep trying to adapt. Activation of the dopaminergic reward system, involving circuits in the amygdala and nucleus accumbens, among others, is linked to humor, optimism, and numerous other aspects of positive emotion and motivation associated with resilience (Feder et al., 2011). Dopamine release in the brain is associated with exploratory behavior, motivation, and learning about rewards. It also appears to play a central role in the Big Five trait of "openness to experience" discussed above as a correlate of resilience. Variants in two genes associated with dopamine in prefrontal function were associated with individual differences in the proclivity for cognitive exploration indexed by this personality trait, both in children and adults (DeYoung et al., 2011). The dopaminergic reward system, however, also has been linked to less adaptive behavior in the context of addiction, suggesting that reward systems can be entrained with maladaptive consequences.

The role of reward systems in resilience is likely to be complex and multifaceted. Nonetheless, is seems clear that the neurobiology of reward is an important avenue for future research.

BIOLOGICAL SENSITIVITY TO CONTEXT AND DIFFERENTIAL SUSCEPTIBILITY

One of the most provocative areas of research in the "fourth wave" to date is focused on the variability observed in responsiveness to experience, including both adverse and positive experiences. This variability, as noted previously in this volume, has been described by a variety of concepts, including "differential susceptibility to experience," "biological sensitivity to context," and "vantage sensitivity" (Belsky & Pluess, 2009; Boyce, 2007; Boyce & Ellis, 2005; Ellis, Boyce, Belsky, Bakermans-Kranenburg, & van IJzendoorn, 2011; Obradović, 2012; Obradović & Boyce, 2009; Pluess

& Belsky, 2013). In discussions of brain function or development, this variability is often described in terms of varying "plasticity," referring to the capacity for change in brain structure or function contingent on experience.

These concepts all have interesting implications for resilience theory and research because the functional significance of the attribute or state of the organism depends on the nature of experiences or context. The phrase "for better *and* for worse" in the title of a seminal paper by Belsky, Bakermans-Kranenburg, and van IJzendoorn (2007) captures this significance well. General sensitivity could be advantageous in a favorable environment or disadvantageous in a negative context. This would mean that the same characteristic could pose vulnerability during periods of adversity and a protective influence when the environment improves, either naturally or through intervention. However, it is also possible that there are individual differences that consistently relate to sensitivity only for positive features of the context or sensitivity exclusively for negative experiences.

For some time, resilience theorists have tried to underscore the idea that a protective factor is defined functionally and not absolutely, even though some protective factors, such as capable parents and good problem-solving skills, have positive functions in many contexts (Masten, 2012a; Rutter, 1987). They also have argued that the same attribute could be protective for one outcome and risky for another, or change in function from one period of development to another, or vary in its functional significance from one culture to another. The idea of differential susceptibility drives home the functional dependence of so-called protective factors on the situation or context. It also underscores the population-level advantages of individual differences in a world fraught with diverse dangers and ever-changing opportunities.

Another provocative aspect to this new conceptualization of adaptive variation is the idea that sensitivity itself may be susceptible to change from experience, and particularly for experiences occurring when adaptive systems are organizing (Boyce, 2007). Early exposure to adversity combined with low protection is hypothesized to shift the organism toward greater sensitivity as a protection from danger. But rearing in more advantaged, low-adversity circumstances also shifts the organism toward greater sensitivity, preparing the child to take advantage of greater resources. As a result, Boyce has suggested that the relation of early experience to sensitivity is a U function (Boyce, 2007). This programming of the organism based on experience, including prenatal experience, it is argued, enables individual adaptive systems, such as the stress or immune systems, to be organized or calibrated for better adaptation to the likely environment.

These biological models of differential sensitivity or susceptibility offer a new, context-dependent perspective on the function of traits in the individual and their development. From a population level, these ideas highlight the advantages of variation in adaptive success and the tuning of the organism to the expected environment. Moreover, emerging science on epigenetic processes offers biologically plausible models of how differential sensitivity might emerge and be transmitted. This work underscores the perspective that efforts to understand and promote resilience will need to consider developmental and ecological context, and long, as well as short, time horizons. Resilience will depend on the present concatenation of adaptive processes and their suitability for the current situation, but also the processes linking the organism to successful adaptation in a particular context, not only now, but in the organism's developmental history. Most interestingly, the concept of differential sensitivity suggests that individuals who respond with maladaptation to poor environments due to their greater responsiveness to experience may also respond favorably to improved or favorable environments. This thesis is supported by experimental prevention and intervention research for high-risk children, discussed in Chapter 11.

GENETIC AND EPIGENETIC RESEARCH

As indicated throughout this volume, new tools and knowledge in molecular genetics have precipitated growing interest in the genetic and epigenetic processes that may be involved in resilience

(Cicchetti, 2013; Feder et al., 2009; Kim-Cohen & Gold, 2009; Kim-Cohen & Turkewitz, 2012; Raby & Roisman, 2013; Russo et al., 2012; Rutter, 2006). This work, both in theory and empirical research, has taken a variety of forms. These include studies of specific genes or polymorphisms of genes with protective effects in particular contexts, such as the gene for alcohol sensitivity reducing the risk for alcohol dependence. There also are studies of moderating effects of individual genes or gene clusters on outcomes in extreme adversity situations, including a growing body of research indicating moderating effects of the serotonin transporter gene, dopamine receptor, and other genes in contexts of severe child maltreatment (Cicchetti, 2013). Some findings suggest moderating effects of genes on protective systems, such as the moderating role of the oxytocin receptor gene on the role of social support in stress responses, described above. Genes indexing sensitivity to experience or plasticity are under study as moderators of response to intervention, either in isolation or in combination, including the serotonin transporter, dopamine receptor, and brain-derived neurotrophic factor (BDNF). There is intriguing evidence that variations in the *BDNF* gene moderate effects of stress or interact with other genes to confer vulnerability or protection. For example, *BDNF*-moderating effects were found in a recent study of adolescents who experienced Hurricane Ike (La Greca, Lai, Joormann, Auslander, & Short, 2013). There is research on the protective effects of telomeres for DNA integrity or longevity and the effects of chronic stress on telomeres, noted above. The effects of parenting quality on gene expression are under widespread investigation, including the effects of parenting quality on methylation of specific genes implicated in adaptive behavior, such as the glucocorticoid receptor (Hackman et al., 2010; Zhang, Labonté, Wen, Turecki, & Meaney, 2013).

Evidence mounts that diverse but widely observed gene × environment effects suggesting "maternal buffering"—protective effects of competent parenting—for human children, rat pups, and rhesus monkeys (for example) in the context of genotypes or biological markers that confer risk for behavioral problems may be mediated by epigenetic effects (Cicchetti, 2013; Meaney,

2010; Suomi, 2011; Rutter, 2012b; Zhang et al., 2013). New studies also have shown that genetic variations linked to differential sensitivity may moderate response to intervention in prevention experiments (e.g., Bakermans-Kranenburg, van IJzendoorn, Pijlman, Mesman, & Juffer, 2008; Brody, Beach, Philibert, Chen, & Murry, 2009).

It is now conceivable that interventions could be personalized or tailored at a genetic level, akin to genetically personalized chemotherapy (Brody, Chen, & Beach, 2013). However, as knowledge expands, it becomes increasingly clear that elucidating genetic processes involved in resilience is a complex undertaking. The science is exciting but just getting under way.

SUMMARY

Research on the neurobiology of resilience is burgeoning (Cicchetti, 2010, 2013; Feder et al., 2011; Hughes, 2012; Karatsoreos & McEwen, 2013; Russo et al., 2012; Rutter, 2012b). This fourth-wave surge undoubtedly was spurred by tremendous advances in technologies and knowledge of the dynamic role in adaption and development of genes, epigenetic change, brain function and development, and many adaptive systems within the human organism (such as the HPA system), along with increasingly better animal models of stress and resilience. The early picture is one of dynamic and developmental complexity. Yet goals that once seemed completely elusive now are gaining traction. The next decade promises to illuminate many aspects of resilience at a neurobiological level. At the same time, this area of investigation already underscores the importance of an integrated understanding of resilience across levels, in context, and over time. The capacity for human resilience cannot be understood in its entirety if science is limited to levels within the functioning of a single human individual.

CHAPTER 8

RESILIENCE IN THE CONTEXT OF FAMILIES

The family as a system and context for human development and adaptive function has played central roles in the science on risk and resilience—in theory, empirical studies, and intervention. Child development is embedded in the family, initially as a fetus in utero and then in the rearing family. Eventually, most individuals find a partner to form a new or extended family, often rearing their own children, in a family life-cycle process that has been the focus of extensive comment in family systems theory and practice (Goldenberg & Goldenberg, 2013). The roles of family have been considered in theory, research, and practice from multiple perspectives, as a source of risk, a key protective influence, and a key socializing agent for the development of a child's human capital potential. Parents also are viewed as key brokers of a child's access to social capital.

The family itself has been studied as a system that develops, shows health and competence (or problems), and is threatened, vulnerable, or resilient in ways that parallel these concepts in individual development (Becvar, 2013; Goldenberg & Goldenberg, 2013; Patterson, 2002; Walsh, 2006, 2011). Resilience theory and applications in family systems have roots in general systems theory (von Bertalanffy, 1968), as well as family systems theory and therapy (e.g., Bowen, 1993; Goldenberg & Goldenberg, 2013; Minuchin & Minuchin, 1974; Nichols, 2013; Walsh, 2006), and specific roots in the work of McCubbin, Patterson, and their colleagues on family stress and adaptation (e.g., Boss, 2001; McCubbin & Patterson, 1982). Theory, research, and therapy focused on the family underwent a shift toward strength-based approaches and attention to positive adaptation in the aftermath of crisis similar to the broader resilience literature (Patterson, 2002). The concepts of competence, threats and disturbances, vulnerability, and resilience have all been applied to the function of the family system.

In this chapter, I discuss family function and adaptation in relation to risk and resilience in the individual child. In the first section, I describe risk arising in the family that threatens child development. Subsequently, I review work on healthy families and family resilience, followed by a section about the ways families protect children, and child development, with implications for intervention. Finally, I consider how communities, cultures, and societies support and protect family roles in the lives of children.

RISK ARISING IN THE FAMILY

Some of the most dire threats to child development arise within the family itself, in the form of abuse, neglect, and interparental conflict. Others have their influence through their effects on family function because they harm or degrade the positive function of parents or family in promoting child development or protecting children from harm. Children also biologically inherit genetic or epigenetic liabilities from their parents, with concomitant risks for psychopathology, compromised adaptive systems, or sensitivity to negative experiences. There is an extensive literature on all of these possibilities. In this section, I address some of the most influential ideas and findings on family-based risks and vulnerabilities that pose significant threats to child development.

Genetic or Epigenetic Vulnerability

Genetic risk and vulnerability is one of the fundamental ways that families convey hazards to their biological children. Studies of risk based on genetic relationships were one of the early pathways to research on resilience, as scientists followed "high-risk" children to learn about the origins of illness. Initially, scientists recognized that some problems ran in families, and then they did more systematic research to document the elevated risk that could be associated with the probabilities of shared genes. The role of experience, often in the role of external adversities interacting with presumed genetic vulnerabilities, was the next wave of science, giving rise to the diathesis–stress models. Now, it is possible to measure genes and gene patterns, as well as whether genes are "expressed" or not. Investigators are beginning to document consistent patterns of risk or vulnerability or reactivity to experience related to particular genetic patterns (Gottesman & Hanson, 2005; Kim-Cohen & Turkewitz, 2012; Rutter, 2009; see also Chapter 7).

Children of parents with partially heritable mental health problems may face a kind of double jeopardy, when genetic vulnerability or sensitivity to experience is combined with stressful experiences or poor parenting related to their parents' problems. They may also be exposed to developmentally toxic levels of stress or drugs during fetal development as a result of parental stress or substance abuse. Genetically vulnerable or sensitive children, on the other hand, may develop into healthy and adaptive adults under more favorable conditions. These complex processes of biological and experiential risk and protection in family systems, including intergenerational transmission of risk or vulnerability, are the focus of considerable attention in the fourth-wave studies of resilience (see Chapter 7).

Erosion of Family Function by Adversity: Mediated Risk

Children also are threatened when adversities harm family function, and especially the quality of parenting. Many risks for children are mediated by family or parent function. Glen Elder's (1999) studies of the Great Depression, and his work with Rand Conger and colleagues on the Iowa farming crisis (Elder & Conger, 2000), demonstrated how economic crisis can impact the family and in turn the children in those families. Conger and colleagues (Conger & Elder, 1994; Conger, Reuter, & Conger, 2000) developed the family stress model to account for the effects of economic deprivation on children through their effects on the parents in these families. In the model, economic hardship and deprivation generate persistent strains and pressures that influence the emotions and function of the family, interfering with parental effectiveness and contributing to child problems. This model is consistent with many studies of extreme poverty and parenting (McLoyd, 1998; see Chapter 4). Similarly, disasters, war, and terrorism can cause death and irreparable harm to families, as well as overwhelming stress that could undermine parental function (see Chapter 5).

Interparental Conflict and Divorce: Family Function as Stress Generating

Extensive research also documents the role of family in generating stress for children when there is interparental conflict (Cummings, Davies, & Campbell, 2000; Kouros, Cummings, & Davies, 2010). Conflict predicts child adjustment problems over time in multiple domains, perhaps because early antisocial behavior—strongly associated with interparental conflict and violence—tends to cascade into other areas of function, such as academic and social competence. Elegant experiments by Cummings and his colleagues have shown that children, even quite young children, respond to observed anger and conflict between adults in a laboratory experiment, even adults they don't know (see Cummings, 2006). Unresolved anger and conflict, in particular, appear to distress children.

Thus, it is not surprising to find that studies of divorce also indicate considerable stress for children before, during, and after divorce, sometimes for long after (Amato, 2010). The risks of divorce for children have been linked, in part, to conflict between the parents, before and after the divorce itself (Amato, 2010; Cummings, 2006). However, divorce is a prolonged and complex process that often involves multiple risks for children and parents, including economic hardships, the stressors of moving or changing schools, and depression in the parents. In some cases, divorce may substantially reduce a child's exposure to interparental conflict, which can be better than exposure to ongoing conflict in a marriage. Evidence has accumulated over the years that many influences contribute to the effects of divorce on child development, including the broader context of divorce, reflected in ongoing relationships and risks, as well as societal norms and expectations; the timing for all the members of the family; and the vulnerabilities and protections present in the lives of children exposed to divorce.

Maltreatment, Neglect, and Abandonment: When Family Fails

The greatest direct threat to children arising in the family is neglect or child maltreatment, particularly when the source is the primary attachment figure. A large literature has documented the risks to children of child abuse and neglect (Cicchetti, 2013; Dubowitz & Poole, 2012). As in the case of war and other complex forms of trauma faced by children, maltreatment typically occurs in a context of repeated and mixed forms of maltreatment, and also in the context of many other risk factors for child development, including poverty and interparental conflict, unsafe neighborhoods, and inadequate nutrition and health care. The complexity of the cumulative risk makes it very difficult to isolate the nature of unique risks posed by specific forms of maltreatment and the processes involved. The intensity and duration of maltreatment may often create a situation of overwhelming stress associated with potentially toxic and persisting effects on brain development and adaptive function (Shonkoff et al., 2009). Memory and cognitive development can be disturbed. Early-occurring maltreatment also may alter the development of stress-regulation systems (Cicchetti, 2013; see Chapter 7) as well as the attachment system. Severe maltreatment by the primary caregiver is associated with the D pattern of disorganized attachment, which is a risk factor for later mental health and relationships (Cicchetti, Toth, & Lynch, 1995; Main, 1996).

Thus, maltreatment not only causes immediate physical and emotional harm, it also can disturb the development of major adaptive systems that promote competence and resilience, including cognitive skills, the stress response systems, and the capacity for close and secure relationships. Therefore, it comes as no surprise that maltreatment is associated with diverse and cascading problems in development. Nonetheless, some children show resilience, and over the years, the focus on resilience in maltreated children has increased (Cicchetti, 2010, 2013). Many of the implicated protective factors in the literature on maltreated children are familiar, including positive relationships with a caring adult, good cognitive skills, and self-control. There is also great interest in genetic moderators of maltreatment risk, spurred by landmark research (e.g., Caspi et al., 2002) suggesting that some children may be more genetically vulnerable or sensitive to maltreatment (Cicchetti, 2013; see Chapter 7).

Child abuse is clearly harmful, but so is neglect, which is far more common (Dubowitz & Poole, 2012). Pervasive effects of neglect on development have been well documented. Adequate care is essential for brain development and acquiring the skills for learning and adaptation.

Sometimes neglect is a by-product of mental health problems or illness in parents who become functionally disabled. Depression or substance abuse in a primary caregiver, for example, can undermine the ability of the parent to provide consistent basic care, emotional support, or stimulation to an infant or child, with potentially profound consequences on development. Thus, screening and intervening to treat depression or addiction in parents can be extremely important. A report from the American Academy of Pediatrics (Early, 2010) described the protective potential for child development of pediatricians and other primary care providers routinely screening mothers for depression during prenatal and early well-baby checkups. Numerous investigators over the years have called for efforts to treat or reduce depression in parents as a prevention strategy for healthy child outcomes (Beardslee, Gladstone, & O'Connor, 2011).

Child Protection, Foster Care, and Adoption: Solution or Added Threat?

The burden of suffering and costs associated with maltreatment and neglect has produced many systems of child protection and intervention around the world, designed to provide better care for children at risk due to maltreatment, neglect, or abandonment (Flynn, Dudding, & Barber, 2006; Gilbert, Parton, & Skivenes, 2011; Zeanah, Shauffer, & Dozier, 2011; Yates & Grey, 2012). Good foster care, crisis nurseries, adoption, and child protection systems clearly save lives and promote better development for some children. Unfortunately, the child welfare systems intended to protect children and their development from maltreatment can also become a source of harm. Out-of-home placements and foster care carry their own risks, especially when the systems are overwhelmed, disorganized, and staffed with poorly trained social workers or surrogate parents. Foster care characterized by multiple placements, abuse, lack of supervision, and/or inadequate monitoring can pose tremendous risks for child development. Replacing the family as a child-rearing system turns out to be extremely challenging, which has led to increased efforts to monitor and improve child welfare strategies and the quality of foster care (Munro, 2011; see Chapter 11).

COMPETENCE AND RESILIENCE OF THE FAMILY AS A SYSTEM

What is a healthy, well-functioning family from the perspective of promoting competence and resilience in children? In this section, I discuss the concept of the competent family, broadly defined in family systems theory and research. The subsequent section focuses on the ways that families foster resilience in children.

Competence and resilience must be defined by criteria, whether one is talking about an individual person, a family, a society, or an ecosystem. With the growing attention to positive models of family systems, family therapists and researchers have begun to delineate these criteria, building on ideas that date back decades in family systems theory (Goldenberg & Goldenberg, 2013; Walsh, 2011). Years ago, Pratt (1976) described the qualities of the "energized family" in fostering the physical health and psychological well-being of family members. Effective families were described as involved, responsive, open, and flexible; connected to the community; active in problem solving; and providing age-appropriate autonomy to their children. The combination of engagement and flexibility is a repeated theme in theory about effective family systems.

The circumplex model has been influential in family systems theory, focusing on family cohesion, flexibility, and communication (Olson, 2000; Olson & Gorall, 2003). The main dimensions of the circumplex model were cohesion (ranging from disengaged to enmeshed) and flexibility (ranging from rigid to chaotic), with good function somewhere in the middle, balanced and well suited to the situation. Communication facilitated the other two dimensions and thus good communication was viewed as a general adaptive quality in a family system. Families challenged by adversity could respond with flexibility while retaining their closeness. Confronted with a developing child, an adaptive family would respond with changes in rules and roles to accommodate development. Thus, an adaptive family would grant more independence to an adolescent than the same child at a younger age.

Families also develop and change, as do individuals. Some family theorists have described developmental tasks of families, which also vary over the family life cycle (see Goldenberg & Goldenberg, 2013). For example, when a couple becomes parents, having or adopting a baby, the expectations for their family change. They are expected to care for the baby and will be evaluated by themselves, their relatives, and friends, and also society according to common expectations for what a parent is expected to do in this regard. As the child develops, the family is expected to socialize the child to behave appropriately for the culture and society. If a child does not meet expectations for social conduct, for example, if they are hitting, lying, or stealing in age-inappropriate ways, parents may be criticized for dereliction in their child-rearing responsibilities. These family developmental-task expectations are cultural, moral, and legal in nature. Parents who neglect or abuse their children by the standards of their community may be criticized, be ostracized, or lose legal custody of their children.

Family Roles and Routines

Families and, more specifically, parents, have numerous roles and regulatory functions that serve to maintain adaptive biological, psychological, and social well-being, and healthy development in family members (Fiese, 2006; Masten & Shaffer, 2006; Pratt, 1976). The family system, usually led by parents, develops roles, rules, and routines that serve to maintain balance and growth, and also restore function when there is a disturbance. Barbara Fiese has written compelling accounts of these routines and rituals, and their effects on individual development, based on her studies of interactions and routines in the daily life of families; she extended the transactional model of human development to the family system level (e.g., Fiese, 2006; Sameroff & Chandler, 1975; Sameroff & Fiese, 2000).

Routines and rituals help maintain the cohesion and stability of the family as a balanced system. Families have routines around mealtime, bedtime, chores, religious practices, and other activities. These routines follow a developmental pattern over the course of the family life cycle, varying when there are young children, adolescents, or an "empty nest." Work life changes, school activities, separations, and divorce will affect these routines, as will seasons of the year. Historical and cultural changes also occur, with intergenerational shifts, as well as the adjustments brought by acculturation in the context of migration.

Fiese (2006) has studied the nature and significance of mealtime routines in family life. There are rules and roles about where each person sits, manners, conversation and turn taking, and attendance. There may be special holiday or birthday rituals and expectations. Evidence suggests that families that practice routines, such as regular mealtimes several times a week, have more competent children and happier marriages. Similarly, in the context of turbulence or trauma, maintaining or reestablishing routines appear to serve a protection function for children, as observed in the disaster literature discussed in Chapter 5.

Akin to individuals, families develop over the course of family life cycles as they form, have children, die, divorce, or otherwise change membership and age. They also face the challenges of unexpected tragedies and trauma. Members of a family are continually interacting with one another and others outside the family through complex transactions. Change, slow or abrupt in one family member, will influence all the other members of the family as they assimilate or accommodate these changes.

Coregulation and the Development of Resilience Capacity

In developmental theories of attachment and socialization, parents or the extended family also train self-regulation through a process of coregulation, where adults serve as external modulators of arousal, emotion, and behavior of young children until they can regulate themselves (see Gross, 2007, 2008). Beeghly and Tronick (Beeghly & Tronick, 2011; Tronick & Beeghly, 2011) have argued that the mutual coregulation experienced in parent–infant interactions serves to shape regulatory capacity that is essential for later competence and resilience. Through many everyday interactions, adjusting for routine disturbances, the child develops regulatory and resilience capacity, as well as a sense of agency and pleasure in mastery. This may come in the form of arousal games that sometimes upset the baby because they get too intense (e.g., tossing a baby into the air, peek-a-boo), or other forms of play, as well as routine soothing when a child takes a tumble or gets frustrated. Successful interactions of this kind are accompanied by very positive affect. It is noteworthy that the child is believed to learn through experiencing disturbances and recovery, not simply from total harmony of interactions: Infants learn that "we can repair mismatches" from the experience of mismatch and recovery (Tronick & Beeghly, 2011, p. 9). They also gain a sense of security and meaning in the context of these interactions that shapes attachment relationships, trust, and meaning-making capacity well into the future.

Sensitive and Authoritative Parenting

Positive parent–child interaction has been elucidated in developmental theory and research for many decades. In attachment theory, sensitive and responsive caregiving promotes secure attachment with caregivers, which is carried forward in models and expectations about interpersonal relationships into future relationships with peers and romantic partners (Bowlby, 1982; Cassidy & Shaver, 2008; Sroufe et al., 2005). Effective parenting also has been studied in relation to competence in children, in an effort to understand how parents promote competence or resilience (Masten & Coatsworth, 1998).

Authoritative parenting style has long been linked with competence in children (e.g., Baumrind, 1966, 1991; Steinberg, 2001). Authoritative parenting is often characterized by a balance of responsiveness and demandingness, or a combination of high warmth, structure, and high expectations. In contrast to permissive, authoritarian, or totally disengaged parents, authoritative parents are engaged and accepting, but also expect responsible behavior and achievement from their children. This combination is consistently associated with success in age-salient developmental tasks, such as academic achievement and prosocial behavior, particularly in modern Western societies (Masten & Coatsworth, 1998). Some investigators have challenged whether authoritative parenting is always optimal, particularly in harsh or dangerous environments, or in authoritarian-style cultures (see Baumrind, 1996, for a discussion of the issue). For example, it has been noted that parents of children living in dangerous environs are much stricter than parents of those living in safe environs. However, they are not usually perceived as harsh or rejecting; in this context, strictness may be perceived as protective. It seems likely that effective parents generally adjust their values and expectations based on their knowledge of what promotes success in a given time and culture, and also based on their knowledge of what an individual child needs at a given time in development.

Family Resilience

Resilience can be conceptualized and studied at the level of the family system, as noted above. In their early work on the double ABCX model of family crisis and adaptation, McCubbin & Patterson (1983) described patterns of adaptation (from "bonadaptation" to "maladaptation") in families over time, analogous to pathways delineated in Chapter 2 with respect to adaptive function in individuals. In recent decades, Froma Walsh (2006, 2011) has been highly influential in defining resilience at the family level and applying a resilience framework to family practice. Family resilience focuses on the adaptation and recovery of the whole family as a unit, rather than the individual, and builds on family systems theories concerned with stress and coping described in the opening section of this chapter. The functioning of the family is situated dynamically in culture, history, and time, showing trajectories over the family life-cycle course of development. There is considerable attention to risk and cumulative risk, as well as protective influences on the quality of the family's function, and also the ways that larger systems, like communities, can support family resilience through policy, services, or practice. McCubbin and Patterson (1983) described how demands on families can pile up, and Patterson (2002) subsequently noted that families, like individuals, can face a sequence of interrelated hazards that pose great strain on system functioning. Repetti, Robles, and Reynolds (2011) have suggested that "risky" families may mediate adversity through biological pathways, spreading the effects of allostatic load in one or more family member to others in the family system.

Walsh (2011) has identified nine processes for family resilience in three domains of family function (family beliefs, organization, and communication). She argues that these processes can be assessed and targeted in interventions. The protective processes for family resilience delineated by Walsh show some parallels to the adaptive systems implicated in the individual-focused resilience literature (described in Chapter 6). Family belief systems, for example, are believed to foster adaptive function in the family in ways similar to meaning making or religious beliefs in the individual literature. Families can foster a sense of coherence, hope, and optimism. Walsh also identifies family flexibility and connectedness as key protective processes for family resilience, which parallel the roles of cognitive skills and attachment relationships in the individual literature. Families can mobilize social and economic resources that afford vital help during periods of crisis or strain.

At the same time, there are some notable differences in family-level protective processes. For example, Walsh emphasizes the importance of family communication and collaborative problem solving in resilience. Families can provide respite, empathy, and humor in one another's lives. They also can teach and support conflict management, negotiation skills, and collaborative decision making. Moreover, like other family systems theorists and practitioners, Walsh emphasizes how families can manage disturbances and crises by maintaining a sense of security, nurturing children in troubled times, maintaining or restoring daily routines and rituals, and drawing on extended social networks for emotional or economic backup.

The family practitioner plays a facilitative role to support and bolster these protective processes in family systems. Overall, the implications of a resilience-based framework of family function for intervention are similar in theme to the implications discussed in Chapter 11 for a resilience framework for practice. At the level of family, rather than individual, Walsh (2006, 2011) underscores the importance of a dynamic, systems view, with a focus on family strengths and a developmental perspective. She also sets forth guidelines to strengthen family resilience that emphasize identification and focus on family strengths, building family supports, and facilitating positive adaption, recovery, growth, and mastery.

HOW FAMILIES PROMOTE RESILIENCE

Given the central roles accorded to families in child adaptation and rearing, there has been great interest in the ways that families promote resilience in their children. These include active strategies to control the level of exposure to adversity, attempts to mitigate the effects of adversity, and the nurturing of individual adaptive systems strongly implicated in resilience (see Masten & Monn, in press).

Preventing and Moderating Exposure to Adversity

One of the basic jobs assigned to parents in most cultures is monitoring dangers to their children and taking action to prevent or mitigate harm. According to attachment theory, this expectation has biological roots in a system evolved for the purpose of protecting children from harm. Perceived danger on the part of either partner will activate attachment behaviors, such as seeking proximity. Parents have much more responsibility in an attachment relationship for monitoring dangers to children, especially very young children who cannot monitor dangers on their own. Thus, parents are expected to keep infants away from cliffs, traffic, fireplaces, and household dangers, through supervision and "child proofing" their homes. In dangerous environments, including neighborhoods, effective parents might be expected to be more vigilant or cautious and to shift parenting strategies, for example, by becoming stricter and monitoring their children more closely. There is evidence consistent with the idea that perceptions about the neighborhood influence parent behavior, although causal influences are difficult to establish (Dumont, Ehrhard-Dietzel, & Kirkland, 2012).

There is considerable evidence linking the quality of parental monitoring or knowledge of child whereabouts and safety to better child outcomes, particularly in risky environments, although it is not always clear whether monitoring is actually what is providing the protection, rather than the quality of the relationship itself (Dishion & McMahon, 1998; Masten & Shaffer, 2006; Stattin & Kerr, 2000). Interventions to prevent antisocial behavior or substance use in risky environments often emphasize the importance of parental vigilance or monitoring. In the Strong African American Families intervention, for example, designed to prevent substance use, reduce risky behaviors, and promote competence in African American youth, the prevention program focuses on boosting parent vigilance and monitoring (Brody et al., 2004; Murry, Berkel, Gaylord-Harden, Copeland-Linder, & Nation, 2011).

Good parenting, on the other hand, does not mean eliminating child exposure to adversity. On the contrary, as discussed previously in this chapter, some exposure to risk and adversity is essential to normal development. The concepts of steeling effects and stress inoculation discussed elsewhere in this book also suggest that adversity exposure can promote the capacity for resilience and adaptability. Children need experience with managing stress, recovering from manageable disturbances, and learning how to solve problems on their own. As they grow more skilled, their parents need to pull back so that children gain confidence and self-efficacy along with skills in adapting to adversity. The challenge for parents is knowing how much exposure is going to be overwhelming or harmful in a continually changing child.

Buffering the Effects of Adversity

Parents also take action to reduce the negative effects of adversity. They hug, soothe, and support, for example, in direct efforts to help a child regulate arousal or fear. They physically help injured children and they also seek professional help as needed for medical or psychological care. Most fundamentally, however, parents in a secure attachment relationship with a child have considerable power to calm a child through simple proximity.

The buffering effect of parents on fear and anxiety, as well as the stress hormone cortisol, has been demonstrated in classic studies of children during inoculations and experiments where the infants or toddlers were approached by strangers or potentially scary toys or animals (Gunnar & Donzella, 2002). Stress and fear reactions are attenuated by the proximity of the parent for children in secure attachment relationships, presumably because they have a strong history of responsive care and comforting by the caregiver. Experiments with nonhuman primates also show the powerful buffering effects on stress conferred by the presence of the mother.

Children also judge danger through the reactions of adults and especially their attachment figures, a phenomenon sometimes called *social referencing* (Carver & Cornew, 2011; Hornik & Gunnar, 1988). Infants, for example, in classic "visual cliff" experiments, looked to the parent for cues, particularly in situations set up for ambiguity (e.g., Sorce, Emde, Campos, & Klinnert, 1985). In the visual cliff, the infant was placed on what looked like an edge with a drop-off (actually a safe surface). The height of the cliff could be adjusted. With a very high-looking cliff, infants did not cross; with very low cliffs, most infants did cross. In the uncertain range, however, infants were particularly responsive to the emotion conveyed by mother's emotion: if it was fear or anger, they did not cross; if it was positive, they did. Later studies of social referencing have shown that many aspects of the context and the individuals involved can influence these processes. A bold toddler, for example, may be less influenced than a timid toddler by anxious signals from a parent.

Although social referencing research has focused on infant behavior, people of all ages undoubtedly use this kind of emotional information to judge danger and safety, and the reactions of trusted people, including family members, would be expected to carry more weight. In applied work on disaster and terrorism, parents are advised to keep in mind that they are communicating terror through their own emotional reactions. Terror is contagious in humans and many other species. Parents are conduits of fear for children and it is easy to understand why this would evolve as adaptive. However, since parents often mediate and communicate stress and fear to their children, it is important for parents to be aware of their own responses and control them appropriately, either to alert or buffer their children in regard to pending danger.

Rearing Competent, Adaptive Children

Perhaps the most fundamental role of families in resilience is their diverse roles in supporting the development of competence and adaptive capacities (see Clarke-Stewart & Dunn, 2006; Guerra, Graham, & Tolan, 2011; Lewis & Feiring, 1998; Masten & Monn, 2015). Many of these roles have already been described throughout this volume. Parents and other family members participate in coregulation processes that contribute to the development of self-regulation skills. Infants have limited capacity to control their own arousal levels, emotions, and behaviors. Over time, aided by growing cognitive capacities, and the experience of many interactions with other people, most particularly their family members, children learn better self-control. Cognitive skills are facilitated by interactions of family members with children, including conversations, reading, and games. Families also convey social and cultural norms and expectations through modeling, teaching, discipline, and many other activities (Harkness & Super, 2012; Masten & Monn, 2015; Ungar, Ghazinour, & Richter, 2013).

Families provide the physical needs for their children, but also opportunities and social resources. They play a key role in facilitating education and extracurricular activities like sport or music through financial support and engagement. The social networks of the family provide children with many adult role models and potential opportunities.

All of these roles can contribute to the development of competence and adaptive skills and relationships that have been implicated as the primary source of resilience capacity. Thus, family systems contribute to child resilience in two primary ways: by their own actions to influence the interactions of children with stressful experiences and through their influences on the development of adaptive capacity in the course of child rearing. Like a pediatrician who is responsible for looking after a child's health, parents are charged with doing something about threats to the child's well-being in a crisis but also with fostering healthy development more generally.

For a family to fulfill these crucial roles in protecting and promoting resilience in children, the family itself must have the capacity for resilience. Numerous interventions have been developed to support family resilience, often targeting parents. Additionally, communities and societies have a considerable stake in the resilience of families and their capabilities for rearing children with good adaptive capacity. Thus, larger social systems also have developed strategies and policies to support families.

Interventions to Support Family Function for Resilience of Parents and Children

Numerous interventions have been designed to improve family function, parenting, or the quality of parent–child relationships or interactions as a means for promoting resilience in children at risk due to adversity or economic hardship (Sandler et al., 2011). These include home-visiting programs, interventions targeting parent–child interactions, and efforts to help families dealing with divorce or bereavement. Additional intervention strategies are discussed in Chapter 11.

Home-visiting programs for high-risk families (see Howard & Brooks-Gunn, 2009) have been effective and popular. The best known and documented of these is the Nurse–Family Partnership (see Olds, 2006, or the Nurse–Family Partnership website: *www.nursefamilypartnership.org*). Trained nurses visited first-time mothers during pregnancy and through the child's first 2 years of life to support and guide mothers and promote healthy development in the child. Several large RCTs have demonstrated positive effects of this program on parenting and other family outcomes.

Interventions have also been developed to prevent child maltreatment and promote child welfare through improving the quality of parent–child interactions. Child–parent psychotherapy (CPP) is a promising strategy developed by Alicia Lieberman and grounded in theory on parent–child relationships, attachment, and mental health (Lieberman & Van Horn, 2011). CPP has been tested in RCTs with parent–child dyads in families at risk for child maltreatment (Lieberman & Van Horn, 2011; Toth & Gravener, 2012). In this approach, used with both infants and toddlers in parent–child treatment dyads, the therapist works with the dyad to foster sensitivity and understanding by the parent, provide developmental guidance, and encourage age-appropriate expectations. The therapist also takes action to model protective behavior during the sessions.

Parent–child interaction therapy (PCIT) is another approach to dyadic intervention, focused on reducing negative interactions between parent and child in families with very high risk for child abuse. With both direct teaching and coaching of live interactions, parents are taught to improve management, sensitivity, and enjoyment of interactions with their children. This method also has shown effectiveness in reducing abuse and improving observed parental sensitivity in high-risk parent–child dyads in RCTs (Chaffin et al., 2004; Thomas & Zimmer-Gembeck, 2011).

A number of family interventions have focused on helping families through the challenges of divorce, separation, or bereavement, among other adversities (Sandler et al., 2011). Here again, RCTs support the effectiveness of these programs, particularly the parent-focused components. The New Beginnings program, for example, was designed to help families of 9- to 12-year-olds coping with divorce (Sigal, Wolchik, Tein, & Sandler, 2012; Wolchik et al., 2002). In this experiment, investigators compared parent-only group intervention with parent-plus-child groups and a control condition provided with literature about divorce. For parents, the manualized intervention focused on improving the mother–child relationship, effective discipline strategies, engaging fathers, and reducing interparental conflict (Wolchik et al., 2002). Both the parent-plus-child treatment and the parent-only treatment groups had better outcomes in the short and long term compared with the control group. There were lasting positive effects on child outcomes, mediated by improvements in parent–child relationships and discipline.

HOW COMMUNITIES, CULTURES, AND SOCIETIES SUPPORT AND NURTURE FAMILIES

Families are nested in cultures, communities, and societies that play numerous roles in supporting or undermining family function (Becvar, 2013; Conger & Elder, 1994; Masten & Monn, 2015; Panter-Brick & Leckman, 2013; Walsh, 2006). Most societies have policies and practices designed to support families in their role as caregivers of children, although there are wide variations in the kinds and levels of support provided. Norway, for example, provides far greater support to families with children than the United States, through more generous maternity leave policies and better access to high-quality early childhood education, as well as free health care. Yet the United States does have tax policies intended to offset some of the costs of child rearing, including the deductions for dependent children and the Earned Income Tax Credit for low-income working families. And these policies matter. Research has shown that the Earned Income Tax Credit has a measurable benefit on the likelihood of children's academic success (Duncan, 2012).

Communities support families in good times and bad, including practical everyday necessities such as clean water, public safety, and medical facilities, as well as emergency services. The role of communities in disaster response underscores the multiplicity of ways that individual and family resilience depend on community resilience (Masten & Narayan, 2012; Masten et al., 2015; Norris et al., 2008), as highlighted earlier in Chapter 5.

Research on how immigrants fare in different receiving countries also reflects different levels of support to families in various nations (see Masten, Liebkind, & Hernandez, 2012b). Based on analyses of income supports for immigrant households with children in rich countries, Smeeding, Robson, Wing, and Gershuny (2012), for example, suggest that national policies regarding family supports to reduce the impact of poverty have more influence on child outcomes than immigrant status per se. Countries with better welfare supports for families, including northern Europe and the Scandinavian nations, generally have better economic outcomes for children, whether native or immigrant. The United States, in contrast, has very high poverty rates for children, both native born and immigrant children, accompanied by lower prospects for achieving economic success than their more affluent peers.

Nonetheless, the United States continues to be a desirable destination for many migrating families, particularly for refugees

(Beck & Tienda, 2012). The general wealth of the country, free public education, and opportunities for gaining citizenship, among other qualities, continue to attract immigrant families.

Tensions can arise in immigrant families that move into cultures with different values and expectations for children as their children try to navigate different values and expectations at home and school or in the community (Fuligni & Telzer, 2012; Motti-Stefanidi, Berry, Chryssochoou, Sam, & Phinney, 2012). Indeed, resilience among immigrant youth often has been associated with competence in navigating multiple worlds and roles (see Chapter 10). Developmental task expectations for children may differ between the immigrant family culture and the receiving culture. Immigrant youth also may find themselves serving as language and cultural brokers for the family, with potentially positive or negative consequences (Fuligni & Telzer, 2012). These roles can be a source of burden as well as pride, and may not be fully appreciated by the receiving community.

The "immigrant paradox" also raises some interesting issues pertinent to the role of family and culture in resilience. This concept (discussed further in Chapter 10) refers to the observation that immigrant youth sometimes show better health and well-being than native-born youth or subsequent immigrant generations that remain in the receiving nation. Garcia Coll and colleagues (2012), in their analysis of the immigrant paradox, suggest that immigrant families may import positive values and cultural capital that is subsequently lost to future generations, and that potentially could be supported and sustained to the benefit of their own descendants as well as the receiving societies.

SUMMARY

Families play multiple roles in risk and resilience for children, transmitting genes and traditions, generating stressors and resources, and acting to protect their children and prepare them for future resilience. Families provide physical, emotional, and spiritual needs and protections for children, but also opportunities for children to gain experience and confidence in their own adaptive skills. Given the central and pervasive nature of their roles in the lives of children, both present and future, effective families are vital to child resilience. As a result, among the most devastating dangers faced by children are circumstances that destroy or damage the availability or function of families, or dangers from family members themselves. In such circumstances, it is imperative for child well-being to restore or establish effective family care.

One of the most important ways to foster resilience in children is to support good family function and care. This fundamental lesson has been learned in the aftermath of disaster or war, as well as situations of divorce, maltreatment, or bereavement. Consequently, it is dangerous for any community, culture, or society to neglect or undermine the capacity of families to nurture resilience capacity in their children.

CHAPTER 9

RESILIENCE IN THE CONTEXT OF SCHOOLS

Beyond the family, school is the most organized system in which most children around the world spend most of their time as they grow up (Eccles & Roeser, 2012). In most societies, the education system is charged with preparing children for citizenship and diverse future roles in society, including the workforce. Thus, one would expect education systems to have crucial and multifaceted functions in resilience theory and research. Schools nurture many of the adaptive systems in the individual that generate capacity for resilience over the course of development, while also affording opportunities for relationships with adults and peers beyond the family. These relationships contribute to resilience capacity building but also provide additional social capital. Schools also are a powerful symbol of normal life in societies, which heightens their significance in the aftermath of disaster or tragedy, as discussed in Chapter 5. Schools can provide an island of tranquility and routine, a secure base for children whose lives are chaotic or dangerous. They also can be the location where communities provide children with food, medical care, and safe places for activities outside of the regular school day. At the same time, school can be a context of fear, exposing individuals to bullying and victimization, discrimination, poor-quality education, or mind-numbing boredom.

The lives of children in most societies are embedded in school, which is one of the major "microsystems" described by Bronfenbrenner in his ecological model of human development (Bronfenbrenner, 1979; Bronfenbrenner & Morris, 1998). Figure 9.1 illustrates a model of embedded systems, including school, inspired by Bronfenbrenner's theory. This figure spans levels from individual child to microsystems and macrosystems in which the child's life is embedded. In this illustration, the child is embedded in three microsystems: family, school, and peer group. In Bronfenbrenner's theory, children interact directly with other people in their microsystems. The child is part of a classroom that is embedded in a school, which is in turn embedded in other larger systems at the community, state, or national level. Macrosystems, such as national policies, influence the child indirectly through their influence on the state or school system. In contrast, the classroom teacher influences the child directly. The teacher also communicates with the parent of the child, forming one of the connections among the child's microsystems that comprise what Bronfenbrenner termed the "mesosystem." The child also belongs to several peer groups, which might be neighborhood friends or a group brought together in the community to perform or compete in sports. In Figure 9.1, the child has a friend in the peer group who does not go to his or her school.

The workplace of the child's parents also influence development, though usually indirectly, through effects on the parents' psychological function or the family budget. Thus, effects of workplace on the child are typically mediated by effects on the parents' behavior or the family system as a whole.

Schools and the interactions of schools with other systems have enormous influence on the course of children's lives. As a result, schools can play a major role in risk and resilience, exacerbating or mitigating risk in the lives of children, shaping resilience capacity, and restoring a sense of normalcy after disaster. In this chapter, I highlight briefly some of the risks experienced by children in the school context and the burgeoning literature on school competence and resilience, while focusing the most discussion on roles of schools in the resilience of individual children

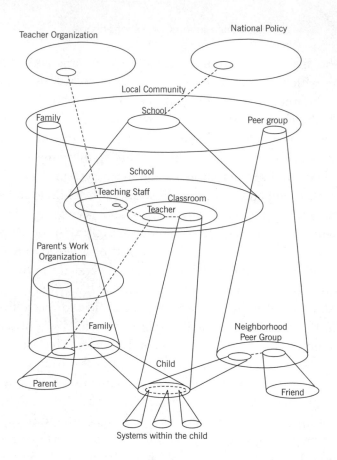

Teacher Organization

National Policy

Local Community

Family

School

Peer group

School

Teaching Staff

Classroom

Teacher

Parent's Work
Organization

Family

Neighborhood
Peer Group

Child

Parent

Friend

Systems within the child

FIGURE 9.1. Illustration of embedded systems based on Bronfenbrenner's (1979) ecological model that could directly or indirectly influence a child's life, highlighting connections to school. The child interacts directly in this example with people in three "microsystems": family, peer group, and school. The child is part of a classroom that is part of a school that is part of a community and also connected to larger "macrosystem" organizations and systems that influence the school, including a teacher's organization and national (or state) policymaking systems. The child is part of the family system that also is embedded in other systems, only one of which is illustrated, a parent's workplace. For the child, the parent workplace is an "exosystem" that indirectly affects the child through influences on parents and family well-being. The child's parent communicates with the teacher at school, linking these two microsystems, illustrating one of a network of links among systems in the child's life, comprising the child's "mesosystem." The child is also part of a peer group in the neighborhood that includes friends who may or may not attend the same school. Systems within the child (e.g., cardiovascular system, stress response system, immune system) are indicated only very generally. From Masten (2003, p. 170). Copyright 2013 by the National Association of School Psychologists. Bethesda, MD. Adapted with permission of the publisher. *www.nasponline.org.*

who attend those schools and interventions to promote resilience enacted in or by schools.

RISKS ARISING IN THE SCHOOL CONTEXT

Analogous to family life, a child's life at school can pose serious hazards for development. These dangers include bullying, sexual harassment, discrimination, and the corrosive effects of "educational neglect" in the form of poor teaching quality or low expectations.

Egregious cases of bullying by school peers have captivated public attention in recent years, often in the aftermath of a tragic suicide. Examples in the United States include 15-year-old Phoebe Prince, who killed herself in January 2010 after severe and prolonged bullying by peers in South Hadley, Massachusetts, and 14-year-old Kenneth Weishuhn, Jr., persecuted by classmates after he came out as gay in a small Iowa community. His death on April 14, 2012, coincided closely with the premier of the documentary *Bully* that was filmed with help from a nearby school district. On April 22, 2012, the *Sioux Falls Journal* published a full-page editorial on the newspaper's front page calling for action to stop bullying. The editorial received widespread coverage in the news and social media.

Extreme school violence, including rampage shootings perpetrated by students, such as the incidents in Columbine, Colorado, and Red Lake, Minnesota, are extremely rare. In contrast, bullying and sexual harassment are very common. Surveys often indicate that around 20 to 30% of students in middle and high school have experienced physical bullying on school grounds, with larger proportions experiencing verbal attacks (e.g., Centers for Disease Control and Prevention, 2012; Williams & Guerra, 2007). Bullying through the Internet and mobile phones (often among school peers) appears to be rising rapidly, though it is difficult to track electronic bullying with the speed of changing technologies and extraordinary expansion in the use of texting and social media among youth. Rates of sexual harassment at school also are very high (Hill & Kearl, 2011). Concerns about all these forms of aggression in the school context have given rise to numerous intervention and prevention programs to reduce the prevalence of these adversities in schools and to protect current or potential victims, discussed further below.

A different kind of danger to child development is posed by poorly managed schools, poor teaching, or school contexts that are poorly suited to the needs of their students. Over the years, the effectiveness of schools has come under growing scrutiny as societies, communities, and parents try to figure out "what works" for the education and well-being of their children, particularly in a world of globalized competition. "No Child Left Behind" and "Race to the Top" efforts in the United States reflect this concern, which has drawn increasing attention to the competence of schools and teachers, particularly for high-risk children.

EFFECTIVE SCHOOLS

School effectiveness is the equivalent of competence in an individual. As noted above, schools are charged by most societies and cultures with the task of educating and socializing their students, and they can be evaluated on how well they are doing their job. As in the case of competence for individual development, the criteria for judging school effectiveness would be expected to vary, by grade level and also by culture, community, nationality, and historical timing. In the United States and many other modern economies, the criteria for effective schools often include graduation rates, college placement rates, attendance, and performance on achievement tests standardized by state, nation, or international standards.

Schools also can be evaluated relative to other schools serving high-risk students by similar criteria. Much as resilient children can be diagnosed by criteria for competence despite exposure to high risk, schools can be evaluated with respect to school-level resilience in terms of producing higher rates of learning or greater success than schools of comparable risk, in challenging neighborhoods or serving large proportions of high-risk students (Anderson, 1994; Edmonds, 1979). Books on this theme include *No Excuses: Lessons from 21 High-Performing, High-Poverty Schools* (Carter, 2000) and *Good Schools in Poor Neighborhoods* (Clewell, Campbell, & Perlman, 2007).

Frequently identified qualities of effective schools and classrooms include positive school climate (a welcoming and supportive environment), strong leadership, and effective classroom teachers, as well as engaged students and parents (Bandura, 1997; Cohen, 2012; Doll, 2013; Doll, LeClair, & Kurien, 2009; Gettinger & Stoiber, 2009; National Research Council and Institute of Medicine, 2004; Rutter & Maughan, 2002). Effective teachers often combine good classroom management skills with warmth and high expectations, qualities that resemble characteristics of effective parents (Brophy, 2010; Masten, Herbers, Cutuli, & Lafavor, 2008). Effective schools simultaneously reduce disruptive and other antisocial behaviors that interfere with learning while they advocate the individual cognitive and social skills that promote learning and positive development (Doll et al., 2009; Masten et al., 2008).

At the core of most of these effective school qualities are positive relationships and expectations that communicate to children and their parents a caring and invested community for learning. Effective principals and teachers provide strong leadership, while they also form positive relationships with students, families, and colleagues. Effective schools and classrooms promote competence while they also build capacity for resilience in their students and teachers alike.

DEVELOPMENTAL TASKS IN THE SCHOOL CONTEXT

For school-age children in societies around the world, many of the central developmental tasks defining competence in childhood and adolescence refer to success in the school context, both academic and social. Children in modern societies are expected to attend school and to learn the reading, mathematics, writing, and social skills required for adult roles in their society. Implicit in these tasks are the fundamental behaviors required for learning itself and for fitting into group instructional settings, including expectations for self-regulation of attention, emotion, impulses, behavior, and the motivation to implement these self-control skills (Blair, 2002). School readiness can be assessed in regard to these multidimensional domains of function, including a range of knowledge about letters and numbers; EF skills such as paying attention, inhibitory control, and remembering rules or instructions; and the social skills of getting along with other children and listening to the teacher.

Once formal schooling begins, success becomes an extremely salient and multidimensional developmental task domain that holds considerable importance for multiple stakeholders in the society and family. As indicated throughout this volume, a large body of evidence attests to the importance of academic achievement and social adjustment at school for short- and long-term development (Masten, Burt, et al., 2006; Masten et al., 2008). Academic achievement and social behavior at school have been implicated as predictors many years later in adulthood of mental health, work success, civic engagement, and social competence in relationships with friends and one's own family. Moreover, early success or problems in school appear to have particularly important consequences, cascading across the years with a kind of snowball effect on later adaptation (see Chapter 3). Thus, the early school years play a foundational role for later school-based developmental tasks, which in turn are important for success in the developmental tasks of adulthood in many contexts.

For children whose development is jeopardized by poverty, family problems, and other adversities, school success is also likely to be jeopardized. Yet, school may also play a crucial role for pathways to resilience. When the family does not or cannot adequately protect development for children threatened by adversity, school is likely to serve as the most important context for promoting resilience. As a result, many studies of naturally occurring resilience have focused on the school context for assessing competence and studying protective processes. And, for similar reasons, efforts to promote resilience through intervention also have frequently focused on the school context.

HOW SCHOOLS PROMOTE RESILIENCE

In most contemporary societies, schools are assigned a unique role in the nurturing of human capital, teaching children academic skills, and the imparting of a body of knowledge about government, culture, and history viewed as important for socialization in a particular community or society. In their education role, schools play a vital part in the development of resilience capacity through the fostering of basic adaptive systems. As a key context of development outside the family, schools also can meet or supplement basic needs for nutrition and health care, provide opportunities for relationships with supportive adults and peers, serve as a secure emotional base, and generate opportunities for nurturing specific talents or work skills.

There is growing momentum for a more comprehensive approach to educational success for disadvantaged children, recognizing that support for learning and human capital development necessitates a broader view of education that begins early in human development and recognizes that the health and well-being of the whole person must be nurtured to foster learning and address achievement disparities. This momentum is exemplified by the campaign for a "broader, bolder approach to education," which was kicked off by print ads in *The Washington Post* and *The New York Times* in 2008, signed by a high-profile group originally convened by the Economic Policy Institute (see *http://boldapproach.org*).

Human Capital Development

The primary task assigned to schools is education, with a focus on individual children. In this role, schools nurture domains of human capital that play a central role in resilience. For children at risk due to poverty or other family-related adversities, cognitive skill development in the form of literacy and numeracy skills, critical thinking, problem-solving skills, and other aspects of academic achievement are extremely important. Virtually every study of resilience in low-income children implicates cognitive capabilities as promotive or protective (see Chapter 6). Early reading skills, for example, predict later learning in both math and reading, but they appear to be even more important as predictors for very poor children than they are for more advantaged children (Herbers et al., 2012). As noted previously, precursors to achievement disparities between more and less advantaged children arise early in development, calling for greater investment in early childhood. Nonetheless, effective schools can build capacity for resilience through facilitating the cognitive know-how and knowledge of all children, some of whom are facing adversity now and others who may face adversity later in life.

Social and emotional know-how also are fundamental aspects of human capital nurtured in school. Classroom adjustment requires self-regulation of emotions or impulses and social skills for getting along with others (peers and authority figures) that are important for success in many later developmental tasks in other contexts, including the workplace. Educational practitioners and scientists have increasingly recognized the importance of promoting social–emotional learning and intelligence in the school context, along with traditional cognitive skills and knowledge (Blair, 2002; Elias, Zins, Graczyk, & Weissberg, 2003; Galassi & Akos, 2007; Greenberg, 2006).

Nutrition and Health Care

Schools also can promote resilience through nutrition and health care programs for low-income students. One of the oldest national intervention efforts in the United States implemented in the school context is the National School Lunch Program and related efforts to provide free or low-cost food to children at school. With food insecurity a persistent risk factor for American children living in poverty (see Chapter 4), free and reduced-price meals and snacks are a very basic strategy for promoting and protecting human capital. This food program reached over 31 million children in 100,000 schools and child care institutions in 2012 (United States Department of Agriculture Food and Nutrition Service, 2013).

Since the 1980s, the number of school-based health centers has shown rapid growth, with support from federal and state governments and private foundations. One of the four priorities recommended in the "broader, bolder approach to education" statement (mentioned above) was increased health services, particularly with clinics located in schools. For disadvantaged families with poor access to health care and children at greater risk for numerous health problems, a school-based health clinic may provide crucial monitoring and services for children with health problems that could easily interfere with learning. For example, in our research with homeless families, we observed very high rates of asthma in the children, much higher than the prevalence for the state of Minnesota (Cutuli, Herbers, Rinaldi, Masten, & Oberg, 2010). Similarly high rates of asthma are typical among very disadvantaged children in the United States. Moreover, many of the children we have observed in shelters over the years with chronic health problems, such as asthma, appear to have poorly managed health maintenance related to a complex combination of factors, including stress, instabilities in daily life, inadequate health care access, and overwhelmed caregivers. Stable monitoring of health by school-based medical personnel for chronic health problems like asthma could make a big difference for these high-risk children, reducing absenteeism and emergency room visits, while enhancing lung function and cognition.

Relationships with Competent and Caring Adults

Studies and case reports of resilience in children and youth, described throughout this volume and many others, underscore the role of relationships with teachers, administrators, coaches, and other school personnel as protective influences. Outside the family, teachers are frequently cited as the source of support among resilient children (Doll et al., 2009; Theron & Engelbrecht, 2012). Schools provide extensive opportunities for children to form relationships with adults who can function as positive role models, mentors, purveyors of social capital, and otherwise as generally knowledgeable resources, particularly for young people who may not have adequate opportunities for relationships with competent, caring, and responsible adults at home. Even for children who have close attachment bonds with a parent at home, teachers may offer disadvantaged children important access to opportunities or high-quality guidance and support for pursuing higher education or developing talents that low-income or poorly educated parents may not be able to provide despite wanting the best for their children.

Positive relationships with teachers appear to have a particularly important role for high-risk children in the early school years, when teachers often get to know students well (Pianta, 2006). Research suggests that children who experience more conflict or disadvantages in the home environment benefit the most from supportive relationships with teachers (Doll et al., 2009; Pianta, 2006).

What are the processes by which positive teacher–student relationships promote resilience? There are many possibilities, just as there are for effective parent–child relationships. Teachers can be role models and provide the emotional security that comes with attachment bonds. They can keep an eye out and open doors for opportunities, report suspected abuse or bullying, or arrange for extra resources of many kinds. Through their teaching skills, expectations, and encouragement, teachers also can influence the motivation to achieve as well as contribute to the self-confidence and self-efficacy of their students.

Theron and colleagues (see Theron & Engelbrecht, 2012) conducted a qualitative study of resilience-promoting transactions between teachers and young people at risk in South Africa, focused on students ages 14–20. These young people were invited to write a narrative about the ways one or more teachers helped them do well during a difficult time in their lives. These disadvantaged students described the following ways: a parent role that included providing basic needs as well as caring; a mentoring role, providing guidance and knowledge; refuge ("healing spaces"); advocacy on behalf of the youth; and belief in the young person ("I know someone believes in me").

Bonnie Bernard, who has written extensively on resilience for practitioners, coined the term *turnaround teachers* to describe the powerful role that teachers can play in the resilience of young people (Bernard, 2003). The turnaround teacher promotes resilience by providing a student *caring and support, high expectations,* and *opportunities for participation and contribution.* Both Bernard (2003) and Henderson (2012) have described a number of ways that turnaround teachers communicate and facilitate caring, expectations, and opportunities. Their lists are consistent with findings from research on effective teachers and schools, as well as research on resilient youth, such as the qualitative study above.

Motivation and Self-Efficacy

One of the most powerful engines for adaptation in human development is the motivation associated with agency and pleasure in the effort to master the environment (see Chapter 6). Teachers and other adults in schools play a major role in providing opportunities for children to experience success at school in some of the most important developmental tasks of childhood, and concomitantly in stimulating and reinforcing the efforts of children to learn and engage with challenges. As a result, they influence the self-efficacy as well as the achievement motivation of their students.

One of the arts of teaching lies in individualizing the experiences of each child so that there is an effective balance of challenge and support that builds skills along with agency. Too much scaffolding can undermine confidence, whereas too little can engender defeat or demoralization. Low expectations can be a subtle but pernicious form of discrimination and powerful drag on the development of agency and self-efficacy. On the other hand, excessive expectations, including performance demands far beyond the developmental capabilities of a child, can have a similarly devastating impact on perceived agency and intrinsic motivation. Similarly, extrinsic rewards and effusive praise can have negative consequences on motivation or self-confidence. Striking a "just right" balance in teaching for individual learning and fostering self-efficacy is not an easy task for teachers, and the target zone for each child is continually changing as a result of both development and learning.

Numerous books and guidelines for educators on motivating students have been published over the years (Brophy, 2010; National Research Council and Institute of Medicine, 2004; Stroud & Reynolds, 2009). Theories and strategies vary, with recommendations for teachers focusing on the quality of the teacher–student relationship, as well as strategies for building motivation to learn at both the level of the whole classroom and the individual student. Though recommended strategies vary, they often involve role modeling, scaffolding, individualized goal setting, intrinsic rewards, and guided mastery experiences. Bandura (1997) emphasized the role of teachers' perceived efficacy in creating learning environments that motivate students to learn. Teachers with high perceived efficacy create more mastery opportunity experiences for their students. Moreover, effective schools are more likely to attract and nurture teachers with high self-efficacy.

Extracurricular Activities

Schools also can provide access to a wide variety of opportunities to develop skills, leadership, and experience mastery in activities outside the traditional curriculum. These include sports, music, art, clubs (e.g., chess, dance, community service), student government, and similar "extracurricular activities." Each of these contexts affords possibilities for diverse students to connect with potential mentors, develop an area of expertise or talent, and experience leadership. These activities are sometimes viewed as frills in the school context, especially when money is tight. However, these opportunities may play a vital role in retaining students at risk for dropping out of school and also for promoting motivation and competence in young people at risk.

Longitudinal studies of school-based extracurricular activities show generally positive links to school engagement, educational attainment, and later achievement in other competence domains, such as work or civic engagement (Eccles, Barber, Stone, & Hunt, 2003; Mahoney, Larson, & Eccles, 2005; Obradović & Masten, 2007). These activities could foster affiliation with prosocial peers, attachments to competent adults, skill acquisition, and mastery motivation, all of which could enhance resilience capacity for young people experiencing adversity. However, it is also possible that the positive links between extracurricular activities and later achievement in developmental tasks are mediated by the competence of those who self-select into these activities. Moreover, extracurricular activities may not always promote positive outcomes, because the values and behaviors of adults involved in these groups, peers participating in them, nature of the activities, and culture of the groups vary. Intervention experiments with randomized trials provide a revealing strategy for testing the causal nature of the links between extracurricular activities and positive development or resilience.

SCHOOL-BASED INTERVENTIONS TO PROMOTE RESILIENCE

Children spend so much time in schools and they have such multifaceted roles and services that many of the interventions designed to promote resilience in children at risk for various reasons have been implemented in the context of schools. These include efforts to improve school effectiveness; efforts to boost academic achievement through curriculum changes, teacher training, or tutoring; mentoring programs; programs to prevent school dropout and other forms of disengagement; and programs to reduce problem behaviors that disrupt learning or school climate. Schools also have developed systematic programs to prepare for disasters and respond to bullying and school violence. Examples highlighted here are highly congruent with a resilience framework (see Chapter 11) or clearly target a fundamental adaptive system to promote success among children at risk for school problems related to adversity.

Strength-Based School Counseling

The movement toward a strength-based model of school counseling illustrates in a school context the profound shift toward competence promoting and away from deficit-based models of intervention that has been spurred by resilience research. Galassi and Akos (2007) described this transformation in a book on strength-based school counseling (SBSC), which was followed by a special issue they edited of the American School Counselor Association's flagship journal *Professional School Counseling* (Akos & Galassi, 2008). Galassi and Akos (2007) delineated six major principles of SBSC, emphasizing the promotion of strengths in students and school environments, along with evidence-based practices. These principles and the recommended methods for applying a SBSC model were highly congruent with the broad framework emerging from resilience science as applied in a school context (Masten et al., 2008; see Chapter 11). The SBSC approach emphasizes positive goals, models, measures, and methods, with practitioners targeting positive change in the school climate as well as individual students. Mentoring and promoting self-efficacy are important, as are fostering a caring school community. The transformation in the profession of school counseling has been accompanied by a shift in professional identity about the nature of school counseling as a profession. There is an increased emphasis for school counselors on facilitating positive development in students and schools, rather than fixing deficiencies and problems.

After-School Programs

Among the most popular approaches for promoting resilience in high-risk students in the school context but outside of regular school hours are after-school and summer programs (Durlak, Weissberg, & Pachan, 2010; Mahoney et al., 2005; National Research Council and Institute of Medicine, 2002). From their early days, many of these programs were designed to prevent substance abuse, conduct problems, or school dropout, or to provide remedial education. In recent years, many of these programs have been designed to promote cognitive and social competence, school engagement, and social skills, as a means to closing achievement gaps, preventing school dropout, or in other ways ameliorating risk for youth. Many of the characteristics associated with successful programs reflect the broad adaptive systems highlighted throughout this book, such as relationships with competent adults and prosocial peers and opportunities for mastery experiences, as well as specific skill-building activities. These programs are often implicitly or explicitly designed to initiate a positive ripple or snowball effect that will spread to achievement and greater success in the regular school day.

There is now enough research that it is feasible to conduct meta-analyses of the findings on the success of such programs. A meta-analysis by Lauer et al. (2006) that was focused on high-risk students included both after-school and summer programs. Results indicated a positive overall effect of these programs on achievement. More recently, Durlak et al. (2010) completed an analysis of 75 after-school programs designed to boost personal and social skills (though some also focused on issues such as obesity). Compared with control groups, these programs had an overall favorable and significant effect on student behavior, both with respect to increasing positive behaviors and reducing negative behaviors. Programs with the following "SAFE" features (often recommended for skill-focused programs) were particularly effective: *sequential* (step-by-step, coordinated skills-building), *active* (hands-on, with students actively engaged), *focused* (in terms of time and attention; dose), and *explicit* (those with specific learning objectives).

Prevention Programs

Many of the interventions implemented in schools are focused on risk reduction for health and behavior problems of great concern to societies, such as antisocial behavior, bullying, smoking or drinking, sexual behavior, or suicide. Some are universal, targeting the whole population, whereas others are targeted to higher-risk groups. Some are evidence based and many are not (Durlak, 2009). Some have an explicit focus on promoting competence in high-risk students as a strategy for reducing later problem behavior, or on facilitating protective factors to mitigate the effects of adversity.

Extensive evidence has accrued on the effects of prevention programs, with good evidence supporting the value of many programs, including reports on RCTs and meta-analyses of higher-quality studies (Durlak, 2009). The evidence suggests general conclusions about the nature of programs that work, summarized by various authors over the years (Bond & Hauf, 2004; Durlak, 2009; Nation et al., 2003). These conclusions bear a striking resemblance to the qualities of effectiveness in parenting and teaching that promote positive child development, including the following: well timed and developmentally appropriate; fostering connections to adults and prosocial peers; and fitting the needs, preferences, and values of the target population (see Durlak, 2009, Table 42.3, p. 911). Many successful programs also promote competence or skills valued by multiple stakeholders, including the child (Durlak, 2009; Masten, Burt, et al., 2006). And there is clearly value in targeting change at the level of microsystems (family, classroom, school) as well as the individual. Some of the most successful programs target multiple levels for change.

The Life Skills Training (LST) program (Botvin & Griffin, 2004; Botvin & Tortu, 1988), designed to prevent substance abuse in adolescents, is typically implemented universally with young adolescents in a school context. LST is widely regarded as one of the best preventive interventions available, with strong evidence of effectiveness in reducing substance use and enhancing positive behaviors. This prevention program is built around competence enhancement, with a focus on building skills in self-management, general social competence, and specific skills and attitudes for resisting drug use (Botvin & Griffin, 2004). It is typically implemented by teachers in grade 7 with a standardized curriculum over 1 year of school with booster sessions in the following 2 years. Evidence has also accrued on the mediating role of competence skills and their effects on perceived well-being and attitudes as important in the process by which the program has its effects on drug use.

The Seattle Social Development Project (also known as the Skills, Opportunities, and Recognition program), developed by Hawkins and Catalano with their colleagues (Hawkins, Kosterman, Catalano, Hill, & Abbott, 2005) also is built on a model of prevention with a focus on promoting positive changes in a key mediating pathway, which in this case is positive bonding to school (and family). The full program, implemented throughout elementary school, includes classroom and family components. Teachers are trained in mastery teaching strategies, learn how to improve classroom management, and teach social skills in the classroom. Parents are trained in effective parenting techniques, such as monitoring and consistent discipline. Long-term results provide good evidence of substantial effects of this program on developmental task achievements, as well as reductions in antisocial behavior and other negative outcomes.

Check and Connect is another school-based intervention with strong evidence of effectiveness based on experimental data that builds on a resilience framework (Anderson, Christenson, Sinclair, & Lehr, 2004). Check and Connect was developed by Christenson and colleagues (2008) to reduce school dropout by promoting school engagement during the elementary and middle school years. This program emphasizes positive relationships, assigning a "monitor" to support the student through interactions with student, family, and school. This monitor is a paid professional whose job is to stay in touch and foster school engagement. The monitor "checks" and "connects," but also provides a persistent relationship for the student. The quality and closeness of the relationship of monitor to student as perceived by both also relates to engagement.

Each of these three school-based prevention programs focused in a major way on building positive processes believed to mediate and promote success while reducing risk for key problems (drug use, antisocial behavior, dropout). They all adopted a competence- or resilience-framed model to accompany a theory of risk and protective processes. Each was well informed by an understanding of the developmental pathways involved in the problems of concern and all were very well timed and developmentally appropriate.

In many cases, however, there is considerable evidence that the best timing for prevention is well before formal compulsory schooling begins. Moreover, as noted elsewhere in this volume, there is good evidence for high return on investment in very early educational child care and preschool settings.

Preschool Prevention Programs

Thus, it is not surprising to find growing evidence supporting the effectiveness of preschool-based interventions. Programs like Head Start can be viewed as resilience-promoting efforts by communities and societies that support such prevention programs to enhance later success in school. Though Head Start is a very broad program, with diverse ingredients and qualities that are inherently difficult to evaluate, there have been efforts to improve the quality of Head Start in specific ways that can be tested with great effectiveness.

Head Start REDI provides one example (Bierman, Domitrovich, et al., 2008; Bierman, Nix, Greenberg, Blair, & Domitrovich, 2008), with REDI standing for "research based and developmentally informed." This program has a strong focus on positive skills development, both in the curriculum and teacher training implemented in the "treatment" classrooms and in the materials sent home for parents. The program aimed to promote social–emotional competence, literacy, and language development, and succeeded in changing some of the targeted domains of competence compared with "preschool-as-usual" control classrooms.

The Chicago School Readiness Project was also implemented in preschool Head Start classrooms but this program was more specifically designed to target self-regulation skills in children as a strategy for improving school readiness (Raver et al., 2011). Teachers were trained in classroom management and stress-reduction strategies. This intervention is a highly promising example of recent interventions focused on self-regulation skills during a developmental window of opportunity, the preschool years when there is rapid development of EF and brain function supporting cognitive self-control (Diamond & Lee, 2011; Zelazo & Carlson, 2012).

Promoting Resilience in Teachers

Some of the interventions mentioned above recognize explicitly that teachers need support in very high-stress schools or classrooms (e.g., Raver et al., 2011). Burnout is a major concern in stressful classrooms from preschool through high school, leading many teachers to leave or interfering with effective teaching and a positive climate in schools (Fleming, Mackrain, & LeBuffe, 2013). Moreover, it is reasonable to assume that stress can interfere with self-regulation in teachers, which in turn interferes with teachers modeling or fostering self-regulation in their students, and their availability to participate emotionally in the quality of relationships that many children need. Concomitantly, it is conceivable that interventions engaging and supporting teachers may work in part because they lower stress, and improve well-being and self-regulation in the teachers, whether these are explicit goals or not. More attention to stress reduction and resilience promotion for teachers and other staff in schools may be an important strategy for promoting resilience in individual students as well as the school context as a whole.

Disaster and Emergency Planning

Schools are frequently called upon to respond to disasters, terrorism, and other crisis events. In the disaster literature (see Chapter 5), teachers and other school personnel have come to be viewed as first responders. Consequently, schools in many communities and societies have developed (by mandate or voluntarily) a crisis plan and response system. These systems include plans for specific emergencies (fire, terror, natural disaster, etc.) and an organizational system for emergency response, often with a command and communication structure (Sandoval & Brock, 2009). In the aftermath of Columbine and other mass-casualty events unfolding during the school day, as well as natural disasters like Katrina, schools have been called on to prepare for emergencies. They have evacuation and lockdown drills, and send emergency notifications to parents. The December 2012 tragedy at Sandy Hook Elementary School in Newtown, Connecticut, motivated many communities and schools to reevaluate and enhance their emergency preparedness.

Schools also play a vital role in recovery from disasters of many kinds, because school appears to be a powerful symbol of recovery and resilience to children, parents, and the community at large. The importance of restoring school operations in the aftermath of disasters or mass-trauma events is widely recognized by governments, nongovernmental organizations (NGOs), and local communities through their actions, as well as by reviewers of the literature (American Psychological Association, 2010; Masten & Narayan, 2012; Masten & Osofsy, 2010).

SUMMARY

Schools, like families, play vitally important roles in child development and resilience. Families and schools are charged with many aspects of nurturing human development, which includes building capacities for success in society. Schools are instrumental in fostering many of the adaptive systems that have been implicated for resilience capacity, including cognitive skills, self-regulation skills, mastery motivation, and relationships with competent, prosocial adults and peers. Schools can compensate to some degree for deprivation in the home context by providing extra nutrition, adult guidance, attachment relationships, monitoring, and access to health care.

Schools are expected to educate and socialize children for a successful life in the community or society and their competence in these tasks can be evaluated. School effectiveness is often measured by child achievement and knowledge, as well as the rates of graduation and conduct of their students. There is particular interest in what might be called resilient schools, meaning schools that succeed in very difficult situations, such as schools with high-achieving children in high-risk neighborhoods where many schools fail, or schools that recover well from disasters. Effective and resilient schools share many of the qualities identified in healthy or resilient families, such as warmth, structure, routines, strong leadership, and high expectations.

Schools can play a central role in disaster preparedness and response. First, because children spend so much time in the school context, school personnel need to be viewed as first responders. Second, for the same reasons, schools need emergency procedures and routines for responses that are well rehearsed. Third, schools are a powerful symbol of normal life to children and adults in communities. Establishing or reestablishing school routines and functions is widely recognized as both a symbol and strategy of recovery.

Schools are a major context for interventions to promote resilience. It is an accessible and familiar context for children and parents where extra resources can be provided and programs can be located. The goals of schools overlap to a large degree with the goals of programs aiming to promote resilience, because education is centered on building competence and adaptive skills that are fundamental to resilience capacity as well as success in developmental tasks.

Finally, schools are a context where many of the most influential systems and people for human development intersect or interact, including the family, education, and peer systems, but also the values and cultures of a society. Schools are highly complex organizations that shape and are shaped by their constituent students, their families, the community, and society. Schools and their staff interact in many ways with individual children and families, as well as larger societal systems. As a result, schools have the potential to play a variety of roles in the development of capacity for resilience in individual students and the larger society.

CHAPTER 10

RESILIENCE IN THE CONTEXT OF CULTURE

Children develop in the context of culture, often multiple cultures, as well as families and communities. Although culture can refer to nearly anything that is transmitted across generations through nongenetic means, I focus here on the more organized aspects of culture reflected in religion, ethnic or national heritage, and enduring community values and practices. The lives of children are deeply embedded in cultural contexts and their development is influenced by the traditions, values, rituals, practices, and beliefs shared by groups of people across families. Cultures influence concepts of "doing well in life" and concomitantly the expectations for individual behavior across the lifespan. Cultures also provide guidance about how to rear a good child and rituals for dealing with many of the adversities of life.

Culture always has been implicitly part of defining resilience, since the criteria for good adaptation always have a cultural as well as a historical context. However, explicit attention to culturally-based promotive and protective influences was neglected in early work on resilience (Luthar 2006; Masten & Wright, 2010; Spencer et al., 2006). That neglect is now changing (Masten, 2014). There are books on the social ecologies of resilience, emphasizing culture as well as family, increasing cross-cultural or multicultural studies, and greater attention to religious and other cultural practices in research on resilience (see Ungar, 2012; Ungar et al.,

2013). Studies of migrant populations also have drawn increasing attention to acculturation processes in relation to resilience in youth (Masten, Liebkind, & Hernandez, 2012b). In 2012, the World Bank published a review of the global evidence on risk and protective factors for children in the context of economic shocks (Lundberg & Wuermli, 2012).

Earlier in this volume, I assert that the major adaptive systems that yield most of the capacity for human resilience evolved over many generations, through a combination of biological and cultural evolution. Cultural ideas and traditions that promote resilience would be expected to endure and become instantiated in systems of belief and traditions transmitted over generations. In this chapter, I highlight briefly how cultural systems, including religion, have shaped the definition of resilience, and contributed to the capacity of individuals, families, and larger social groups to adapt in the face of adversity. While studies of resilience across cultures reveal interesting differences in the concepts and ways of promoting resilience, there also are remarkable consistencies that, once again, underscore the fundamental nature of human adaptive systems. Religious practices, for example, often engage the same adaptive systems discussed throughout this volume as promotive and protective for human development.

RESILIENCE ACROSS CULTURES

There are a variety of ways to study cultural similarities and differences in resilience. One approach begins with individual studies that focus on resilience in a specific cultural context, studying promotive or protective factors in that context. A wide variety of such studies can then be reviewed to observe commonalities and differences. This approach is typical of the available research on children in war and disaster (see Chapter 5), where it would be extraordinarily difficult to set up a single cross-cultural study. Nonetheless, evidence drawn from diverse studies across cultures and communities of resilience in war or disaster consistently points to the importance of attachment figures, problem-solving skills, and hope or faith, among other commonly identified protective factors. Studies of war and disaster also underscore culturally-based differences in risk and resilience, such as the stigma attached to rape of child soldiers for girls compared with boys in Sierra Leone (Betancourt et al., 2010). However, generally speaking, the differences across these investigations, in methods and situations, as well as cultural context, tend to highlight general similarities across context, rather than differences.

In their volume reviewing a host of global programs to reduce risk and promote resilience in children enduring the current economic crisis, the World Bank was able to draw on many examples from research they have funded on interventions around the world (see Lundberg & Wuermli, 2012). They emphasize the role of context and culture in the successful design of these programs and their effectiveness. Examples from their work include an array of interventions implemented in diverse contexts around the world, ranging from macroeconomic policies to interventions focused directly on schools or families. Interventions in response to economic crisis might include expanding national safety nets, preserving health care systems, increasing cash transfers, broadening public works programs, scholarships or conditional cash programs to support education, boosting food distribution to students in schools or mental health resources for parents, increasing support to after-school and mentoring programs for youth, community-based parenting interventions, and targeted jobs or unemployment programs for young people as well as adults.

Another approach to the study of resilience in multiple cultures is to set up a large-scale, cross-cultural study through a collaboration of investigators who develop methods together and try to identify similarities and differences using the same methods in multiple contexts. This is a challenging undertaking for different reasons, because measurement equivalence is not easy to establish and there are truly formidable challenges inherent in building the relationships and funding to implement such a study.

The International Resilience Project and subsequent Pathways to Resilience Project offer examples of such efforts by an international team of investigators led by Michael Ungar and colleagues

(Ungar, 2008; Ungar & Liebenberg, 2005; Ungar et al., 2013; see also the website for the Resilience Research Centre at *http://resilienceresearch.org/*). Their goal was to understand globally general and contextually specific features of resilience and related adaptive processes across cultures. A multinational team developed a new measure of youth resilience and initiated a study of about 1,500 youth across 5 continents, in 14 communities, using mixed methods. Their methods included qualitative interview methods along with quantitative assessments using their new measure of resilience. The Child and Youth Resilience Measure was administered to young people across all the settings. It is a 73-item self-report measure that includes 15 site-specific items and 58 common items (e.g., "Are religious or spiritual beliefs a source of strength for you?"). The 58 items assessed 32 domains of interest (see Ungar, 2008, p. 227), including culture (e.g., affiliated with a religious organization, being culturally grounded—part of a cultural tradition that is expressed through daily activities), community (e.g., safety and security needs are met, access to school and education), relationships (e.g., quality of parenting meets the child's needs, having a positive mentor and role models), and individual (e.g., problem-solving ability, self-efficacy, sense of humor). The fact that it was feasible to assess common domains across diverse contexts suggests some fundamental commonalities in protective factors across diverse contexts. At the same time, their qualitative interview data revealed cultural specificity and differences. Their findings also emphasized the difficulty of differentiating cultural perspectives from protective roles. An adolescent might endorse the importance of religion in his or her life either because religion is strongly valued in that adolescent's culture or because spiritual practices were important in overcoming a particular adversity in that individual's life, or both.

One of the goals of this work was to glean a qualitative understanding of resilience within distinct cultural contexts. Theron, Theron, and Malindi (2013), as part of the Resilience Pathways Project, contributed qualitative descriptions of resilience in Basotho youth in South Africa. Like many traditional African cultures, the Basotho value what they call *Botho*, which is similar to the philosophy of *Ubunto* in other African cultures. In *Ubunto* philosophy, raising children is a collective responsibility, religion is valued, and reverence is given to human interdependence. Cooperation, harmony, spirituality, and humanitarian practices are highly valued.

Youth identified by adults in the Basotho community as resilient were described as flexible and determined, with good communication skills and positive social support systems. Their supports were not described in terms of individual relationships but rather (in keeping with the *Ubunto* philosophy) in connectedness to a strong community support system. These youth were also described as having vision and goals for the future, and an investment in education. They also showed equanimity, an acceptance of things they could not control, and respect for community values.

Detailed and rich descriptions of resilience conducted within a specific cultural context have the potential to highlight both similarities and differences across cultures in conceptualizations of resilience and protective influences. In the Basotho data, qualities such as good communication skills, future orientation, and flexibility represent examples of widely reported characteristics of resilient youth, whereas stoic acceptance and the collective nature of social support reported in these data are less common.

Another important study of adaptation across cultures that focused on immigrant 13- to 18-year-olds in 13 countries was the International Comparative Study of Ethnocultural Youth (ICSEY). ICSEY examined both developmental tasks and acculturation tasks in over 5,000 youth, along with psychological well-being (Berry, Phinney, Sam, & Vedder, 2006). Although not explicitly about resilience, this seminal study of adjustment across cultures suggested that immigrant youth were usually as well adjusted as native youth, and sometimes better adjusted. Additionally, they found that youth who were biculturally competent in the ways expected by the host culture, as well as in the family culture, were generally more successful in terms of overall developmental task achievement, though they did not differ in well-being.

The discussion that follows draws primarily on conclusions from a diverse world literature rather than international studies of resilience that include multiple cultures and communities. There simply are too few of the latter studies available at this time. Nonetheless, there are impressive commonalities evident in international research, as long as one keeps in mind that the study of cultural differences in resilience remains in its early stages.

RISKS OF CULTURE, RELIGION, AND SPIRITUALITY

Culture, similarly to family and school contexts, can serve as a source of risk and adversity as well as protection and resilience. Ethnic or racial minority youth may face discrimination and threats from negative stereotypes. Discrimination is so widespread in the United States that racial or ethnic socialization is studied as a protective process in minority families (see below). Clashes of cultural values can impose tremendous stress and pressure on young people navigating multicultural worlds. "Acculturation stress" can arise from the perceived difficulties of dealing with cultural differences (Serafica & Vargas, 2006). A Muslim child who moves into a neighborhood or school with no other Muslim families may encounter discrimination and pressure to conform to values that go against his or her traditional family or religious values (Sirin & Gupta, 2012). In a predominantly Muslim country, a Christian child may face similar adversity. Cultural clashes also play a huge role in war and ethnic conflicts that impose overwhelming trauma on children. Horrifying atrocities have been committed in the name of religion for centuries.

Deeply held religious beliefs that provide hope and meaning in life can be shattered by betrayal or disaster. Children have been subjected to devastating physical and sexual abuse under cover of religious practices. In the child abuse literature, betrayal by trusted adults, whether a parent in the home or a priest sexually molesting a child in the church, can have worse repercussions than abuse by a total stranger, in part because of the violation of trust (Crawford et al., 2006). Similarly, natural disasters can also shake an individual's faith in a loving and caring spiritual figure and, concomitantly, the individual's beliefs that life has meaning.

Needs for belonging, attachment, structure, and meaning can also be exploited by gang leaders. Children who feel unsafe, persecuted, and neglected by family or the larger culture may seek refuge or comfort in a countercultural group or antisocial gang; gang involvement may then increase the risk for violent or risky behaviors, dropping out of school, and other dangerous outcomes (Howell, 2010, 2011; Ogbu, 1981; Whitbeck, Hoyt, Chen, & Stubben, 2002).

DEVELOPMENTAL TASKS IN THE CONTEXT OF CULTURE

Expectations about what it means to do well in life, the criteria for evaluating positive adaptation or competence in any given period of development, are deeply influenced by culture. All parents everywhere share some common expectations for development, as do cultures and societies. These universal developmental tasks reflect the human-typical aspects of development, such as learning to walk and talk, forming attachment bonds with caregivers, and following the rules of the social group. However, the expected language or rules to be learned will differ by cultural context. Anthropologist Frank Boas expressed this idea in his 1928 foreword to Margaret Mead's classic volume *Coming of Age in Samoa* in the following way: "Courtesy, modesty, good manners, conformity to definite ethical standards are universal, but what constitutes courtesy, modesty, good manners, and ethical standards is not universal" (in Mead, 2001, p. xxii).

To put it more simply, parents everywhere appear to have no trouble identifying "bad" or "good" children. Such evaluations are universal, though the specific criteria would be expected to vary, and these evaluations may themselves have adaptive origins (Durbrow, 1999). Survival of children depends to some degree on acceptance, support, and investment of the community. Thus, it can be essential for children to conform to community expectations and definitions of good behavior.

Some of the expected developmental accomplishments in a culture strongly reflect local norms and beliefs, as well as the historical and ecological context. In groups where livelihood depends on hunting or weaving, a young boy or girl may be judged by achieving skills in hunting or weaving. In many economically advanced societies, school achievement over many years becomes a highly salient developmental task and dropping out of school is viewed as a serious failure. In ethnic communities organized by a strong adherence to religious practices, there often will be religious tasks to accomplish, and perhaps rites of passage to adult status related to religious ceremonies.

In Chapter 3, I discussed the strategy we developed in Project Competence to ascertain developmental task expectations in different cultures or contexts, working with an anthropologist. Cultural informants are invited to complete a "criteria of competence" interview, asked to think of a person who is doing okay (or doing well, whatever is more culturally suitable), and then to indicate how they can tell the person is doing okay. The statements about how the person is doing are then sorted by independent informants into piles of answers that "go together" to generate data for a co-occurrence matrix that can be factor analyzed. The dimensions by which people are evaluated as competent emerges from this analysis. In one study utilizing this strategy, criteria based on interviews in three different contexts of poverty were compared by Durbrow and colleagues (2001): a Caribbean village, a Filipino village, and a homeless shelter in a midwestern American city. In all the groups, the most common characteristic mentioned for a child doing satisfactorily well was good conduct, though undoubtedly what constitutes "good conduct" varied across these very different contexts. Mothers in each culture also mentioned academic competence, family support (helpfulness), and getting along with peers. Differences also emerged; church attendance, for example, was important for adolescent girls (less so for boys) in the Caribbean village.

In pluralistic societies like the United States, criteria for competence and developmental task expectations can differ within the same community for subgroups of individuals. Even for the same individuals, children who develop in multicultural contexts or move between distinct cultural worlds, from home to school or home to neighborhood, can face conflicting task demands. In the context of diminished opportunities and racism, Ogbu (1981) and others have argued that the criteria for black, inner-city youth were different than the expectations in the mainstream or middle-class-dominated school context. Blocked from achieving in the mainstream, Ogbu suggested that these young people adopt a countercultural alternative set of expectations and goals, sometimes defined by street culture or gang leaders. Burton, Obeidallah, and Allison (1996) described a similar idea in their concept of the "revised American Dream" based on their ethnographic work. Disadvantaged African American youth, faced with limited options for success in mainstream culture, looked for alternatives and new possibilities to define success on their own terms. Teens might focus on having a baby or dressing well, rather than finishing school and going to college.

For young people who live in contexts where they will face racial or ethnic discrimination, racial or ethnic socialization may be an important protective strategy of parents (Hughes et al., 2006; Serafica & Vargas, 2006). Racial–ethnic socialization is a broad concept that encompasses a variety of messages, methods, and goals by which parents prepare children for life as a racial- or ethnic-minority member in society. Parents may teach their children pride in their heritage and also cultural traditions, while at the same time they may prepare them to deal with prejudice, bias, or barriers to opportunity. Trained youth who encounter such challenges could be better prepared, for example, when they encounter bias, because they are more likely to make attributions about their experiences to external causes (discrimination) rather than personal causes. Evidence is mixed, but a number of studies suggest that such training has protective effects on identity, competence, and well-being in minority youth (Evans et al., 2012; Hughes et al., 2006; Motti-Stefanidi et al., 2012; Serafica & Vargas, 2006).

Young immigrants may face a different kind of cultural conflict, where the expectations of their parents and culture of origins with respect to desirable behavior and accomplishments may diverge sharply from what is expected in the receiving culture of school, community, or peer groups. Navigating these cultural differences can be viewed as another developmental task for immigrant children growing up in multiple cultures (Motti-Stefanidi et al., 2012). Successful immigrant youth often appear to find a way to navigate comfortably across their cultural contexts, preserving ties to both cultures (Cooper, 1999). For Muslim American youth, Sirin has described successful young people who reside happily "on the hyphen" (Sirin & Gupta, 2012).

THE IMMIGRANT PARADOX

One of the more intriguing themes in the resilience of immigrant youth is the concept of the immigrant paradox, which refers to the observation that first-generation immigrant youth may be more successful or healthier than later-born generations (Garcia Coll et al., 2012; Garcia Coll & Marks, 2012). It has sometimes been observed that the first-generation immigrants have better achievement, health, and psychological well-being than subsequent generations, even though they may face greater adversity or acculturation challenges. Data continue to be mixed in regard to the immigrant paradox, with stronger evidence for physical health and good conduct than mental health and well-being. Yet there are clearly instances where first-generation immigrants show better adaptation. In the United States, first-generation immigrant children are generally healthier, and in the United States, Europe, and Canada research suggests that recent immigrants show fewer externalizing behavior problems than later generations of adolescents (Garcia Coll et al., 2012). Thus, there is great interest in explaining why. What is the immigrant advantage and how is it lost over time?

One kind of explanation focuses on the exceptionalism of the first generation, self-selected in effect for success and resilience. Migrating individuals often overcome great adversities to make it to a new country, and thus may represent an unusually resourceful, intelligent, energetic, or healthier group of people than a random sample of the population from the country of origin. Buriel (2012) has described the self-selection of Mexican immigrants who migrate to the United States in such terms, resulting in selection for qualities conducive to success in the United States, such as high-achievement motivation, a strong work ethic, a propensity for delay of gratification, and optimism. Buriel argues that over generations, these qualities can erode, unless strong ties are maintained to the traditional culture through bicultural practices including, in particular, the retention of Spanish language fluency.

Another explanation for the immigrant advantage emphasizes cultural influences, suggesting that the first generation holds more strongly to cultural practices in diet, child rearing, and values that promote health or achievement. Over generations, with greater adoption in the United States of an unhealthy American diet and lifestyle, these advantages could be lost. Garcia Coll and her colleagues (2012) also have argued that cultural protective factors may be lost over time as immigrant youth adopt the ways of the receiving culture. Since fluent bilingualism has been associated with better adjustment among immigrant youth, they suggest that these skills may sustain access to a broader network of cultural resources among family and cultural community members.

These observations are consistent with a broader literature suggesting that biculturalism and fluent bilingualism hold advantages for immigrant youth (Han, 2012; Motti-Stefanidi et al., 2012). There may be multiple ways that bicultural and bilingual practices foster resilience. Young people may have the advantages of relationships with extended social networks that translate to greater social (and cultural) capital. They may hold on to the qualities that promoted success in the first generation. Or, they may benefit directly from the cognitive effects of bilingual learning, which is associated with better EF skills (Bialystok & Craik, 2010).

CULTURE AND DEVELOPMENT

Many concepts of culture have been influential in psychology with respect to their role in human development. Harkness and Super (2012) have discussed these concepts in a recent chapter on the cultural organization of children's environments. One of these influential ideas is the differentiation of individualistic and collectivistic cultures, often contrasting Western societies as more oriented to the individual, valuing independence, with societies in other parts of the world, such as Africa and Latin America, viewed as more collectivist in orientation, valuing interdependence and relatedness. Cultural orientation in this regard would be expected to influence parents' ideas about desired achievements and qualities in children and their parenting behavior toward reaching those goals.

For many immigrants who often are migrating from traditionally collectivistic to relatively individualistic cultures, achieving a balanced solution to the values placed on autonomy (in the receiving culture) and interdependence (in the culture of origin) may be crucial. Kağitçibaşi (2012) has argued that autonomy and connectedness are orthogonal values that can be resolved in the "autonomous-related self," where autonomy of action and achievement along with interdependence in closeness to family and culture are both valued. This perspective offers reassurance to immigrant families that their children can be successful in a receiving culture that values autonomy and individual achievement, while also maintaining close ties to the family and their cultural traditions.

Another important concept in cultural psychology is the idea of cultural niche (see Harkness & Super, 2012), variously described as the "ecocultural niche" (Gallimore, Weisner), "developmental microniche" (Worthman), or "developmental niche" (Harkness, Super). These related concepts all reflect integrative conceptualizations for understanding how cultural goals, beliefs, scripts, and routines, often implemented by parents, influence daily life and thereby child socialization and development. The idea of developmental niche encompasses physical and social settings, customs and practices of child care, and the "caretaker psychology" or the theories of parents about what is important for children and rearing them appropriately (Harkness & Super, 2012). Children developing in different cultural niches might be expected to learn different competences and coping strategies for dealing with stress, ideas about desirable behavior, and ways of caring for their own children. Even so, there could be common themes in different cultural niches related to common human capabilities, common challenges in life, or similar geographies.

HOW CULTURE, RELIGION, AND SPIRITUALITY PROMOTE RESILIENCE

All cultures and religions develop and transmit ideas, traditions, and practices for living and confronting the vicissitudes of life. These beliefs and practices evolve over generations to provide guidance and comfort to members of the group. The functions of cultural systems, including religion, in resilience have been neglected to a surprising degree over the years in psychological science, even though faith, cultural beliefs, and related practices come up spontaneously in many accounts of resilience. Emmy Werner repeatedly observed the importance of faith and religious affiliations in the children of Kauai who were resilient, both those who were persistently resilient from an early age and those who turned their lives around after a troubled adolescence (e.g., Werner 1993; Werner & Smith, 2001). These Hawaiian Islanders practiced various religions, including Christianity and Buddhism. Similarly, in our longitudinal study of resilience (see Chapter 3) and our work with homeless families (see Chapter 4), religion and faith often emerged spontaneously in accounts of coping and resilience. Young parents living in emergency shelters, with little or no material resources, especially those who have become disconnected from family of origin and community, often report that their faith keeps them going.

One of the founding fathers of the Black psychology movement, Joseph White, Professor Emeritus of Psychology at the University of California at Irvine, has noted the crucial role of the church and spirituality in the capacity for resilience. In the book *Black Man Emerging* (1999), White and coauthor Cones emphasize the historical importance of the Black church for the resilience of African American individuals and communities, providing a sense of connection, spiritual guidance, and coherence through long years of suffering and discrimination.

Investigators focused on understanding resilience in cultural context have undertaken research on resilience in extremely challenging research environments. The work of Panter-Brick and Eggerman in Afghanistan provides a compelling example (Eggerman & Panter-Brick, 2010; Panter-Brick, Goodman, Tol, & Eggerman, 2011). In a context of chronic conflict, economic distress, and danger, this team was able to carry out a study of over 1,000 adolescent students and their families, involving a student survey of mental health supplemented by interviews and a follow-up of significant subsamples of the cohort. They gathered rich ethnographic information as well as survey data, with extraordinary sensitivity to the culture and historical context. In their publications, this team suggests that the importance of values in Afghan culture on faith, family unity, service, effort, morals, and honor play central roles in the resilience of Afghan families. In a situation fraught with prolonged suffering, these values imbue life for Afghan families with a sense of cohesion and meaning. Eggerman and Panter-Brick (2010) quote the words of two parents to illustrate the salience of hope in resilience as they have observed it in Afghanistan: "Life feeds on hope" (28-year-old mother, p. 71) and "If a person has hope, then he or she can work and acquire knowledge to make their life better" (49-year-old mother, p. 76).

Studies of children in war underscore the importance of religious practices for resilience. In a study of orphans in war-torn Sri Lanka, for example, Fernando and Ferrari (2011) observed that religious practices, both Buddhist and Christian, by children in orphanages were associated with resilience. These included meditation, recitation of stories and scripture, and a philosophy of life that promoted acceptance and peace.

What has been most striking to me about the power of cultural systems and religion is the degree to which religions and ethnic traditions engage what I have described previously as the fundamental adaptive systems for human development and resilience. In the following section, I highlight these parallels, focusing on religion since ethnic cultures often are intertwined with a religious or spiritual belief system.

Cultural Guidelines for Parenting, Conduct, and Moral Values

Cultures and religions prescribe ways of living and rules to live by. These customs and practices may be so integrated into daily life that parents consider them to be natural or obvious ways of doing things or rearing children (Harkness & Super, 2012). Holy texts often codify these rules and include teaching stories or parables that convey values and principles for living. Many religions teach their followers to show compassion, forgiveness, honesty, and other virtues. Parents in studies of resilience have noted the importance of religion for helping them to instill such values in their children (Brodsky, 2000). Many religions also teach forgiveness, which may alleviate suffering and motivations for revenge after horrific trauma experiences (Crawford et al., 2006).

Kirmayer, Dandeneau, Marshall, Phillips, and Williamson (2011), in an article on "rethinking resilience from indigenous perspectives," describe a powerful ritual of reconciliation and forgiveness practiced by the indigenous people of Atlantic Canada, the Mi'kmaq. This practice was used to resolve disputes and restore harmony in this traditional culture, and was employed at the individual, community, and even the national level. Parties involved in the dispute would gather in a circle around a fire, with the "offended" person and supporters on one side and the "offending" constituents on the other side. After prayers to invoke "the spirit of the Wise Council," a ritual process was followed with elements of acknowledgment, discussion of the offending circumstances, apologies, restitution plans, and reestablishing harmony. This article also describes other aspects of indigenous culture that may promote resilience, including cultural values conveyed in creation stories transmitted orally across generations.

Attachment Relationships

In many different ways, religions of the world provide a sense of connection to the divine that is often experienced as a relationship much like an attachment relationship. In some religions, this spiritual relationship is very personal. The individual may speak or pray directly to God (or other spiritual figures), often as a parent figure. This relationship may bring a familiar sense of security, the sense of safety and emotional comfort provided by a secure base figure in attachment relationships. In other religions, the connection to the divine may be much more abstract, experienced as a sense of unity or interconnectedness. In either case, the relationship with the divine can provide a sense of security and transcendence that is not threatened by physical separation and thus can be a comfort at any time in any place or situation.

Positive Role Models and Bonds to Prosocial Mentors and Peers

Religions, as well as ethnic ties, however, also provide relationships with tangible humans who can be a source of tremendous support and guidance to parents and children (King & Benson, 2006). Religious communities provide many opportunities for children to interact with adults and peers outside the family, people who the family approves because they share many of the same values. In a dangerous community or situation, these adults and peers can provide help, mentoring, and prosocial activities that foster competence (as desired by the family) and resilience in times of turmoil. These connections also can provide a deep sense of belonging (King & Benson, 2006).

Self-Regulation Teachings and Practices

Many religions teach self-regulation skills, encouraging prayer, self-reflection, or meditation practices that facilitate EF and also arousal regulation. Various mindfulness practices have been linked to beneficial outcomes for health and well-being, including stress reduction (Shapiro, 2009). There is growing interest in secular mindfulness practice for children, parents, and teachers as a strategy for ameliorating stress and promoting self-regulation skills important for learning and adaptation (e.g., Benn, Akiva, Arel, & Roeser, 2012; Greenberg & Harris, 2012). Recent efforts to train EF skills in children include mindfulness training, through such group activities as martial arts and yoga (Diamond & Lee, 2011).

Meaning-Making Systems of Belief

Religions also offer profound and well-developed world views about the meaning of life, as do cultural communities, often shared through oral and written traditions, stories, and mythologies. Beliefs that life has meaning long have been associated with resilience in the face of adversity, sustaining hope during the bleakest human experiences, including concentration camps or the work camps of the Khmer Rouge, as noted elsewhere in this volume. Of course, traumatic experiences can challenge or shatter belief systems; some Holocaust survivors lost their faith. Yet religious beliefs often persist, providing an anchor of hope in the future or the afterlife for the believer. A transcendent sense of the spiritual or enduring faith anchored in religious beliefs can provide comfort in suffering, whether it is through the belief that there is a higher purpose at work, a view that all life is suffering, expectations that justice will be done in the end, or simply in the realization that there is beauty in the world that cannot be ruined by human evil or controlled by human design.

Opportunities for Mastery

Religions often provide opportunities for spiritual journeys, pilgrimages, and other quests that could engender a sense of challenge and accomplishment. Youth may be encouraged to undertake missions in foreign countries or charitable work near home. Rites-of-passage ceremonies may require lengthy preparations or involve physically challenging rituals that serve to build a sense of self-efficacy and accomplishment. Striving to meet these expectations also is supported by the religious or ethnic community and their achievement is widely recognized and celebrated. For young people experiencing discrimination or religious persecution, the recognition and support of the religious or ethnic community may offer a powerful context of protection and empowerment (Crawford et al., 2006).

Individual and Family Social Support

Religious and cultural traditions also provide direct support to individuals and families in many ways. When a neighbor or community member is sick or dying, it is customary in many communities to offer help, bring food, take care of chores or children, and in other ways convey emotional and concrete support. Similarly, when there is an economic crisis in a family or a disaster in the community, religious organizations often organize economic or material supports to families. Faith communities also offer many kinds of free counseling for individuals or families going through difficult times, through the religious leaders, professional counselors, lay helpers, or self-help groups. These may include support or groups for substance abuse, divorce, chronic illnesses, bereavement, and other common problems in life.

Cultural Identity

Belonging to an ethnic group or religion can also foster a sense of positive cultural identity. Research on both historically oppressed minority groups within a society and immigrant youth new to a society suggest that positive ethnic identity can play a protective role for psychological well-being and general adjustment. Studies of immigrant youth consistently find subjective well-being associated with positive ethnic identity, either in the context of bicultural identity (positive identification with the receiving culture and the individual's ethnic family culture) or a singular ethnic identity. Ethnic identity provides a sense of meaning and belonging, and also has the potential to buffer the effects of perceived discrimination (Sirin & Gupta, 2012; Verkuyten, 2012).

Positive ethnic identity may also co-occur with enculturation and adoption of positive cultural practices that promote resilience. Research on resilience in American Indian youth by LaFromboise, Hoyt, Oliver, and Whitbeck (2006) suggested that resilience, defined by success or lack of problems in multiple domains of adaptive behavior, was related to degree of enculturation, indexed by engagement in traditional Indian activities, identification with traditional culture, and traditional spiritual involvement.

Cultural Practices, Rituals, and Traditions

Finally, cultures and religions transmit many traditions and practices believed to promote positive development and resilience (Gauvain, 2013). Most religions have ceremonies and rituals for all of the major events of human life that can present challenges, including birth, puberty or coming of age, marriage, and death. These rituals often bring community members together, and involve music, prayer, words of wisdom, and other emotionally soothing or supportive activities. These rituals often have evolved over centuries, and thus also can provide a sense of collective continuity as well. Religious organizations also offer religious instruction for adults and children, and sometimes provide a comprehensive educational system designed to convey values as well as academic skills to children.

Dangers of Religion and Ethnic Identity: A Cautionary Note

Although cultural beliefs and practices can serve promotive and protective roles in human function and development, it is also true that crimes against humanity, wars, and acts of discrimination in many forms have been perpetrated over the centuries under the auspices of religious or cultural belief systems (Crawford et al., 2006). Since the science of resilience emerged a half-century ago, millions of children have suffered the direct and indirect consequences of violent conflicts among groups of people with different religious or cultural beliefs, in Northern Ireland, the Middle East, and other regions of the world. Violence, discrimination, oppression, and many other forms of adversity can arise from conflicts based on ethnic-group identity or religious convictions, with children often suffering the consequences in the ensuing conflict and disruption. It is important to remember that although culture and religion can serve powerful roles in human resilience, they also can function to undermine and harm individual development, underscoring once again that the same adaptive systems in human life can function very differently to help or harm.

HOW SCHOOLS, COMMUNITIES, AND NATIONS CAN PROMOTE RESILIENCE THROUGH CULTURAL STRATEGIES

It is clear that racism and ethnic discrimination directed against ethnic minorities or immigrant youth are pervasive and harmful in many schools, communities, and countries throughout the world. At the same time, many communities and nations now recognize the enormous stakes they have in the success of minority and immigrant youth for the future. "Minorities" are rapidly becoming majorities and immigrant children represent a large and growing proportion of the future workforce in many economically developed nations. Consequently, there is great interest in strategies for promoting success in ethnic-minority and immigrant youth and a recognition that those strategies need to be culturally informed (Masten, Liebkind, & Hernandez, 2012a).

Numerous chapters in our recent volume *Realizing the Potential of Immigrant Youth* (Masten, Liebkind, & Hernandez, 2012b) make recommendations for policies and actions at the national or local level to facilitate resilience in immigrant or disadvantaged minority children. At a policy level, these suggestions include general strategies, such as investing in early childhood education, and more targeted strategies, such as promoting positive perceptions in the media of the human and cultural capital represented by immigrant youth.

Schools, in many ways, function as a key "acculturation zone" for children and families from diverse backgrounds (racial/ethnic, socioeconomic, and cultural). Local, school-based approaches for promoting positive acculturation and reducing intergroup conflicts include many strategies for consciously fostering positive interactions and minimizing conflict. Teachers and other staff need to be culturally aware and competent, trained in strategies to reduce intergroup conflict and foster intercultural respect and friendship. Cooperative learning activities and multicultural studies and celebrations can be incorporated into the curriculum. Bilingual skills can be developed and supported for all students, and recognized as an important investment in multicultural capital.

SUMMARY

Human capacity for resilience presumably evolved over many generations through the interplay of interacting cultures, families, and individuals. Individual resilience is deeply embedded in the legacies of cultural evolution passed down in the form of ideas and practices that influence the child's experience in many forms, including parenting, language, education, and community expectations. In contemporary societies, with increasing globalization and intercultural contact, children may encounter many distinct cultures as they develop.

Cultural experiences shape the developmental tasks children face and also the tools, knowledge, and strategies for meeting those expectations, as well as the unexpected adversities of life. Cultures and religions encode and transmit adaptive strategies through their cultural practices, beliefs, and sacred texts. It seems reasonable to assume that strategies and ideas that promote resilience in times of threat and adversity would be noted, valued, and passed on from generation to generation. Some would be unique to the cultural context of a people in time and place, whereas others would be universal to the human experience.

In this chapter, I highlighted some of the ways that culture could be considered in thinking about resilience, with a primary focus on how culture may influence individual resilience in human development. I suspect there may be many observations of effective protective strategies practiced in distinct cultures that could be gleaned from the detailed observations and ethnographies of anthropologists and others who have studied cultures in depth around the world. Explicit studies focused on resilience in the context of culture, or multicultural studies of resilience, remain quite limited at this time. But there are hopeful signs of a new wave of culturally expanded and informed research on resilience.

PART IV

MOVING FORWARD

Implications for Action
and Future Research

CHAPTER 11

A RESILIENCE FRAMEWORK FOR ACTION

The resilience pioneers had a fundamentally practical goal, which was to improve the odds for positive development in young people whose lives were threatened by risk. They hoped to learn about resilience in order to promote it for those who would not be able to make it on their own. They were a rigorous group who held the highest standards for scientific evidence, and they knew that good science takes time. At the same time, they knew that children in danger *now* could not wait for science to provide all the definitive answers. Thus, from the outset, it was important to glean knowledge, however limited, to guide efforts to promote resilience even as the research continued.

The same imperative exists today. Around the globe, children are threatened by war and natural disasters, family and community violence, or poverty and homelessness. Immediate action is required and there is a growing body of knowledge about resilience to guide practice and policy. Certainly caution is called for as well as more science. But there is a reasonably good consensus emerging about how one might promote resilience in children, reflecting a profound transformation in thinking about intervention. This chapter presents a general resilience framework for action, highlighting how thinking has changed and also providing concrete examples of strategies built on a resilience frame of reference.

It could be argued that resilience research itself has had a transformative effect on the conceptual frameworks of practice in multiple fields concerned with human well-being. Many applied fields have shifted away from deficit-based models about symptoms and treating problems to focus on strengths and methods to facilitate success and adaptive processes. This shift is evident across many fields of practice: in prevention science increasingly focused on promoting wellness or competence (Cicchetti, Rappaport, Sandler, & Weissberg, 2000; Gest & Davidson, 2011; Greenberg, 2006); in family therapy (e.g., Goldenberg & Goldenberg, 2013; Walsh, 2006); in training and services for military soldiers and families (e.g., Cozza & Lerner, 2013; Park, 2011; Saltzman et al., 2011); in the positive youth development movement and related out-of-school programs such as 4-H, Big Brothers/Big Sisters, or scouting (Lerner, 2009); in the strength-based school counseling movement (Akos & Galassi, 2008; Masten et al., 2008); in child welfare reform (e.g., Flynn et al., 2006; Masten, 2006b); in social work (e.g., Anthony, Alter, & Jenson, 2009); in nursing (e.g., Szanton & Gill, 2010) and medicine (e.g., Southwick et al., 2011); and in the policy and practices of humanitarian organizations (e.g., Ager, 2013; Lundberg & Wuermli, 2012).

The resilience framework presented below has five components, which might be called the "Five Ms": mission, models, measures, methods, and multilevel/multidisciplinary approaches. Additional lessons gleaned from the science to date with implications for action are also discussed, including strategic timing and targeting. Finally, the concept of translational synergy is discussed, focusing on the simultaneous benefits to science and practice when scientists and practitioners collaborate fully in the design and implementation of interventions to promote resilience.

MISSION: FRAME POSITIVE GOALS

One of the most basic but important consequences of the shift in focus that characterized a resilience framework was the influence on the goals and objectives of intervention. The resilience investigators wanted to know how to promote positive outcomes and much of their work focused on predicting those positive criteria. They were not satisfied with preventing problems, seeking to elucidate as well how competence or success was achieved in spite of risk or adversity. Health and success, in their view, represented more than an absence of symptoms. In prevention science, a dual focus evolved on promoting the positive and preventing negative behavior and this dual focus continues to flourish (Gest & Davidson, 2011; Masten, Burt, et al., 2006). Moreover, research findings suggested that promoting positive function and development often reduced the risk of psychopathology without the potential risk of stigmatization associated with problem-focused intervention, particularly those that identify a "high-risk" target group.

Framing positive goals also had "marketing" benefits that have been anecdotally reported (e.g., Flynn et al., 2006), though these are difficult to document systematically. It is easy to understand why parents would be more interested in signing up for a program to promote success than one to prevent problems in their children. Similarly, children in the child welfare system would rather discuss their progress toward positive achievements than their shortcomings on a list of problems. Parenting training interventions designed to improve child behavior through behavioral techniques often begin by having parents "catch your child being good," reinforcing positive behaviors with small but immediate social reinforcements. This focus serves to shift the overall tone of the parent–child interaction away from negative interactions. The power of positive goals, of course, has been much touted in the popular literature on organizational and personal success for many years.

Most concerns can be stated, refocused, or reframed in terms of positive objects. This is easy when the goals are focused on achieving widely expected developmental tasks, such as succeeding in school, making friends, getting a good job, or effective parenting. Common targets of prevention, such as reducing violence, symptoms, or risky behaviors, also can be reframed in terms of promoting behaviors incompatible with those problems, including competence in developmental tasks, but also conflict resolution skills, healthy relationships, or self-regulation. Negative criteria can be assessed along with positive criteria, but efforts to set and state positive goals may enhance enthusiasm, buy-in, and the likelihood of noticing progress in positive domains.

MODELS: INCLUDE POSITIVE FACTORS, INFLUENCES, AND ACTIONS

Models to guide practice and policy based on a resilience framework include positive ingredients and processes, expanding well beyond models limited to risks and vulnerabilities that lead to problem outcomes. Positive outcomes are targeted or added while not forgetting that exposure to risk, vulnerabilities, and problems also matter. Assets and resources are added to supplement risk factors. Protective influences are considered as well as vulnerabilities. Intervention itself can be conceptualized in terms of averting or ameliorating risk; adding, enhancing, or protecting key assets and resources; and restoring, protecting, or mobilizing positive adaptive systems.

Figure 11.1 depicts some of the multiple ways that one could think about actions to foster resilience in general terms. One approach is to prevent a well-known risk factor from occurring at all (risk *a* in the figure). Another approach is to mitigate the effects of a risk factor (risk *b*). A third approach is to prevent or reduce the harm a risk factor (risk *c*) may have on a key positive resource or influence in a child's life (illustrated by asset *b*). In many cases, risk factors harm children indirectly through their harmful effects on other people, most notably parents. This kind of risk to children is *mediated* by negative effects on the positive factor (illustrated by asset *b*). Protecting key resources and protective factors for human development is an important strategy for intervention. Additionally, one can aim to add resources or assets to the lives of children, aiming to improve function or development, illustrated by asset *a*. This model is not exhaustive. Specific examples of these various approaches are provided in the section below on methods.

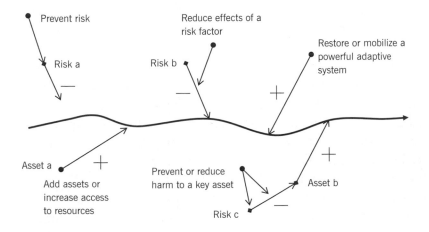

FIGURE 11.1. Model illustrating different ways to conceptualize interventions to foster resilience.

MEASURES: TRACK THE POSITIVE AS WELL AS THE PROBLEMS

Resilience-based approaches underscore the importance of assessing positive aspects of intervention and outcome, along with any negative predictors or outcomes that are being tracked, and potential mediators of change. When clinicians and scientists began to study resilience, they quickly realized that measurements of symptoms, problems, and risk factors were more plentiful and advanced than the measures of strengths, assets, positive physical or mental health, and other positive aspects of development. Many clinical measures considered only symptoms and deficits, giving little attention to measuring competence or progress in developmental task domains such as friendship, prosocial behavior, or civic engagement. An exception was academic achievement, which had long been a concern of communities and nations invested in public education. As noted previously, considerable progress has been made in developing measures of positive function in individuals, families, and other systems.

In the international child welfare reform movement called Looking After Children (see Flynn et al., 2006; Masten, 2006b), a decision was made in multiple countries to transform child welfare systems by adopting a positive mission with positive goals, articulated and measured in terms of progress on multiple domains of human development. These domains included "seven developmental dimensions of well-being." This required developing a set of measurement tools, called the Assessment and Action Record for documenting child well-being and tracking progress. One of the most interesting changes noted by advocates of this reform system was the positive effects not only on the welfare system itself but also on child clients, foster parents, social workers, and others within the system as they focused their attention on clear positive objectives and measures of child well-being (see Klein, Kufeldt, & Rideout, 2006).

A similar measurement effort was required by the shift in school counseling away from a deficit-based model and toward a strength-based model, discussed in Chapter 9 (Galassi & Akos, 2007). The American School Counselor Association (2005) reframed their national goals in terms of building a set of competences in all students. In response, proponents of the new model had to operationalize how the standards would be met and develop reliable and valid assessments for each domain of competence (Akos & Galassi, 2008).

It is also quite conceivable that interventions that will lead to goals like reduced violence, delinquency, substance abuse, depression, suicide, or other mental health problems may begin with observable improvements in *positive behaviors* by children or parents that then cascade forward. Some interventions now are designed to propagate such cascades (see Masten & Cicchetti, 2010a, 2010b, 2010c). Moreover, it is also possible to miss where the action is (how exactly an intervention is working) by focusing too narrowly on either negative or positive domains of behavior.

METHODS: PREVENT, PROMOTE, PROTECT

Interventions require strategies for change as well as strategic planning in terms of timing and levels to target. Resilience research suggests three basic strategies to promote resilience in diverse contexts of threat or risk to human development: focusing on risk, resources, or adaptive systems. Resilience research also provides ideas for strategic timing, pointing to opportunity windows when the conditions for change are more favorable.

Risk Focused: Prevent or Reduce Risk or Adversity

Resilience-based approaches include risk-focused strategies. Naturally occurring resilience also involves risk-targeted strategies. Effective parents and friends often attempt to lower the dose of trauma or risk exposure of people they care about, in multiple ways. Part of a parent's job is to keep an eye on what is coming that may be harmful to his or her children, whether it is the immediate threat of a large dog approaching a toddler on the playground, or the potential threats posed by gang recruiters in a dangerous neighborhood. At the same time, parents know that children need to learn how to manage adversities without always running to their parents; thus they often are making judgments about their child's capabilities for handling the situation as well as the potential danger. Friends also keep an eye out for impending danger, whether it is to warn of an approaching bully in an ordinary high school or an approaching bomb in a war zone. If a serious threat cannot be avoided, parents and friends can act to provide support or help to mitigate the impact of the threat. Similarly, societies and international agencies can intervene to prevent or lower risk exposure and/or attempt to reduce its impact.

One of the basic conclusions across many studies of risk and resilience is that *dose matters*. Thus, it makes sense to focus on reducing exposure dose for children—by actions taken before, during, or after trauma and disaster strike. Many recommendations on dose reduction can be found in the literature on trauma and disaster described previously. These include, for example, training parents and teachers, as well as public officials and broadcast journalists, to monitor media exposure of children to terrorism and mass-trauma events.

Preventing a risk factor or tragedy from occurring is a powerful strategy of intervention. Modern societies invest in prenatal care as a public health intervention to prevent low birth weight (LBW) and premature birth in the population (Alexander & Kotelchuck, 2001). This risk-reduction strategy is widely supported because of its value in terms of public health and well-being and a highly favorable cost-to-benefit ratio. There can be huge costs associated with preventable disabilities and treatments related to LBW or prematurity.

The costs of allowing a child to grow up in poverty with insufficient food, health care, child care, and education also are enormous (Alderman, 2011; Duncan, Ziol-Guest, & Kalil, 2010; Yoshikawa et al., 2012), which has led many wealthy countries, such as Norway or France, to provide extensive social welfare benefits to their residents in an effort to reduce or mitigate the risks posed to human development by the risks of poverty or privation. The toxic levels of stress endemic in the lives of the millions of children living in poverty in the United States jeopardize not only the health and brain development of these individual children (Shonkoff, 2011) but also compromise the human capital of the nation. Impressive evidence indicates the solid return on investment for programs focused on reducing or mitigating risk in low-income children (Heckman, 2006; Heckman, Moon, Pinto, Savelyev, & Yavitz, 2010; Reynolds, Temple, White, Ou, & Robertson, 2011). Yet, despite a strong consensus on the hazards of poverty, especially early in development, and the value of prevention efforts, as well as the advocacy efforts of nonprofit groups such as the Children's Defense Fund, there continues to be limited investment or coordinated policy. The global recession that began around 2007 did not help the situation. Nonetheless, recent attention to the effects of stress and poverty on brain development, combined with evidence on the benefit-to-cost return on investment in early childhood programs, promises to shift the equation toward action, especially in the context of economic recovery.

Many examples of specific, risk-focused interventions also can be considered. Just a few examples illustrate some practical and symbolic lessons. First, it makes no sense to build a new school on the grounds of a former war zone without checking for land mines. Second, hungry children cannot be expected to concentrate on learning, even with wonderful teachers. Third, the best parents in the world cannot compensate for the risks posed by gunfire on the way to school. Fourth, it is nearly impossible to comfort children who can see that their parents are terrified. Fifth, first responders who have good reason to believe that their own children are drowning or otherwise in imminent danger cannot be expected to perform their jobs well.

Finally, in considering strategies for risk-focused interventions, it must be remembered that exposure to milder and manageable adversities may be important for developing self-protection systems and skills. The literature on stress inoculation and steeling effects suggests that some exposure and experience in regard to engaging with challenges or adversities is important for the development of adaptive capacity, as well as self-efficacy concerning one's capabilities for handling adversity.

Resource Focused: Increase Assets

Another basic strategy for intervention is adding resources or access to resources. Emergency relief efforts often take this form, providing water, food, shelter, medical care, and other basic necessities in the aftermath of disaster. Typically, in disasters, these emergency resources are provided until regular systems for acquiring essentials are restored or created anew.

Many social welfare programs, governmental and nongovernmental, designed to aid disadvantaged children and families take this form as well, providing food, temporary or longer-term shelter, medical care, child care, or money to help purchase these necessities.

More targeted efforts to promote success also have focused on adding resources or assets to the lives of children. Efforts to close the "achievement gap" between advantaged and disadvantaged children, for example, often include adding access to preschool, after-school programs, tutoring, or computers. "Reach Out and Read" is a national effort to promote early literacy and school readiness by giving away books in pediatricians' offices across the country. This effort began at Boston City Hospital in 1989. Now, this nonprofit effort is active in all 50 states, giving away millions of books every year to low-income children.

Another approach within this asset-targeted category is to enhance the quality of the assets available. Efforts to improve teacher quality or the training for Guardians *ad litem*, for instance, or to improve quality of computers or tutoring, are all examples of efforts to improve outcomes by bolstering assets.

Sometimes the problem is not the availability of resources, but *access* to existing resources. There may be barriers to access or simply a lack of knowledge or skills to gain access. A homeless and highly stressed parent may not know where or how to get help that is available, or may be too exhausted to figure out a complex bureaucratic system. Adding an advocate or case manager to smooth access to resources can be a highly effective way to increase resources for families.

Adaptive System Focused: Restore, Harness, or Mobilize the Power of Human Adaptive Systems

The third major strategy is to focus on restoring, harnessing, or mobilizing the most powerful known adaptive systems for human resilience and development. This approach is based on the core insight from resilience science that most resilience arises from the operation of the fundamental adaptive systems that are the legacy of human biological and cultural evolution. These systems and their effective operation are a priority for human development. Thus, for example, in the aftermath of disaster, in addition to ensuring basic survival needs (water, food, medicine, shelter, etc.), it is also essential to make sure that young children have a functional caregiver on hand. Similarly, it is important to support good function of systems that support child development, including not only families but also schools and cultural practices. Indeed, the operation of basic community and societal support systems for children and families are so fundamental to human well-being that it can be reassuring for survivors to see evidence that they are resuming. It is not a coincidence that devastated communities will go to great lengths to begin even a makeshift school, provide opportunities to play, or hold culturally important ceremonies. All of these activities send a strong, symbolic message of hope that *recovery is under way*. Whether it is family routines or community routines or national routines, efforts to mobilize adaptive systems not only begin to actually foster adaptive function, they also inspire hope.

In situations of individual or family disaster, these fundamental systems also are a priority. In the case of Sara described previously (Chapter 2; see also Masten & O'Connor, 1989), the team recommended an all-out attempt to facilitate recovery by providing the single most powerful adaptive system for a child's life, which is a loving and capable family. Then we stepped aside to observe what this powerful system could do for Sara. The intent of many interventions to place children with new families is similar, to improve the quality of caregiving and attachment bonds with capable parent figures. These programs include domestic and international adoption, as well as foster care for children who have been orphaned, abandoned, profoundly mistreated, or neglected by their own parents.

Compelling studies have demonstrated the relative advantage of foster care in a family over institutional care. One of the most important demonstrations of foster care as an intervention was provided by the Bucharest Early Intervention Project (Nelson et al., 2007; Zeanah et al., 2011). This study represents an extraordinarily rare effort to test through an experimental design (with random assignment to treatment) the effects of foster care on human development. Young children living in institutions in Bucharest (ages 6–31 months) were randomly assigned to usual care (continued institutional care) or foster care in families that were specially selected and trained by the study team. These children have been followed forward over time (through age 12 as of this writing) and, as is usual in longitudinal studies, the purity of the experiment was affected by naturally occurring changes in status (such as individuals in the care-as-usual group moving into foster care or back to families). Dramatic differences in cognitive development and brain function were evident in early follow-ups, with some persisting differences documented after 8 years (so far).

Research also demonstrates that efforts to improve the quality of foster care through training foster parents can have beneficial effects on foster children. Mary Dozier has developed and tested in convincing experiments the Attachment and Biobehavioral Catch-Up Intervention (Dozier et al., 2006; Dozier, Peloso, Lewis, Laurenceau, & Levine, 2008) to help foster parents nurture foster children and help them regulate their behavior. Philip Fisher and his colleagues (2011) have shown that training foster parents to improve their quality of care has a beneficial effect on the stress regulation of children placed in their care, indexed by the diurnal patterns in their cortisol levels. This experiment was a planned trial to promote resilience to the stress of placement changes in foster care by boosting a key protective system (parenting in the receiving foster parents) that was expected to regulate stress response in the foster children. Both of these studies indicate that effective parenting plays a role in a child's capacity for regulating stress, and serves to validate the role of parenting in resilience (Fisher, Gunnar, Dozier, Bruce, & Pears, 2006).

Many children endangered by risk within the family, including neglect or abuse, are not placed out of home. Instead, an attempt is made to improve the quality of attachment and parenting for an existing caregiver–child dyad. Gold-standard evidence (randomized experiments) shows efficacy for a number of these interventions to promote resilience within families at risk due to maltreatment or neglect, including child–parent psychotherapy (CPP) and the Incredible Years Parenting Skills training program (see Toth & Manley, 2011).

A less intensive strategy that also is focused on relationships with capable adults is to foster mentoring relationships for children at risk for various reasons. This strategy turns out to be more challenging than one might expect from observing naturally occurring mentoring relationships. There are many issues related to match making, protecting children from predators, training mentors, and sustaining these relationships over time. Nonetheless, there is evidence that mentoring programs for disadvantaged young people, such as "Big Brothers/Big Sisters of America," benefit the young people they are designed to help (DuBois, Holloway,

Valentine, & Cooper, 2002; Grossman & Tierney, 1998). DuBois and colleagues conducted a meta-analysis of 55 studies of mentoring, finding a modest but significant positive effect.

Interventions that target individual capabilities can be viewed as targeting a fundamental adaptive system within the child. As noted previously, there is currently considerable interest in interventions to promote self-control (self-regulation, EF) skills in children at risk for school problems. Capabilities to control one's own attention, thinking, and behavior have been widely implicated as helpful for maintaining or recovering adaptive function in stress-provoking and hazardous situations, as well as in the course of normal life across the lifespan. Self-control has been broadly implicated as a correlate and long-term predictor of better adaptation, both in children and adults (Bandura, 1997; Moffitt et al., 2011; Ryan & Deci, 2000; Tangney, Baumeister, & Boone, 2008; Zelazo & Carlson, 2012). Self-control training is central in many forms of intervention for children, applying diverse methods that range from meditation to martial arts to memory games (Diamond & Lee, 2011; Zelazo & Carlson, 2012). Methods to train parents in better child-management skills often emphasize the importance of parents regulating their own emotions and stress (Sanders, 2012). The current "mindfulness" training movement across many fields, including education and medicine, emphasizes the practice of attending to the present moment as a strategy for developing self-awareness and self-control skills. There is a growing body of work on mindfulness training in children (Zelazo & Lyons, 2011).

Many other examples could be viewed as efforts to mobilize adaptive systems. These include efforts to build a sense of self-efficacy or promote experiences of mastery through opportunities to develop and demonstrate physical skills or artistic talents. Opportunities for experiencing success through applied effort, perceived success, and the concomitant activation of the reward–effort feedback loop are associated with mastery motivation (see Chapter 6). After disasters, disheartened adolescents have been engaged effectively to help with rebuilding or supervising younger children in learning or community projects. The benefit is twofold: Community recovery efforts are bolstered at the same time that individuals gain meaningful experiences of contribution and accomplishment that nurture their own hope and motivation. Similarly, efforts in the wake of disaster to foster cultural practices of the affected population, including traditional holiday meals, dancing, music, or religious rituals and ceremonies, also represent examples of restoring or mobilizing protective systems, aimed at different levels of action.

MULTIPLE LEVELS, APPROACHES, AND DISCIPLINES

As emphasized throughout this volume, resilience research has increasingly encompassed a multiple-levels perspective, recognizing that individual development unfolds from the interactions of many systems across levels, both within and outside the individual. The life of an individual is embedded in many other systems and all of these are continually interacting. These ideas reflect the central themes of general systems theory and development (e.g., Lerner, 2006; Overton, 2013; Zelazo, 2013). Implicit in the growing attention to multiple, interacting systems is the possibility that interventions directed at individual resilience can target change in higher-level systems (e.g., families or schools) and, concomitantly, that efforts to promote resilience at the community or national level can target change at the individual or family level. Most interventions would be expected to target only a few levels of interaction, at most. Yet even the simplest multiple-levels perspective on resilience begs for involvement of multiple disciplines, in order to have the necessary expertise on hand.

Some of the best examples of efforts to build a multiple-level, multidisciplinary approach to resilience have been motivated by disasters, potential disasters, terrorism, and efforts to plan for resilience in advance of such calamities. Concerns about flu pandemic, climate change, and terrorism, for example, have sparked international conferences on resilience, such as Resilience 2008 in Sweden, Resilience 2011 in the United States, Resilience 2014 in France, the First World Congress on Resilience held in France in 2012, the Second World Congress on Resilience in Romania in 2014, and motivated dialogue among international coalitions of scientists such as the Resilience Alliance, which also publishes the open access journal *Ecology and Society*. That journal has published a series of special features and articles aiming to bridge disciplines to address the topic of resilience in the face of global problems like climate change or terrorism (e.g., Gunderson, 2010; Longstaff & Yang, 2008; Masten & Obradović, 2008; Herrfahrdt-Pähle & Pahl-Wostl, 2012). Disaster preparedness is increasingly conceptualized from a resilience perspective (Brown & Westaway, 2011; Norris et al., 2008). Large centers established to address mass trauma and disaster, such as the National Child Traumatic Stress Network (NCTSN), include interdisciplinary scientists.

Recent efforts to promote educational success among low-income children and address the intransigent and pernicious achievement gaps that leave so many disadvantaged children behind also illustrate the power of an integrated, multisystem approach to resilience. *Whatever It Takes*, Paul Tough's (2009) book on the Harlem Achievement Zone, chronicles Geoffrey Canada's vision for transforming the ecology, development, and prospects of children residing in one of the most disadvantaged neighborhoods in America to foster adult success through high school and college graduation. Tough describes how Canada's vision emerged and how he went about the complex and bumpy process of making ambitious goals into reality. That process required radical rethinking about how to mobilize the systematic and sustained resources and partnerships that were needed for the children in the Zone to succeed.

Canada's strategies are now receiving a broad national test in multiple cities across the United States through President Obama's Promise Neighborhood initiative. In the Twin Cities, a team led by Sondra Samuels won a grant to implement the Northside Achievement Zone, or NAZ, which has the goal of college readiness for every child in a part of Minneapolis known more for abysmal graduation rates and street violence than academic achievement. NAZ has built a network of partners to coordinate opportunities and services, and a family "connector" to facilitate access for the NAZ families. NAZ makes a commitment to stay the course and do whatever it takes to foster academic success. One of their signature programs for young families is the Family Academy, a 14-week program to build skills for parenting young children. The mayor and many other community leaders in Minneapolis attend the graduation ceremonies, where the achievements of parents are applauded and each child receives a T-shirt with their anticipated college graduation date ("Class of . . ."). NAZ collaborates with dozens of partners to build a climate of support and success, including public and private schools, afterschool programs, affordable housing agencies, and many others. They want every parent and child to know that someone has your back. Like Canada, their goals are ambitious, including college readiness for every child and a transformed community.

The recent focus on resilience in U.S. military training and family policies also illustrates a shift to resilience models that are inherently multilevel and multidisciplinary (Cornum, Mathews, & Seligman, 2011; Cozza & Lerner, 2013; Masten, 2013a; Saltzman et al., 2011). The modern U.S. military appears to recognize that the resilience of soldiers and military operations are interdependent, and also influenced by the well-being not only of individual soldiers and commanders but also of their families. Military research on resilience spans levels from the molecular biology of resilience to the resilience of units and military organizations on much larger scales.

A new horizon for interventions spanning multiple levels is represented by new research on personalized interventions, such as cancer treatments tailored to an individual's genotype or the genetic nature of the cancer. In the field of prevention for children, there is growing interest in the possibility of tailoring treatments (medications or interventions) to fit individuals in much the same way. In one of the first efforts to test a gene × environment interaction hypothesis, Brody and colleagues (2009) found that a family-focused intervention was more effective for young people who had a particular genetic variation of the serotonin transporter gene (5-HTT) that may index sensitivity to experience. This kind of research is still at an early stage but advances in molecular genetics and intervention science are motivating investigators to refine their approaches to figure out what strategies work best for whom.

The interest in spanning levels of analysis and disciplines is also spurring collaboration in interventions. This trend is discussed at the end of this chapter.

WINDOWS OF OPPORTUNITY: STRATEGIC TIMING

Resilience findings also suggested that timing as well as targeting of interventions could be important. The apparent consequences of adversity and protective influences studied in the literature varied as a function of developmental timing and also timing with respect to the threat itself. In other words, observations of naturally occurring resilience suggest that interventions could be timed and targeted strategically. Tailoring interventions to optimize developmental timing is likely to be more successful (Toth & Cicchetti, 1999).

When do conditions converge for resilience? From a systems perspective, conditions may be conducive to change when systems are unstable, or responding to disturbances. Thus, adversity itself may present a window of opportunity as well as vulnerability. Systems responding to disturbances, especially major disturbances, may be able to reorganize more easily than stable systems. Dynamic systems can be quite resistant to change due to powerful self-regulatory mechanisms that tend to keep the system operating within stable parameters.

Developmentally, periods of transition characterized by multiple-level changes in the organism or the context or both may afford windows of opportunity for change. The transition years when children enter preschool and primary school (around ages 3–7), early adolescence, and the transition to adulthood have all been characterized this way in modern societies (Dahl & Spear, 2004; Masten, 2004; Masten, Obradović, et al., 2006). Each period shows rapid changes in the organism and interactions with others.

There are new opportunities and challenges posed by changes in biology, cognition, and/or context.

In the developmental literature on growth and change in the structure and function of the human brain, these same transition periods have been described as periods of high plasticity. Developmental periods of heightened neural plasticity have been termed *sensitive periods*. Some of these occur prenatally or in very early development. Others are later. The early childhood years represent a period of rapid improvements in EF capabilities that depend in part on brain development (Zelazo & Carlson, 2012). Early adolescence often is viewed as a vulnerability window because so many problem behaviors begin to rise at this time of concentrated pubertal and social changes. Yet, adolescents who have the benefits of caring families and communities and opportunities to develop their talents and apply themselves to meaningful pursuits typically do well and begin to move with passion and energy into the worlds of advanced academics, work, sports, close friendship, and romance (Dahl & Spear, 2004; Lerner, 2009; Steinberg et al., 2006). The transition years spanning adolescence and early adulthood also are associated with systematic changes in brain development accompanied by changes in cognitive control skills, which seem to facilitate more mature aspects of planning and complex decision making (Masten, Obradović, et al., 2006; Somerville & Casey, 2010).

Timing considerations also indicate what protective system to target when. In early childhood, for example, it is crucial to protect or restore the caregiving function of parents. Later in development, attachment relationships will still be important, but the focus of intervention might be on relationships with mentors, friends, or romantic partners rather than parent figures. Similarly, strategies to protect children from the amplification effects of media exposure on trauma after highly publicized events would differ developmentally. Parents of young children would be advised to monitor exposure very closely, to reduce exposure dose. For older children, it may be more developmentally strategic to encourage parents to watch with their children and educate them to be wise consumers of media coverage of events. Older children may also be able to use social media as a means to help others or themselves.

One of the most provocative ideas in intervention pertinent to resilience is the possibility of reopening plasticity windows or inducing plasticity through some sort of intervention. This possibility might make it feasible to "reprogram" maladaptive systems that were not optimally organized, for example, due to toxic stress exposure at the wrong time in early development, or to induce a state of high plasticity prior to exposure to some kind of favorable experience, including therapy or training.

TESTING RESILIENCE THEORY THROUGH INTERVENTION: MOVING TOWARD TRANSLATIONAL SYNERGY

Wave three of resilience research turned attention to intervention studies as a means of testing causal ideas about resilience. As wave four unfolds, investigators are expanding interventions to consider multiple levels of function (molecular to social) and the interplay across systems and system levels. In both cases, well-designed intervention experiments (ideally with randomized control groups) can inform theories about resilience in addition to best practices.

Translational synergy refers to the mutual benefits that accrue to both science and practice, and the scientists and practitioners engaged in these activities, when interventions are developed and tested collaboratively by representatives from both sides of the translational bridge (Masten, 2011). Practitioners grew tired of the long wait for guidance on what to do to promote resilience. Meanwhile, intervention scientists grew frustrated with the failures of their beautifully designed interventions to work as well when they were taken out into the field or taken to scale.

Collaboration offers a solution to both issues. Practitioners who help design interventions from the outset can bring wisdom from the field on what is important, practical, and feasible. They also build buy-in for a new approach. Scientists who collaborate in a transactional design process bring knowledge from the literature and their research experience, including strategies for measurement and evaluation that will be compelling to funders and credible to other scientists. Some compromise is inevitable in this kind of process, but the benefits are potentially huge in cutting the time for translation of knowledge to application in the field and also in developing interventions that have ecological validity and practical appeal that will actually work in the real world. The young people and families these interventions are designed to help also are often engaged in this collaborative research, in early focus groups for input on design, and then also in the process of evaluation and feedback as iterations of an intervention are tested.

Multiple partners from the academy and community, perhaps including policymakers as well, each bringing distinct expertise, are required for this kind of synergistic, practical but theory-informative intervention. The challenge is to maintain rigorous science standards while developing more practical and feasible interventions. Community-based research centers, such as the Mt. Hope Family Center in Rochester, New York, are leading the vanguard of this approach. Funders are also are getting on board, investing more often in collaborative research characterized by an iterative process of development. Federal programs like the Promise Neighborhoods and Race to the Top, especially when they require strong evidence of efficacy, can be viewed as part of this trend.

Our research to develop prevention interventions for homeless and similarly mobile, disadvantaged children, described in Chapter 4, was designed collaboratively from the outset with the goal of translational synergy. Our aim is to foster academic success during a window of opportunity, focused on a strategic target for change: EF skills in preschool-age children. This window is believed to be a period of high neural plasticity for the development of these neurocognitive skills. The design team is working collaboratively, with expertise from scientists who study neurocognitive development and resilience, preschool teachers who develop curriculum and train early childhood educators, and community staff who know the families very well (Casey et al., 2014). Families provide input through focus groups and evaluations. It remains to be seen whether the strategies will work to promote resilience, but we are confident that they will be feasible and appealing to the children, teachers, and parents involved.

SUMMARY

Children cannot wait for scientists to learn everything important there is to know about resilience and how best to protect or promote human development. Scientists were well aware of this dilemma from the earliest days of resilience research. When disaster strikes, when a child is in imminent danger, or when a child soldier is rescued, those charged with responding must act on the basis of what is currently known and feasible. Ideally, they will consider the best and most pertinent evidence available, be aware of its limitations, and also respond with knowledge about the nature of the children, family, community, culture, situation, and resources at hand. Developmental scientists can help by participating in the process, shaping general guidelines based on extant knowledge, and communicating what is known and the limitations about that knowledge base in ways that inform without overwhelming or misleading responders and policymakers.

Research on resilience has had a transformative influence on many fields of practice concerned with intervening in response to crisis or adversity or preparing for future response. The fundamental models in many fields have shifted from a deficit-based model to a strength-based perspective, grounded in more positive conceptualizations of adaptive systems.

In this chapter, I have outlined a general resilience-based framework for action based on conclusions and observations rooted in decades of research on resilience in children and youth by many scientists, but also informed by many commentaries and interactions with practitioners and policymakers who had to make decisions and take action with incomplete knowledge and many practical constraints. The goal here was to present a general way of thinking about action from a resilience-informed perspective. Specific guidelines and applications would require much more specific knowledge and experience with the situation, people, and context involved.

The resilience framework for action described here emphasized positive perspectives with respect to five components:

1. Mission: Frame positive goals.

2. Models: Include strengths, resources, positive outcomes, and adaptive processes.

3. Measures: Assess strengths, resources, positive outcomes, and adaptive processes.

4. Methods: Reduce or mitigate risk, boost resources and adaptive capacity, and mobilize adaptive systems.

5. Multiple systems: Consider possibilities at multiple levels with expertise from multiple disciplines.

This approach does not exclude or overlook the importance of considering risks and vulnerability processes, but instead highlights the importance of including and emphasizing the adaptive capabilities and capacities of living, dynamic human systems.

This approach also recognizes the embeddedness of human life, with an individual's development influenced by and influencing many other systems. This means that the best leverage for positive change might be at the level of individual behavior or it might be at the level of biology within the individual, or at the level of parent–child interaction and other aspects of family system function. The leverage for change also could be at the level of school system, culture, or national policy, or some combination of multiple system levels.

Strategic timing is important in this framework, because developing human systems go through periods when the individual, family, or community is more open to change. Early developmental timing may be particularly important because so many of the most fundamental adaptive systems in a human individual are programmed and organized early in development. Nonetheless, there are good reasons to believe that there are many other windows of opportunity for change, some developmentally based and some triggered by changes in context or by crisis itself.

CHAPTER 12

CONCLUSIONS AND FUTURE DIRECTIONS

The science on resilience in young people was motivated by the idea that understanding pathways of positive adaptation and development among individuals threatened by hazardous life circumstances would provide knowledge about the processes leading to resilience. This knowledge was expected to inform efforts to promote resilience and prevent or mitigate the consequences of adversity for development. What have we learned after half a century of effort by numerous investigators and what are the implications for science and action? What do we need to know? What are promising directions for future research? In this concluding chapter, I present a summary of major lessons and enduring controversies gleaned from the research to date on resilience in children and youth, and their implications for practice and policy. In closing, I comment on new horizons.

LESSONS FROM RESEARCH ON RESILIENCE IN YOUNG PEOPLE

The science on resilience in development is always growing, of course, but it is useful to take stock periodically on progress and conclusions, as well as the gaps and controversies. What follows is my take on major "lessons learned" as of this writing based on the resilience research discussed in this volume and the broader developmental science on resilience in young people.

Resilience Is Common

Evidence of human resilience is readily observable in all but the most dire circumstances, across diverse situations and cultures. Certainly, there are situations so extreme that no child develops normally. Yet under many challenging conditions, resilience is widely observed in human development and typical after short-lived, acute traumatic experiences that do not compromise fundamental adaptive systems. This observation surprised many of the early investigators, perhaps because research on risk had so often highlighted the bad outcomes. Many children recover from traumatic experiences, overcome socioeconomic disadvantages to do well economically, or become effective parents despite their own experiences of neglect or abuse.

Resilience appears to be the norm when children have access to typical human adaptive systems and when the threat is within the bounds of human capacity for response. The greatest dangers to children for lasting harm arise when prolonged, extreme threats exhaust all capacity for resilience and persist for too long or damage key adaptive systems beyond recovery. There is evidence of enduring consequences when developmental timing is bad, altering the organism in ways that compromise future development. Indeed, there is great interest among current investigators in delineating the parameters of severity, cumulative risk, and timing that determine the boundaries for resilience and recovery in human development.

Resilience Depends on a Multitude of Ordinary Adaptive Systems

Positive adaptation and development in the aftermath of adversity in children and youth are common under all but the most extreme situations because resilience depends on ordinary human adaptive systems that are characteristic of human organisms, cultures, and societies. These can be described at many levels from the molecular to the societal. Fundamental psychosocial systems for resilience include attachment relationships and families; neuropsychological systems of learning and problem solving, self-regulation, mastery motivation, and meaning making; and cultural traditions or organizations that nurture these systems, such as religions or schools. These systems have evolved and changed over many generations of human evolution, and now are species typical, though varied. Some of these systems, such as the neurocognitive systems involved in thinking or meaning making, operate within the individual person, though all of them have been influenced more or less by many interactions of the individual with his or her context over time. Other systems function in relationships, particularly in the relationships that children or adults have with attachment figures and caregivers, including family members, friends, romantic partners, mentors, and others (living and spiritual). Additional capacity arises from adaptive systems that people have created over time in cultures, communities, organizations, and societies, in many forms, ranging from emergency response systems to cultural practices.

The capacity for adaptation in adversity is distributed across many interconnected systems, within individuals, in relationships, families, and many other systems. As a result, building resilience for individuals involves attention to systems beyond the individual. For the resilience of young children, for example, it is vital to attend to caregiving systems.

There is considerable redundancy in the complex network of adaptive systems in the lives of children, although clearly some children have greater depth or more backup systems than other children. A child living in an isolated and impoverished region when disaster strikes is likely to have less immediate access to resources and emergency services than a child in a more populated, wealthier region. Similarly, children embedded in large and close kinship or cultural networks where people routinely help one another are likely to have more resources available in a crisis than less well-connected children.

Adaptive Systems Can Be Hijacked

The adaptive systems that comprise "ordinary magic" for children, including attachment relationships and reward systems for learning and succeeding, systems that generate much of the adaptive capacity associated with better function and recovery from adversities, can be "hijacked" or diverted for purposes and goals that others could judge as negative or evil. Human skills and capabilities can be utilized for many purposes. The motivation to succeed that sees a child through hardships at home to academic success could also be directed at criminal success. Reward circuits that produce pleasure in accomplishments can become dependent on drugs. Friendship that affords social support during adversity could also lead to gang activity.

In other words, adaptive systems can be directed in ways that would not result in outcomes approved of by parents, communities, or societies. Some young people flounder because they do not have adequate capacity to overcome the challenges facing them. Others have the capabilities for overcoming adversity but they have chosen to go down a path or adopt goals at odds with those of their families or communities. It is interesting to observe in community disaster situations when young people who are viewed as "bad" or maladaptive pitch in to help and apply their capabilities for the common good. Such circumstances may represent an opportunity to recover the talents of disillusioned youth by reengaging them in mainstream society.

There Are Many Paths of Resilience

Given that many systems are involved in adaptive function and response to adversities, there are many ways that resilience can emerge and many paths of resilience. This observation is congruent with the view in ecology that the "key to resilience in social–ecological systems is diversity" (Resilience Alliance, 2002). Just as every person has a unique course of development due to myriad interactions over time across many levels of function that shape a human life and personality, there are diverse ways for individuals to adapt successfully to adversity. The adaptive systems that support resilience are continually changing and the developing individual is continually changing, resulting in many possibilities for reactivity and response to threats over the life course. Nonetheless, there are regularities observed in patterns of manifested resilience and in the adaptive systems implicated most often in research on resilience, just as there are regularities in human development and personality. These regularities have made it possible to draw conclusions about resilience and depict trajectories of resilience in the aftermath of disaster and other adversities.

Resilience Frameworks for Action Include Risk Prevention and Mitigation

Preventing or mitigating risk is an important aspect of a resilience framework for action, whether preparing for expected disasters or risk factors, such as hurricanes or terrorism or premature birth, or responding to unexpected shocks. As repeatedly observed in the resilience literature described in this book, dose matters, and focusing on resilience does not mean ignoring risk. Attention to risk prevention or mitigation is important for preparing individuals, families, or communities for resilience in adversity.

There is rising international concern about the numbers of children globally exposed to "toxic stress" in the form of experiences that can alter development in lasting and negative ways. These include prenatal stress, child abuse and neglect, and malnutrition. Toxic stress experiences threaten the development of multiple adaptive systems in children. Moreover, there appear to be sensitive periods when children are more vulnerable to the effects of these adversities.

Developmental Timing Matters

Research on risk and resilience has made it clear that timing matters. During gestation, the timing of exposure to radiation, malnutrition, or stress can alter the course of development in different ways. Developmental timing can influence the nature of toxic stress exposures as well as the nature of coping skills and the protective relationships available.

Capacity for adaptive function changes for many reasons, including development itself. Resilience is dynamic and the capacity of an individual to manage similar kinds of threats and stressors would be expected to vary over the life course. Typical patterns of development in cognitive skills, for example, would alter perceptions and responses to potential danger. Advances in knowledge and thinking skills may simultaneously increase awareness of threats and their long-term significance, increasing stress, while also improving cognitive skills for problem solving and planning. Consequently, a developmental approach is important for preparing families or communities for disasters and other adversities.

Resilience Can Be Promoted

Diverse experiments to prevent problems and promote competence indicate that resilience can be promoted by many different strategies. Promoting general resilience in individuals—the capacity for effective handling of variable adversities—is akin to promoting healthy development or normal operations across multiple systems in the individual, family, and community. Nurturing and protecting brain development and function in a child to foster the capabilities of the human central nervous system, for example, requires many years of effort by a family and community, with a combination of water, nutrients, caregiving, discipline, education, medical care, and other experiences, including experience handling adversity. The resilience of children, as noted throughout this volume, depends on the resilience of other systems, and particularly the resilience of families.

Fostering resilience with respect to specific adversities or threats also is feasible. In this case, preparation focuses on bolstering the specific systems that will be taxed by the expected nature of the adversity and in many cases practicing specific skills and stockpiling particular kinds of expertise or resources. In "tornado alley" regions, it makes sense to prepare specifically for tornadoes by practicing what to do when a tornado is imminent, conducting regular school tornado drills, teaching children a family safety plan, building safe rooms, installing warning systems, and ensuring adequate responders and equipment will be available for the anticipated nature of the damage. These preparations are expected to enhance resilience for tornadoes in tornado-risky areas, but they would not make sense in a community where tornadoes rarely if ever occur. Knowledge of risk and vulnerabilities, whether at the individual, family, or community level, is vital for specific, strategic investments in resilience.

Preparing children for particular adverse experiences is similar to disaster planning. Many families and classrooms actively and specifically prepare children to handle bullying, racism, aggression, and sexual harassment. Schools increasingly train teachers and children about what to do in the event of terror attacks and shootings. Yet, even as they prepare children to respond, families and communities also act to prevent or reduce exposures to dangerous situations of violence or other controllable dangers. There are hazards so damaging and toxic that no children should ever have to face them.

No Child Is Invulnerable

Resilience research illuminates human capacity for adaptation and recovery, while also revealing the boundaries and limitations of resilience. Development is undermined by extreme or prolonged adversities, and particularly the experiences of abuse, neglect, and life-threatening violence. At very high levels of adversity, the frequency of children who fare well generally falls, and there are conditions so adverse for human development that children cannot flourish. Many tales and legends have echoed the lesson of Achilles: No human individual is invulnerable.

IMPLICATIONS FOR PRACTICE AND POLICY

Resilience science has yielded ideas and findings with numerous implications for practice and policy. Some of these implications are specific to a narrow age band or a specific kind of threat, and others are broad, with applications in multiple adverse situations. The latter are emphasized here.

Resilience Frameworks

Resilience science has had a transformational effect on frameworks for practice and policy. A profound shift has occurred in multiple fields of practice, with parallel shifts emerging in policies at local, state, and national levels. For children, this shift is evident in the models of practice and training for school counseling, social work, family therapy, special education, nursing, pediatrics, and child psychiatry (see Chapter 11). For example, the focus on facilitating resilience, enhancing strengths, and promoting health or competence can be observed in policies and practices designed to support military families (Cozza & Lerner, 2013) and the effectiveness of fighting forces in the military (Cornum et al., 2011). Prevention frameworks for reducing various risky or undesirable behaviors, including addiction, delinquency, and school dropout, have shifted or broadened their focus to encompass the promotion of positive development. New questions have come to the fore: What works? Who succeeds and how? What can be done to improve the odds of success for these children at risk?

At a global level, there are many signs that international agencies concerned with the well-being of children have expanded and refocused their efforts on positive development. There are numerous meetings and books that reflect a shift toward resilience promotion as a goal of policy and practice: reforming child welfare to focus on the development of competence (e.g., Flynn et al., 2006); promoting human development in the context of global economic crisis (e.g., Lundberg & Wuermli, 2012); building the wealth of nations through investments in early childhood, which was the theme of a 2010 UNESCO conference; fulfilling the potential of immigrant youth (e.g., Masten, Liebkind, & Hernandez, 2012b); and advancing the positive development of children through early childhood policies and interventions (e.g., Britto, Engle, & Super, 2013). Agencies once concerned primarily with the survival of children are raising the bar to promote human potential and life-long health.

Competence Cascades

There is growing awareness that competence begets competence, in the sense that the achievements in one period of development scaffold achievements later in development in new domains of function (Heckman, 2006; Masten, Burt, et al., 2006). Thus, investments and interventions in one period of development can be viewed as efforts to generate a positive cascade of effects on future development (Masten & Cicchetti, 2010c). The acquisition of skills in one period of development become the tools for building competence in new areas. There appears to be a high return on early investments in child development in part because of these cascading positive effects. Success in key developmental tasks also reduces the odds of later problems, because children end up on different pathways, in better contexts, with more resources and relationships with prosocial adults and friends, and with more opportunities.

Strategic Targeting and Timing

Growing evidence on what matters for whom and when in the developmental science on resilience has additional implications for policy and practices aiming to improve competence and reduce problems in development. There are some windows of opportunity and vulnerability in development when positive or negative experiences have more lasting consequences, and some windows when certain adversities are more likely to occur and thus more vigilance is required to protect children. Radiation is a physical stressor that can have dire consequences on the health and well-being of any human individual, but it has particular effects on a developing fetus, depending on timing as well as dose. We are learning that emotional stressors for a pregnant mother alter the physical environment of the developing fetus, with potentially lasting consequences for health and development.

There also are sensitive periods in the development of adaptive systems when experience has a large impact on the development and nature of a key adaptive system itself. The development of language and the immune system provide examples. Given suitable experiences at the right time in development, children become more adapted to the context in which they are developing, learning the language of the family and community or adapting to the microbes in the environment. However, the window of sensitivity, when the organism easily adapts itself to the environment, may close, making it more difficult to adjust if a child moves to a new location to learn a new language or avoid asthma and gastrointestinal issues.

Some adversities are more likely to occur during particular periods of development or affect older and younger children differently. Infants are less exposed than teenagers to many adversities, due to differences in their cognitive abilities, competence capabilities, mobility, and social relationships. Exposures to specific kinds of abuse or bullying, recruitment as a child soldier, and many other specific adversities vary in relation to age, and prevention efforts can be targeted to those risk patterns as well as the capabilities of children at different ages for getting help or helping themselves. Infants are very dependent and often more protected by adults than teenagers, although this makes them more vulnerable than older youth to loss of caregiving. Adolescents are more politically motivated than children, which also alters their risks of exposure.

The cascade literature suggests that timing is important for interrupting negative cascades as well as generating positive consequences. After negative effects have spread to new areas of function, solving the original problem (such as aggressive behavior) may not undo the damage in other domains (such as school or peer relations). At the least, more effort may be required to get development back on course if multiple domains of function have been negatively affected.

Similarly, there are windows of opportunity for change implicated in the resilience literature, when it appears to be easier to redirect the course of development. Some are early and others are later in development. These appear to be periods of system instability and change, either in the organism, in the context, or both, when human plasticity is high and there is potential to shape development through experiences. When living systems are destabilized by various kinds of perturbations, vulnerability may rise but also potential for positive change. Preschool, early adolescence, and the transition to adulthood, for example, appear to be periods with high potential for shaping development through intervention or enrichment. Societies implicitly acknowledge these windows with special activities to direct development, such as rituals and rites of passage or special training opportunities (e.g., preschool, apprenticeship).

Priorities: Nurture, Protect, and Restore Fundamental Adaptive Systems

The resilience literature also suggests priorities for investment and response, focused on fundamental adaptive systems that support or protect human resilience. Children need water, food, shelter, safety, and medical care, but they also need attachment security, family, opportunities to play and learn, and a meaningful place in society. Protecting brain development, supporting family resilience, emergency services suitable to children, and access to education are all examples of high priorities for building or restoring child resilience.

Disaster response and planning highlight the importance of priorities for children (see Chapter 5). For example, in the report of the National Commission on Children and Disasters (2010) and a follow-up workshop (Institute of Medicine, 2013), priorities were discussed for children that align well with a resilience framework. These include ensuring that appropriate pediatric medical equipment and procedures are available in emergency response vehicles and hospitals, training first responders about children, supporting families, keeping children and attachment figures together, reestablishing routines like school, and mitigating risk, including media exposure.

At a global level, the U.N. Convention on the Rights of the Child implicitly conveys endorsement of similar priorities, although these are expressed in terms of the human rights of children. The Convention, for example, includes a set of rights to life, development, and reaching one's full potential, as well as rights to care, family, nationality, and protection from harm.

CAVEATS: ENDURING CONTROVERSIES AND ISSUES IN RESILIENCE SCIENCE

Over the decades, as resilience science expanded and matured, numerous criticisms and controversies arose (Cicchetti & Garmezy, 1993; Egeland et al., 1993; Luthar et al., 2000; Masten, 1999; Rutter, 1987, 1990). Some waxed and waned, while others have endured or resurfaced in a new form (Masten, 2012a, 2013b, 2014). Key enduring issues are highlighted here.

Definitional Problems: What Is Resilience?

Many of the criticisms of resilience science have focused on definitional issues. Some of these problems probably stem from using a term from common language applied to disparate phenomena in everyday life. Resilience connotes the springing back of a rubber band, the bouncing back of a ball, the hardiness of a weed, the strength of galvanized steel, the buoyancy of a life raft, the pluckiness of an impoverished child, and underlying strengths of a business or market economy, as well as the recovery of a person from shocks or setbacks. Other issues probably derive from the challenges of defining behavior or operations of complex, dynamic systems. There were debates about whether resilience is a process, an emergent property resulting from many processes, a positive outcome under difficult circumstances, a life-course pattern, a trait, or all of these (Luthar, 2006; Masten, 1999, 2012a; Schoon, 2006).

The early investigators also faced the challenge of operationalizing the concept of resilience through measures and analytic strategies. Some began by identifying resilient individuals, often operationalized in terms of individuals who showed good function or development (by some criteria) in combination with a history of risk or adversity exposure. As discussed in earlier chapters, these individuals were typically compared to other people with comparable risk or adversity who were not faring as well. Thus, resilience was studied by comparing people who had a track record of success by some criteria of interest despite high-risk status or high-adversity exposure with others in similar situations who were maladaptive. Their resilience, in other words, had been demonstrated in observable, measureable ways. Some of the early investigators argued that the "resilience" in these individuals varied among the members of the groups, could result from many processes, and might be transient. Others viewed resilience more like a personality trait, like hardiness, that was enduring.

Adding to the definitional struggles was the duality of adaptive function in living systems, which can be evaluated with respect to internal function or external adaptation (Masten & Coatsworth, 1995). A human individual must succeed in maintaining his or her equilibrium internally (e.g., body temperature, emotional well-being) and also interact effectively with the world (e.g., finding food, getting along with other people). In resilience theory, scholars debated whether to include internal well-being in the definition of "doing well" or just focus on domains of external competence (e.g., school success). Should happiness always or ever be a criterion for resilience?

Over the years, most definitions of resilience have shifted toward a systems perspective, referring in some way to adaptive processes or the presumed capacity for adaptive responses to challenges in life. There seems to be a consensus that many processes at multiple levels of organization are involved in responding effectively to challenging life circumstances. Yet, there is still no consensus on how exactly to operationally define and study resilience. As a result, it rarely has been feasible to conduct meta-analyses of research on resilience, because there is not enough consistency in measures or analyses to compile the necessary data for such an aggregate analysis. Nonetheless, as noted numerous times in this volume, the conclusions from this rather large body of research continue to show considerable consistency despite the struggles with definition.

Measurement Problems: Who Decides on the Criteria?

Efforts to study resilience require measurement along with conceptual definitions. Whether investigators began by identifying groups of resilient children or used a variable-focused approach to understand good outcomes in the aftermath of adversity, they had to delineate criteria for defining the aspects of positive adjustment, adaptation, or development of interest in their studies. As described in the first section of this book, early investigators took different approaches to defining "doing okay." Some focused on achievements in age-salient developmental tasks and others focused on avoidance of psychopathology. In any event, it was clear that to start learning about resilience, one had to make decisions and judgments about both components typically used to define resilience for research: adaptive behavior and risk. These choices raised a host of issues about "who decides" the criteria. Pragmatically, of course, investigators decide, often with approval of granting agencies and internal review boards that monitor responsible conduct of research at universities. But their choices can be challenged, and often were.

Some of the critiques about the criteria for measuring resilience focused on the internal–external criteria issue noted above, while others focused on cultural issues. The criteria for assessing success in life are always culturally influenced, though this was not often acknowledged in early research. Investigators simply adopted the cultural criteria of their own majority culture (and historical context). But even at the outset, there were scholars pointing out that the criteria for positive adjustment or development varied across cultural contexts, even within the same community or society. For young people living in multicultural contexts, including many immigrants or youth from religious or ethnic-minority families, their adaptive success might be evaluated by different criteria at home and at school, or by their success at navigating these multiple expectations.

The Pollyanna Problem: Is Resilience More Than Positive Reframing of Risk and Vulnerability?

One of the earliest controversies in resilience science spoke to the "glass half full or half empty" issue, whether the positive focus characterizing resilience studies was really something new or a change in wording. This issue also could be called the "Pollyanna" issue, where critics dismissed the new approach as a simplistic reframing of old research on risk and vulnerability that provided nothing truly new and different. Like Pollyanna of the popular children's book and film, were resilience scholars just looking on the bright side of what was known already based on risk research? Critics argued this case (e.g., Tarter & Vanyukov, 1999), and early reviews of the new field by pioneers articulated the issue (e.g., Rutter, 1987). Scholars countered that resilience perspectives shifted the focus of attention to include different people, processes, and goals, with beneficial effects on both quality of research and its applications, while also mitigating some of the hazards of exclusively risk-focused research (Luthar, 2006; Masten, 2007, 2011; Rutter, 1990, 2006). This issue is currently being revisited in the context of the emerging neurobiology of resilience, as scientists search for processes that promote positive adaptation or mitigate risk independently of the processes that confer risk or vulnerability. Similarly, efforts to promote positive development through interventions or enrichment among children at risk for poor developmental outcomes, discussed in the previous chapter, are seeking to foster competence or bolster adaptive systems using strategies that deviate considerably from efforts to remove risk or prevent psychopathology (Masten, 2011). There is growing attention to the possibility that interventions focused on promoting competence and resilience, particularly if timed and targeted strategically, offer high benefit-to-cost returns and potentially more cascade effects than efforts focused exclusively on reducing problems (Heckman, 2006; Masten, Long, Kuo, McCormick, & Desjardins, 2009).

The Right Stuff: Is There a Resiliency Trait?

One of the most enduring issues in the resilience literature concerns the question of resiliency as a trait (Masten, 2012a; Rutter, 1979). This idea is likely a natural outgrowth of the term itself, in that resilience could be viewed as a trait of an object like a rubber band. We even talk about rubber bands losing their resiliency as they get dried out and brittle. Additionally, the notion of a trait of "hardiness" (Kobasa, 1979) or "ego resiliency" (Block & Block, 1980) came to this literature from theories (mostly adult-derived) of personality. However, there is very little evidence to support the supposition that there is a general trait of resilience (Panter-Brick & Leckman, 2013). And there is considerable risk of "blaming the victim" of adversity who does not manifest this purported trait.

The idea that there is a general trait of resilience is akin to arguing that there is a general trait of "healthiness." Like health, resilience arises from many influences across levels of organisms and their environments. While some individuals may be blessed with more positive resources, families, or immune systems that contribute to their adaptability, much more than any single trait is involved in either health or resilience.

Assuming that there is a trait of resilience that can be strengthened generates a serious ethical risk for concluding that children or adults who do not fare well in response to adversity are somehow deficient or do not have the "right stuff." There is no right stuff for every situation and no single trait for coping well with adversity. Many resources and systems are involved in adaptive behavior and recovery of children at risk for different reasons, and many of them are not "in" the child. Thus, I think the idea of a resilience trait is misguided. At the same time, I would agree that the capacity for positive adaption to adversities can be strengthened in a variety of ways.

Does Resilience Exact a Toll? Is There a Price for Resilience?

Another intriguing question that has been asked for decades about resilience is whether it comes with a cost. This idea has two forms. One is that individuals who endure great adversity do not come away from these experiences without some kind of scarring or lasting effects. The "girl in the picture," Kim Phuc, provides a powerful image of this form of cost, with her scars from napalm burns. In this form, cost is attributable to adversity rather than resilience. Similarly, in our studies of Cambodian youth who survived the killing fields of Pol Pot (see Chapter 5), we observed high rates of recurrent PTSD and depression, although most of these individuals as young adults were doing well by many of the criteria we used to judge resilience, such as academic and work achievement and good social functioning.

The other form of cost actually stems from positive achievement itself, in the sense that striving to overcome adversity could be taxing or stressful. In a chronically stressful environment, resilience could require enormous effort and generate additional stress. One of the classic studies of resilience, following the children of Kauai over the decades, raised the possibility of a cost to resilience in the midlife follow-up report (Werner & Smith, 2001). These investigators observed that individuals in the resilient group in midlife manifested more health problems than expected, and more than their high-risk but less adaptive peers. These health problems, such as back problems and problems with weight, appeared to be stress related.

This issue has reemerged recently in a study of allostatic load among successful African American youth who are part of a longitudinal study (Brody et al., 2013). In a provocatively titled report ("Is Resilience Only Skin Deep?"), these investigators found that the young people from high-risk backgrounds (high cumulative SES-related risks) who were judged competent in early adolescence and reassessed at age 19 showed a combination of good psychosocial adjustment but high allostatic load. Allostatic load indicators, such as high blood pressure and body mass index, are associated with a history of prolonged stress and future risk for health problems. The authors suggest that resilience among these youth came with a price related to the stress of success in a context of economic adversity and racism, in the form of physiological wear and tear. It is not totally clear whether the "price" resulted from the added strain of success-related stressors, and replication is in order, but the multilevel assessments of adaptive well-being represented by this study illustrate some of the interesting new directions of contemporary resilience science. This new work promises to illuminate old issues and raise new ones.

NEW HORIZONS

The fourth wave of resilience science is well under way as investigators pursue knowledge on adaptive processes and strategies for promoting resilience at multiple levels of analysis. Half a century of research has indicated "hot spots" for further research even as developments in science and technology open up new horizons (Masten, 2007). Intensive research is under way to gain a better understanding of change processes, developmental timing, and individual differences in sensitivity to experience, including brain plasticity, related to resilience. Improved methods are rapidly becoming available for studying processes at many levels of analysis that shape child development in relation to adverse experiences. These range from assessments of gene expression to statistical modeling of recovery trajectories following a natural disaster. There is a keen interest in the processes and experiences that shape adaptive systems fundamental to health and positive development and central to resilience. Many of these systems appear to undergo "programming" through experiences that hone them for the expected environment. Sometimes this tuning of organism to environment goes awry. There already is discussion about the possibilities of protecting children from negative programming effects or recalibrating adaptive systems.

There is considerable interest in the idea of differential sensitivity to experience, both in regard to whether this sensitivity itself is shaped by early experiences and to its significance for intervention. This set of ideas, articulated by Belsky, Boyce, Ellis, and numerous others (see Chapter 7 and elsewhere in this volume), has revolutionized thinking about how interventions might be tailored to individual differences. Sensitive children may be more responsive to interventions as well as more responsive to adversity, and less sensitive children may need more intensive or completely different intervention strategies. Moreover, there is evidence suggesting that differential responsiveness may be measurable at a biological level prior to initiating an intervention, so that efforts to promote resilience through training or treatment could be tailored to individual differences. Undoubtedly this line of inquiry will turn out to be more complex than delineated in early work, but it illustrates one of the intriguing new directions of resilience science. It also underscores an old point in the resilience literature: Protective factors are functional; they depend on the context. The same attribute may be protective in one situation and hazardous in another.

Generally, research on the neurobiological systems and processes involved in resilience is expanding rapidly, as highlighted in Chapter 7. There always was interest in these processes among resilience scientists, but the tools for measuring genetic and epigenetic processes, neural function, and many other neurobiological systems, especially in humans, were limited. Advances in brain imaging, mapping the human genome, and noninvasive measures of biological markers and processes have generated a surge of research on neurobiological processes and their interplay with behavioral and social processes in resilience.

Research on cultural processes and resilience in diverse contexts also is burgeoning. As noted in Chapter 10, the lack of attention to culture was criticized in this literature for decades. Now, there is a growing body of evidence as well as interest in cultural perspectives on resilience. Moreover, international concerns about millions of children in developmental jeopardy from trauma and adversity—including disasters, war, maltreatment, exploitation, and extreme poverty—are motivating interest among influential governmental and nongovernmental agencies, policymakers, and

funders in better-quality evidence to inform policies and programs.

Simultaneously, there are rising concerns about climate
change, economic crises, and contagious diseases leading many
sciences and sectors to consider resilience on a global scale around
issues that require integrative thinking and action. Conferences
sponsored by the Resilience Alliance, along with the Stockholm
Resilience Centre and other international organizations, have
drawn international scientists together to integrate ideas and
knowledge on resilience across many levels of analysis and disciplines. Their conferences (e.g., Resilience 2008) and publications
(e.g., *Ecology and Society*) highlight the interdependence of human
and ecological systems and the complexity of social–ecological
adaptive systems. Similar efforts to integrate knowledge and solutions across sectors have focused on resilience in cities. The Rock-
efeller Foundation celebrated its centennial with a call for propos-
als on "The Resilient City," and their vision has been articulated on
their website in terms of resilience: "To build resilience by helping
individuals and communities prepare for, withstand, and emerge
stronger from acute shocks and chronic stresses" (retrieved March
23, 2014 from *www.rockefellerfoundation.org/our-focus*).

These movements to integrate ideas and knowledge about
resilience require shared understanding of terminology and meaning. While there is a surprising degree of similarity across different disciplines in the meaning of resilience, there also are differences (Masten & Obradović, 2008; Zolli & Healy, 2012). Some of
these variations stem from the differences in systems under study
(computer system vs. human child), while others stem from differences in values (the life of an individual organism is likely to
have different value in research on human development as compared with research on the microbiome or fisheries). Nonetheless, there is likely to be some convergence of ideas, meaning, and
methods as the integration of resilience sciences moves forward.
Given the common roots of many sciences in systems theory and
the compelling motivation of global problems to solve, a set of
scalable system concepts seems possible. Ideally, resilience would

be defined in such a way that this concept could be applied across many levels from the molecular to the planetary.

As I bring this book to a close, there is global turbulence of many forms: in the weather, in politics, in the stock market, and in the lives of many individual children who are growing up in chaos or danger. There also is a surge of interest in resilience across many sectors and growing recognition that individual human resilience depends on the resilience of families, communities, and many other systems. The complexity of human life and development can be daunting but there is discernible progress in what we know about specific systems and adaptive processes that influence human development and how to change or shape those processes to improve the odds for positive development. There is a sufficient body of knowledge on resilience in children to guide policy and practice even as exciting new directions of research are pursued.

Children in danger cannot wait for resilience science. Research on resilience will continue to advance, but in the meantime, there is a substantial body of knowledge at hand for guiding efforts to promote resilience in children. It is heartening to observe the progress and consistencies in the extant literature noted throughout this volume. Moreover, it is important to keep in mind the most fundamental lesson from the research on resilience, which is the thesis of this book. Human resilience usually arises from the operation of ordinary and common adaptive systems, both inside and outside of people, and not from rare or extraordinary actions, resources, or processes. Thus, there are reasons for optimism about the possibilities of shifting the odds in favor of success for young people at risk due to adversities past, present, or yet to come. There is an ever-expanding knowledge base that can guide efforts to improve the odds for positive development and there are many pathways to resilience. Evidence mounts that we can foster resilience of children and youth in many ways at many levels of human interaction with investments that have the potential to cascade forward in time to benefit not only young people themselves but also their families, communities, societies, and future generations.

GLOSSARY

Adversity	Experiences that threaten function, development, or survival of an individual or system.
Assets	Advantages or resources associated with positive (desirable) outcomes; predictors of positive outcome.
Competence	Capability for effective function in the environment; manifested capacity for positive adaptation in regard to accomplishing expected developmental tasks.
Developmental cascade	Spreading effects over time that result from interactions in dynamic systems across domains, levels, systems, or generations that cumulatively alter the course of development.
Developmental tasks	Physical or psychosocial milestones or accomplishments expected for individuals in a given period of development in ecological and historical context.
Dose gradient	Refers in resilience science typically to a graph showing a pattern of rising problems or undesirable outcomes as the level of trauma, exposure to disaster, or number of cumulative risk factors increases; in intervention research, this concept refers to rising level of desirable outcomes or falling symptom levels as the exposure to treatment increases.

Human capital	Individual skills and attributes viewed as valuable to economies, families, or societies because they predict productivity or other kinds of success in life.
Late bloomers	Individuals from high-risk backgrounds who begin to manifest resilience later in adolescence or adulthood following a period of maladaptation.
Promotive factor	Predictor of a positive (desired) outcome under both low- and high-risk conditions (associated with statistical main effects).
Protective factor	Moderator of risk associated with better (desired) outcomes when risk is high than when risk is low (associated with statistical interaction effects); a predictor of desirable outcomes particularly in high-risk or adversity contexts.
Resilience	Capacity (potential or manifested) of a dynamic system to adapt successfully to disturbances that threaten system function, viability, or development; positive adaptation or development in the context of significant adversity exposure.
Resiliency	Property of a material, object, or system to withstand stresses or spring back to its original form; sometimes used to describe a human personality trait (of questionable validity).
Resource	Used synonymously in resilience research with an asset or promotive factor.
Risk	Higher probability of a negative (undesired) outcome.
Risk factor	Indicator of risk for a specified negative or undesirable outcome in a group or population.

Risk gradient	Dose gradient showing a rising level of some negative outcome (or falling level of a positive outcome) as a function of higher scores on a risk or cumulative measure; see Figure 2.6.
Social capital	Assets, resources, promotive factors, or protective factors available through a person's relationships and social connections.
Stress	Effects of disturbances in an individual or system that disrupt adaptive functions; response of a dynamic system to challenges or demands.
Stressors	Events or experiences that typically result in stress on a system of interest.
Turnaround cases	Individuals who show a striking change in direction of the life course; in resilience science, referring specifically to positive changes in adaptive function.
Vulnerability	Individual or system susceptibility or sensitivity specific to harmful consequences from threats or disturbances; moderator of adversity or risk that results in higher-than-typical negative effects.

APPENDIX B

ABBREVIATIONS

APA	American Psychological Association
EF	Executive function
HHM	Homeless or highly mobile
HPA	Hypothalamic–pituitary–adrenal axis involved in stress response
LEQ	Life Events Questionnaire
LG	Licking and grooming; referring in this volume to high-LG or low-LG rats that show high or low levels of this parenting behavior with their rat pups
PCLS	Project Competence Longitudinal Study
PTS/PTSD	Posttraumatic stress; posttraumatic stress disorder
RCT	Randomized controlled trial; an experimental intervention with random assignment to treatment and control groups
SES	Socioeconomic status

RECOMMENDED READINGS BY TOPIC

HISTORY OF RESILIENCE SCIENCE

Cicchetti, D. (2010). Resilience under conditions of extreme stress: A multilevel perspective. *World Psychiatry, 9,* 145–154.

Luthar, S. S. (2006). Resilience in development: A synthesis of research across five decades. In D. Cicchetti & D. J. Cohen (Eds.), *Developmental psychopathology: Vol. 3. Risk, disorder, and adaptation* (2nd ed., pp. 739–795). Hoboken, NJ: Wiley.

Masten, A. S. (2012). Resilience in children: Vintage Rutter and beyond. In A. Slater & P. Quinn (Eds.), *Developmental psychology: Revisiting the classic studies* (pp. 204–221). London: Sage.

Wright, M. O'D., Masten, A. S., & Narayan, A. J. (2013). Resilience processes in development: Four waves of research on positive adaptation in the context of adversity. In S. Goldstein & R. B. Brooks (Eds.), *Handbook of resilience in children* (pp. 15–37). New York: Springer.

BIOGRAPHIES AND AUTOBIOGRAPHIES OF RESILIENCE IN YOUNG PEOPLE

Angelou, M. (1970). *I know why the caged bird sings.* New York: Random House.

Beah, I. (2007). *A long way gone: Memoirs of a boy soldier.* New York: Crichton Books.

Chong, D. (2000). *The girl in the picture: The story of Kim Phuc, the photograph, and the Vietnam War*. New York: Viking Penguin.

Comer, J. P. (1988). *Maggie's American dream: The life and times of a black family*. New York: New American Library.

Criddle, J. D. (1998). *To destroy you is no loss: The odyssey of a Cambodian family* (2nd ed.). Auke Bay, Alaska: East/West Bridge Publishing House.

Fisher, A. (with Rivas, M. E.). (2001). *Finding fish*. New York: HarperCollins.

Murray, L. (2010). *Breaking night: A memoir of forgiveness, survival, and my journey from homeless to Harvard*. New York: Hyperion.

Smart, E., & Stewart, C. (2013). *My story*. New York: St. Martin's Press.

CLASSIC PUBLICATIONS ON RESILIENCE (BEFORE 2000)

Anthony, E. J., & Cohler, B. J. (Eds.). (1987). *The invulnerable child*. New York: Guilford Press.

Cicchetti, D., & Garmezy, N. (Eds.). (1993). Prospects and promises in the study of resilience [Special issue]. *Development and Psychopathology, 5*, 497–783.

Egeland, B., Carlson, E., & Sroufe, L. A. (1993). Resilience as process. *Development and Psychopathology, 5*, 517–528.

Garmezy, N. (1985). Stress-resistant children: The search for protective factors. In J. E. Stevenson (Ed.), *Recent research in developmental psychopathology: Journal of child psychology and psychiatry book supplement #4* (pp. 213–233). Oxford, UK: Pergamon Press.

Garmezy, N., & Rutter, M. (Eds.). (1983). *Stress, coping, and development in children*. New York: McGraw-Hill.

Lewis, J. M., & Looney, J. G. (1983). *The long struggle: Well-functioning working-class black families*. New York: Brunner/Mazel.

Masten, A. S., Best, K. M., & Garmezy, N. (1990). Resilience and development: Contributions from the study of children who overcome adversity. *Development and Psychopathology, 2*, 425–444.

Masten, A. S., & Coatsworth, J. D. (1998). The development of competence in favorable and unfavorable environments: Lessons from research on successful children. *American Psychologist, 53*, 205–220.

Murphy, L. B., & Moriarty, A. E. (1976). *Vulnerability, coping, and growth: From infancy to adolescence*. New Haven, CT: Yale University Press.

Rutter, M. (1979). Protective factors in children's responses to stress and disadvantage. In M. W. Kent & J. E. Rolf (Eds.), *Primary prevention of psychopathology: Vol. 3. Social competence in children* (pp. 49–74). Hanover, NH: University Press of New England.

Rutter, M. (1987). Psychosocial resilience and protective mechanisms. *American Journal of Orthopsychiatry, 57,* 316–331.

Werner, E. E., & Smith, R. S. (1982). *Vulnerable but invincible: A study of resilient children.* New York: McGraw-Hill.

CLASSIC STUDIES OF RESILIENCE

High Valley Resilience Study

Hauser, S. T., Allen, J. P., & Golden, E. (2006). *Out of the woods: Tales of resilient teens.* Cambridge, MA: Harvard University Press.

Kauai Longitudinal Study

Werner, E. E. (1989). Children of the garden island. *Scientific American, 260*(4), 106–111.

Werner, E. E., & Smith, R. S. (1982). *Vulnerable but invincible: A study of resilient children.* New York: McGraw-Hill.

Werner, E. E., & Smith, R. S. (1992). *Overcoming the odds: High risk children from birth to adulthood.* Ithaca, NY: Cornell University Press.

Werner, E. E., & Smith, R. S. (2001). *Journeys from childhood to midlife: Risk, resilience, and recovery.* Ithaca, NY: Cornell University Press.

Minnesota Study of Risk and Adaptation from Birth to Adulthood

Sroufe, L. A., Egeland, B., Carlson, E. A., & Collins, A. W. (2005). *The development of the person: The Minnesota study of risk and adaptation from birth to adulthood.* New York: Guilford Press.

Project Competence Longitudinal Study

Garmezy, N., Masten, A. S., & Tellegen, A. (1984). The study of stress and competence in children: A building block for developmental psychopathology. *Child Development, 55,* 97–111.

Masten, A. S., & Tellegen, A. (2012). Resilience in developmental psychopathology: Contributions of the Project Competence Longitudinal Study. *Development and Psychopathology, 24,* 345–361.

Rochester Child Resilience Project

Cowen, E. L., Work, W. C., & Wyman, P. A. (1997). The Rochester Child Resilience Project (RCRP): Facts found, lessons learned, future directions divined. In S. S. Luthar, J. A. Burack, D. Cicchetti, & J. R. Weisz (Eds.), *Developmental psychopathology: Perspectives on adjustment, risk, and disorder* (pp. 527–547). New York: Cambridge University Press.

Cowen, E. L., Wyman, P. A., Work, W. C., & Parker, G. R. (1990). The Rochester Child Resilience Project (RCRP): Overview and summary of first year findings. *Development and Psychopathology, 2,* 193–212.

Wyman, P. A. (2003). Emerging perspectives on context specificity of children's adaptation and resilience: Evidence from a decade of research with urban children in adversity. In S. S. Luthar (Ed.), *Resilience and vulnerability: Adaptation in the context of childhood adversities* (pp. 293–317). New York: Cambridge University Press.

Unraveling Juvenile Delinquency: Glueck Archives and Follow-Ups by Laub and Sampson

Laub, J. H., & Sampson, R. J. (2003). *Shared beginnings, divergent lives: Delinquent boys to age 70.* Cambridge, MA: Harvard University Press.

Sampson, R. J., & Laub, J. H. (1993). *Crime in the making: Pathways and turning points through the life course.* Cambridge, MA: Harvard University Press.

CHILDREN IN POVERTY AND ECONOMIC CRISES

Elder, G. H., Jr. (1999). *Children of the great depression: Social change in life experience.* Boulder, CO: Westview Press. (Original work published in 1974 by University of Chicago Press)

Elder, G. H., Jr., & Conger, R. D. (2000). *Children of the land: Adversity and success in rural America.* Chicago: University of Chicago Press.

Lundberg, M., & Wuermli, A. (Eds.). (2012). *Children and youth in crisis: Protecting and promoting human development in times of economic shocks.* Washington, DC: World Bank.

Schoon, I. (2006). *Risk and resilience: Adaptations in changing times.* New York: Cambridge University Press.

Walker, S. P., Wachs, T. D., Grantham-McGregor, S., Black, M. M., Nelson, C. A., Huffman, S. L., et al. (2011). Inequality in early childhood: Risk and protective factors for early child development. *Lancet, 378,* 1325–1338.

Yoshikawa, H., Aber, J. L., & Beardslee, W. R. (2012). The effects of poverty on the mental, emotional, and behavioral health of children and youth: Implications for prevention. *American Psychologist, 67,* 272–284.

RESILIENCE IN THE CONTEXT OF CHILD MALTREATMENT

Cicchetti, D. (2013). Annual research review: Resilient functioning in maltreated children—past, present, and future perspectives. *Journal of Child Psychology and Psychiatry, 54,* 402–422.

Herrenkohl, T. I. (Ed.). (2013). Developmental foundations of resilience and positive coping in children exposed to violence and chronic stress [Special issue]. *Trauma, Violence, and Abuse, 14,* 191–266.

Kilka, J. B., & Herrenkohl, T. I. (2013). A review of developmental research on resilience in maltreated children. *Trauma, Violence, and Abuse, 14,* 222–234.

Whitelock, C. F., Lamb, M. E., & Rentfrow, P. J. (2013). Overcoming trauma: Psychological and demographic characteristics of child sexual abuse survivors in adulthood. *Clinical Psychological Science, 1,* 351–362.

CHILDREN IN DISASTER, WAR, AND POLITICAL CONFLICT

American Psychological Association. (2010). *Resilience and recovery after war: Refugee children and families in the United States.* Washington, DC: Author.

Barber, B. K. (Ed.). (2009a). *Adolescents and war: How youth deal with political violence.* New York: Oxford University Press.

Betancourt, T. S., & Khan, K. T. (2008). The mental health of children affected by armed conflict: Protective processes and pathways to resilience. *International Review of Psychiatry, 20,* 317–328.

Dimitry, L. (2012). A systematic review on the mental health of children and adolescents in areas of armed conflict in the Middle East. *Child: Care, Health, and Development, 38,* 153–161.

Furr, J. M., Comer, J. S., Edmunds, J. M., & Kendall, P. C. (2010). Disasters and youth: A meta-analytic examination of posttraumatic stress. *Journal of Consulting and Clinical Psychology, 78,* 765–780.

La Greca, A. M., Silverman, W. K., Vernberg, E. M., & Roberts, M. C. (2002). *Helping children cope with disasters and terrorism.* Washington, DC: American Psychological Association.

Masten, A. S., & Narayan, A. J. (2012). Child development in the context of disaster, war and terrorism: Pathways of risk and resilience. *Annual Review of Psychology, 63,* 227–257.

Masten, A. S., Narayan, A. J., Silverman, Q. K., & Osofsky, J. D. (2015). Children in war and disaster. In R. M. Lerner (Ed.), M. H. Bornstein, & T. Leventhal (Vol. Eds.), *Handbook of child psychology and developmental science: Vol. 4. Ecological settings and processes in developmental systems* (7th ed.). New York: Wiley.

National Commission on Children in Disasters. (2010). *2010 Report to the President and Congress.* AHRQ Publication No. 10-M037. Rockville, MD: Agency for Healthcare and Research Quality.

National Research Council (2013). *Preparedness, response, and recovery considerations for children and families: Workshop Summary.* Washington, DC: The National Academies Press.

Norris, F. H., Steven, S. P., Pfefferbaum, B., Wyche, K. F., & Pfefferbaum, R. L. (2008). Community resilience as a metaphor, theory, set of capacities, and strategy for disaster readiness. *American Journal of Community Psychology, 41,* 127–150.

Osofsky, H. J., & Osofsky, J. D. (2013). Hurricane Katrina and the Gulf Oil Spill: Lessons learned. *Psychiatric Clinics of North America, 36,* 371–383.

Werner, E. E. (2000). *Through the eyes of innocents: Children witness World War II.* Boulder, CO: Westview Press.

THE NEUROBIOLOGY OF RESILIENCE

Cicchetti, D. (2013). Annual research review: Resilient functioning in maltreated children—past, present, and future perspectives. *Journal of Child Psychology and Psychiatry, 54,* 402–422.

Feder, A., Nestler, E. J., & Charney, D. S. (2009). Psychobiology and molecular genetics of resilience. *Nature Reviews Neuroscience, 10*, 446–457.

Hochberg, Z., Feil, R., Constancia, M., Fraga, M., Junien, C., Carel, J. C., et al. (2011). Child health, developmental plasticity, and epigenetic programming. *Endocrine Reviews, 32*(2), 159–224.

Karatsoreos, I. N., & McEwen, B. S. (2013). Annual research review: The neurobiology and physiology of resilience and adaptation across the life course. *Journal of Child Psychology and Psychiatry, 54*, 337–347.

Kim-Cohen, J., & Turkewitz, R. (2012). Resilience and measured gene-environment interactions. *Development and Psychopathology, 24*, 1297–1306.

Raby, K. L., & Roisman, G. I. (2013). Gene–environment interplay and risk and resilience during childhood. *Encyclopedia of Early Childhood Development*. Retrieved from *www.child-encyclopedia.com/PDF/Raby-RoismanANGxp1.pdf*.

Russo, S. J., Murrough, J. W., Han, M.-H., Charney, D. S., & Nestler, E. J. (2012). Neurobiology of resilience. *Nature Neuroscience, 15*, 1475–1484.

Southwick, S. M., Litz, B. T., Charney, D., & Friedman, M. J. (Eds.). (2011). *Resilience and mental health: Challenges across the lifespan*. New York: Cambridge University Press.

FAMILY RESILIENCE

Becvar, D. S. (Ed.). (2013). *Handbook of family resilience*. New York: Springer.

Cozza, S. J., & Lerner, R. M. (Eds.). (2013). Military children and families: Introducing the issue [Special issue]. *Future of Children, 23*. Retrieved from *http://futureofchildren.org/futureofchildren/publications/journals/article/index.xml?journalid=80&articleid=587&sectionid=4073&submit*.

Goldenberg, H., & Goldenberg, I. (2013). *Family therapy: An overview* (8th ed.). Belmont, CA: Brooks/Cole.

Henry, C. S., Criss. M. M., Harrist, A. W., & Larzelere, R. I. (Eds.). (2015). Special issue: Interdisciplinary approaches to strengthening family and individual resilience: Conceptual, empirical and practical innovations. *Family Relations, 64*(1), 1–189.

Patterson, J. M. (2002). Integrating family resilience and family stress theory. *Journal of Marriage and Family, 64*, 349–360.

Walsh, F. (2006). *Strengthening family resilience* (2nd ed.). New York: Guilford Press.

RESILIENCE PROCESSES IN EDUCATION

Doll, B. (2013). Enhancing resilience in classrooms. In S. Goldstein & R. B. Brooks (Eds.), *Handbook of resilience in children* (pp. 399–410). New York: Springer.

Durlak, J. A., Weissberg, R. P., & Pachan, M. (2010). A meta-analysis of after-school programs that seek to promote personal and social skills in children and adolescents. *American Journal of Community Psychology, 45,* 294–309.

Fleming, J. L., Mackrain, M., & LeBuffe, P. A. (2013). Caring for the caregiver: Promoting the resilience of teachers. In S. Goldstein & R. B. Brooks (Eds.), *Handbook of resilience in children* (2nd ed., pp. 387–397). New York: Springer.

Galassi, J. P., & Akos, P. (2007). *Strength-based school counseling: Promoting student development and achievement.* Mahwah, NJ: Erlbaum.

Tough, P. (2009). *Whatever it takes: Geoffrey Canada's quest to change Harlem and America.* New York: Mariner Books.

CULTURAL PROCESSES IN RESILIENCE

Crawford, E., Wright, M. O., & Masten, A. S. (2006). Resilience and spirituality in youth. In E. C. Roehlkepartain, P. E. King, L. Wagener, & P. L. Benson (Eds.), *The handbook of spiritual development in childhood and adolescence* (pp. 355–370). Thousand Oaks, CA: Sage.

Kağitçibaşi, Ç. (2007). *Family, self, and human development across cultures: Theories and applications* (2nd ed.). Mahwah, NJ: Erlbaum.

Masten, A. S., Liebkind, K., & Hernandez, D. J. (Eds.). (2012). *Realizing the potential of immigrant youth.* New York: Cambridge University Press.

Panter-Brick, C. (2014). Health, risk, and resilience: Interdisciplinary concepts and applications. *Annual Review of Anthropology, 43,* 431–448.

Ungar, M. (Ed.). (2012). *The social ecology of resilience: A handbook of theory and practice.* New York: Springer.

Ungar, M., Ghazinour, M., & Richter, J. (2013). What is resilience within the social ecology of human development? *Journal of Child Psychology and Psychiatry, 54,* 348–366.

PREVENTION, INTERVENTION, AND POLICY

Ager, A. (2013). Annual research review: Resilience and child well-being—public policy implications. *Journal of Child Psychology and Psychiatry, 54,* 488–500.

Bhutta, Z. A., Chopra, M., Axelson, H., Berman, P., Boerma, T., Bryce, J., et al. (2010). Countdown to 2015 decade report (2000–10): Taking stock of maternal, newborn, and child survival. *Lancet, 375,* 2032–2044.

Britto, P. R., Engle, P. L., & Super, C. M. (Eds.). (2013). *Handbook of early childhood development research and its impact on global policy.* New York: Oxford University Press.

Brody, G. H., Beach, S. R. H., Philibert, R. A., Chen, Y., & Murry, V. M. (2009). Prevention effects moderate the association of *5-HTTLPR* and youth risk behavior initiation: Gene × environment hypotheses tested via a randomized prevention design. *Child Development, 80,* 645–661.

Brody, G. H., Chen, Y. F., & Beach, S. R. (2013). Differential susceptibility to prevention: GABAergic, dopaminergic, and multilocus effects. *Journal of Child Psychology and Psychiatry, 54,* 863–871.

Heckman, J. J. (2006). Skill formation and the economics of investing in disadvantaged children. *Science, 312,* 1900–1902.

Masten, A. S. (2011). Resilience in children threatened by extreme adversity: Frameworks for research, practice, and translational synergy. *Development and Psychopathology, 23,* 141–154.

Nelson, C. A., Zeanah, C. H., Fox, N. A., Marshall, P. J., Smyke, A. T., & Guthrie, D. (2007). Cognitive recovery in socially deprived young children: The Bucharest Early Intervention Project. *Science, 318,* 1937–1940.

Patterson, G. R., Forgatch, M. S., & DeGarmo, D. S. (2010). Cascading effects following intervention. *Developmental Psychopathology, 22,* 941–970.

Rutter, M. (2013). Annual research review: Resilience—clinical implications. *Journal of Child Psychology and Psychiatry, 54,* 474–487.

Shonkoff, J. P. (2011). Protecting brains, not simply stimulating minds. *Science, 333,* 982–983.

REFERENCES

Achenbach, T. M. (1991). *Manual for the Child Behavior Checklist/4-18 and 1991 Profile.* Burlington: University of Vermont, Department of Psychiatry.

Adler N. E., & Ostrove, J. M. (2006). Socioeconomic status and health: What we know and what we don't. *Annals of the New York Academy of Sciences, 896,* 3–15.

Adolphs, R. (2009). The social brain: Neural basis of social knowledge. *Annual Review of Psychology, 60,* 693–716.

Ager, A. (2013). Annual research review: Resilience and child well-being—public policy implications. *Journal of Child Psychology and Psychiatry, 54,* 488–500.

Ager, A., Stark, L., Akesson, B., & Boothby, N. (2010). Defining best practice in care and protection of children in crisis-affected settings: A Delphi study. *Child Development, 81,* 1270–1286.

Ainsworth, M. D. S. (1989). Attachments beyond infancy. *American Psychologist, 44,* 709–716.

Akos, P., & Galassi, J. P. (2008). Strengths-based school counseling: Introduction to the special issue. *Professional School Counseling, 12,* 66–67.

Alderman, H. (Ed.). (2011). *No small matter: The impact of poverty, shocks, and human capital investments in early childhood development.* Washington, DC: World Bank.

Alexander, G. R., & Kotelchuck, M. (2001). Assessing the role and effectiveness of prenatal care: History, challenges, and directions for future research. *Public Health Reports, 116,* 306–316.

Alink, L. R. A., Cicchetti, D., Kim, J., & Rogosch, F. A. (2009). Mediating and moderating processes in the relation between maltreatment and psychopathology: Mother–child relationship quality and emotion regulation. *Journal of Abnormal Child Psychology, 37,* 831–843.

Amato, P. R. (2010). Research on divorce: Continuing trends and new developments. *Journal of Marriage and Family Therapy, 72,* 650–666.

American Psychiatric Association. (1987). *Diagnostic and statistical manual of mental disorders* (3rd ed., rev.). Washington, DC: Author.

American Psychological Association. (2010). *Resilience and recovery after war: Refugee children and families in the United States.* Washington, DC: Author.

American School Counselor Association. (2005). *The ASCA national model: A framework for school counseling programs* (2nd ed.). Alexandria, VA: Author.

Anderson, A. R., Christenson, S. L., Sinclair, M. F., & Lehr, C. A. (2004). Check & Connect: The importance of relationships for promoting engagement with school. *Journal of School Psychology, 42,* 95–113.

Anderson, L. (1994). Effectiveness and efficiency in inner-city public schools: Charting school resilience. In M. C. Wang & E. W. Gordon (Eds.), *Educational resilience in inner-city America* (pp. 141–149). Hillsdale, NJ: Erlbaum.

Angelou, M. (1971). *I know why the caged bird sings.* New York: Bantam Books.

Angold, A., Costello, E. J., & Erkanli, A. (1999). Comorbidity. *Journal of Child Psychology and Psychiatry, 40,* 57–87.

Anthony, E. K., Alter, C. F., & Jenson, J. M. (2009). Development of a risk and resilience-based out-of-school time program for children and youths. *Social Work, 54,* 45–55.

Ayalon, O. (1983). Coping with terrorism: The Israeli case. In D. Meichenbaum & M. Jaremko (Eds.), *Stress reduction and prevention* (pp. 293–340). New York: Plenum Press.

Ayduk, O., Mendoza-Denton, R., Mischel, W., Downey, G., Peake, P. K., & Rodriguez, M. (2000). Regulating the interpersonal self: Strategic self-regulation for coping with rejection sensitivity. *Journal of Personality and Social Psychology, 79,* 776–792.

Baker, D. P., Salinas, D., & Eslinger, P. J. (2012). An envisioned bridge: Schooling as a neurocognitive developmental institution. *Developmental Cognitive Neuroscience, 25,* S6–S17.

Bakermans-Kranenburg, M. J., van IJzendoorn, M. H., Pijlman, F. T. A., Mesman, J., & Juffer, F. (2008). Experimental evidence for differential susceptibility: Dopamine D4 receptor polymorphism (DRD4 VNTR) moderates intervention effects on toddlers' externalizing behavior in a randomized controlled trial. *Developmental Psychology, 44,* 293–300.

Bandura, A. (1982). Self-efficacy mechanism in human agency. *American Psychologist, 37,* 122–147.

Bandura, A. (1997). *Self-efficacy: The exercise of control.* New York: Freeman.

Barber, B. K. (2008). Contrasting portraits of war: Youths' varied experiences with political violence in Bosnia and Palestine. *International Journal of Behavioral Development, 32,* 298–309.

Barber, B. K. (Ed.). (2009a). *Adolescents and war: How youth deal with political violence.* New York: Oxford University Press.

Barber, B. K. (2009b). Making sense and no sense of war: Issues of identity and meaning in adolescents' experience with political conflict. In B. K. Barber (Ed.), *Adolescents and war: How youth deal with political violence* (pp. 281–311). New York: Oxford University Press.

Barber, B. K., & Schluterman, J. M. (2009). An overview of the empirical literature on adolescents and political violence. In B. K. Barber (Ed.), *Adolescents and war: How youth deal with political violence* (pp. 35–61). New York: Oxford University Press.

Baumrind, D. (1966). Effects of authoritative parental control on child behavior. *Child Development, 37*, 887–907.

Baumrind, D. (1991). The influence of parenting style on adolescent competence and substance use. *Journal of Early Adolescence, 11*, 56–95.

Baumrind, D. (1996). The discipline controversy revisited. *Family Relations, 45*, 405–414.

Beah, I. (2007). *A long way gone: Memoirs of a boy soldier.* New York: Crichton Books.

Beardslee, W. R., Gladstone, T. R. G., & O'Connor, E. E. (2011). Transmission and prevention of mood disorders among children of affectively ill parents: A review. *Journal of the American Academy of Child and Adolescent Psychiatry, 50*, 1098–1109.

Beck, A. N., & Tienda, M. (2012). Better fortunes?: Living arrangements and school enrollment of migrant youth in six western countries. In A. S. Masten, K. Liebkind, & D. J. Hernandez (Eds.), *Realizing the potential of immigrant youth* (pp. 41–62). New York: Cambridge University Press.

Becker-Blease, K. A., Turner, H. A., & Finkelhor, D. (2010). Disasters, victimization, and children's mental health. *Child Development, 81*, 1040–1052.

Becvar, D. S. (Ed.). (2013). *Handbook of family resilience.* New York: Springer.

Beeghly, M., & Tronick, E. (2011). Early resilience in the context of parent–infant relationships: A social developmental perspective. *Current Problems in Pediatric and Adolescent Health Care, 41*, 197–201.

Belsky, J. (2012). Quality, quantity and type of childcare: Effects on child development in the U.S. In G. Bentley & R. Mace (Eds.), *Subsitute parents: Biological and social perspectives on alloparenting in human societies.* New York: Berghahn Books.

Belsky, J., Bakermans-Kranenburg, J. M., & van IJzendoorn, M. H. (2007). For better *and* for worse: Differential susceptibility to environmental influences. *Current Directions in Psychological Science, 16*, 300–304.

Belsky, J., & de Haan, M. (2011). Annual research review: Parenting and children's brain development: The end of the beginning. *Journal of Child Psychology and Psychiatry, 52*, 409–428.

Belsky, J., & Pluess, M. (2009). Beyond diathesis stress: Differential susceptibility to environmental influences. *Psychological Bulletin, 135*, 885–908.

Benn, R., Akiva, T., Arel, S., & Roeser, R. W. (2012). Mindfulness training effects for parents and educators of children with special needs. *Developmental Psychology, 48*, 1476–1487.

Benson, P. L., Scales, P. C., Hamilton, S. F., & Sesma, A., Jr. (2006). Positive youth development: Theory, research and applications. In W. Damon & R. M. Lerner (Eds.), *Handbook of child psychology: Vol. 1. Theoretical models of human development* (6th ed., pp. 894–941). New York: Wiley.

Berger, R., & Gelkopf, M. (2009). School-based intervention for the treatment of tsunami-related distress in children: A quasi-randomized controlled trial. *Psychotherapy and Psychosomatics, 78*, 364–371.

Bergman, L. A., & Magnusson, D. (1997). A person-oriented approach in research on developmental psychopathology. *Development and Psychopathology, 9*, 291–319.

Bernard, B. (2003). Turnaround teachers and schools. In B. Williams (Ed.), *Closing the achievement gap: A vision for changing beliefs and practices* (2nd ed., pp. 115–137). Alexandria, VA: Association for Supervision and Curriculum Development.

Berry, J. W., Phinney, J. S., Sam, D. L., & Vedder, P. (Eds.). (2006). *Immigrant youth in cultural transition: Acculturation, identity, and adaptation across national contexts.* Mahwah, NJ: Erlbaum.

Best, J. R., & Miller, P. H. (2010). A developmental perspective on executive function. *Child Development, 81,* 1641–1660.

Betancourt, T. S., Borisova, I. I., Williams, T. P., Brennan, R. T., Whitfield, T. H., De La Soudiere, M., et al. (2010). Sierra Leone's former child soldiers: A follow-up study of psychosocial adjustment and community reintegration. *Child Development, 81,* 1077–1095.

Betancourt, T. S., & Khan, K. T. (2008). The mental health of children affected by armed conflict: Protective processes and pathways to resilience. *International Review of Psychiatry, 20,* 317–328.

Betancourt, T. S., McBain, R., Newnham, E. A., & Brennan, R. T. (2013). Trajectories of internalizing problems in war-affected Sierra Leonean youth: Examining conflict and postconflict factors. *Child Development, 84,* 455–470.

Bialystok, E., & Craik, F. I. M. (2010). Cognitive and linguistic processing in the bilingual mind. *Current Directions in Psychological Science, 19,* 19–23.

Bierman, K. L., Domitrovich, C. E., Nix, R. L., Gest, S. D., Welsh, J. A., Greenberg, M. T., et al. (2008). Promoting academic and social–emotional school readiness: The Head Start REDI program. *Child Development, 79,* 1802–1817.

Bierman, K. L., Nix, R. L., Greenberg, M. T., Blair, C., & Domitrovich, C. E. (2008). Exeuctive funtions and school readiness intervention: Impact, moderation, and mediation in the Head Start REDI program. *Development and Psychopathology, 20,* 821–843.

Blackburn, E. H., & Epel, E. S. (2012). Too toxic to ignore. *Nature, 490,* 169–171.

Blair, C. (2002). School readiness: Integrating cognition and emotion in a neurobiological conceptualization of children's functioning at school entry. *American Psychologist, 57,* 111–127.

Blair, C. (2006). How similar are fluid cognition and general intelligence?: A developmental neuroscience perspective on fluid cognition as an aspect of human cognitive ability. *Behavioral and Brain Sciences, 29,* 109–125.

Blair, C., & Raver, C. C. (2012). Individual development and evolution: Experiential canalization of self-regulation. *Developmental Psychology, 48,* 647–657.

Block, J. H., & Block, J. (1980). The role of ego-control and ego-resiliency in the organization of behavior. In W. A. Collins (Ed.), Development of cognition, affect, and social relations. *Minnesota Symposia on Child Psychology, 13,* 39–101.

Boelcke, K., & Masten, A. S. (2001, August). *How do young adults versus developmental psychologists judge competence?* Paper presented at the annual meeting of the American Psychological Association, San Francisco.

Bokszczanin, A. (2008). Parental support, family conflict, and overprotectiveness: Predicting PTSD symptom levels of adolescents 28 months after a natural disaster. *Anxiety, Stress and Coping, 21*, 325–335.

Bonanno, G. A., Brewin, C. R., Kaniasty, K., & Greca, A. M. L. (2010). Weighing the costs of disaster. *Psychological Science in the Public Interest, 11*, 1–49.

Bond, L. A., & Hauf, A. M. C. (2004). Taking stock and putting stock in primary prevention: Characteristics of effective programs. *Journal of Primary Prevention, 24*, 199–221.

Boothby, N., Crawford, J., & Halperin, J. (2006). Mozambique child soldier life outcome study: Lessons learned in rehabilitation and reintegration efforts. *Global Public Health: An International Journal for Research, Policy and Practice, 1*, 87–107.

Bornstein, M. H., Britto, P. R., Nonoyama-Tarumi, Y., Ota, Y., Petrovic, O., & Putnick, D. L. (2012). Child development in developing countries: Introduction and methods. *Child Development, 83*, 16–31.

Boss, P. (2001). *Family stress management: A contextual approach* (2nd ed.). Thousand Oaks, CA: Sage.

Botvin, G. J., & Griffin, K. W. (2004). Life skills training: Empirical findings and future directions. *Journal of Primary Prevention, 25*, 211–232.

Botvin, G. J., & Tortu, S. (1988). Preventing adolescent substance abuse through life skills training. In R. H. Price, E. L. Cowen, R. P. Lorion, & J. Ramos-McKay (Eds.), *Fourteen ounces of prevention: A casebook for practitioners* (pp. 98–110). Washington, DC: American Psychological Association.

Bowen, M. (1993). *Family therapy in clinical practice*. Lanham, MD: Rowman & Littlefield.

Bowlby, J. (1977). The making and breaking of affectional bonds: 1. Aetiology and psychopathology in the light of attachment theory. *British Journal of Psychiatry, 130*, 201–210.

Bowlby, J. (1982). *Attachment and loss*. New York: Basic Books. (Original work published 1969)

Boyce, W. T. (2007). A biology of misfortune: Stress reactivity, social context, and the ontogeny of psychopathology in early life. In A. S. Masten (Ed.), Multilevel dynamics in developmental psychopathology: Pathways to the future. *Minnesota Symposia on Child Psychology, 34*, 45–82. Mahwah, NJ: Erlbaum.

Boyce, W. T., & Ellis, B. J. (2005). Biological sensitivity to context: I. An evolutionary–developmental theory of the origins and functions of stress reactivity. *Development and Psychopathology, 17*, 271–301.

Boyden, J., & Bourdillon, M. (Eds.). (2012). *Childhood poverty: Multidisciplinary Approaches*. London: Palgrave Macmillan.

Brancucci, A. (2012). Neural correlates of cognitive ability. *Journal of Neuroscience Research, 90*, 1299–1309.

Bretherton, I., & Munholland, K. A. (1999). Internal working models in attachment relationships: A construct revisited. In J. Cassidy & P. R. Shaver (Eds.), *Handbook of attachment: Theory, research, and clinical applications* (pp. 89–111). New York: Guilford Press.

Britto, P. R., Engle, P. L., & Super, C. M. (Eds.). (2013). *Handbook of early childhood development research and its impact on global policy.* New York: Oxford University Press.

Broderick, R. (2003). A surgeon's saga. *Minnesota, 104*(6), 26–31.

Brodsky, A. E. (2000). The role of religion in the lives of resilient, urban, African American, single mothers. *Journal of Community Psychology, 28*, 199–219.

Brody, G. H., Beach, S. R. H., Philibert, R. A., Chen, Y., & Murry, V. M. (2009). Prevention effects moderate the association of 5-*HTTLPR* and youth risk behavior initiation: Gene × environment hypotheses tested via a randomized prevention design. *Child Development, 80*, 645–661.

Brody, G. H., Chen, Y. F., & Beach, S. R. (2013). Differential susceptibility to prevention: GABAergic, dopaminergic, and multilocus effects. *Journal of Child Psychology and Psychiatry, 54*, 863–871.

Brody, G. H., Murry, V. M., Gerrard, M., Gibbons, F. X., Molgaard, V., McNair, L., et al. (2004). The Strong African American Families Program: Translating research into prevention programming. *Child Development, 75*, 900–917.

Brody, G. H., Murry, V. M., Kogan, S. M., Gerrard, M., Gibbons, F. X., Molgaard, V., et al. (2006). The Strong African American Families Program: A cluster-randomized prevention trial of long-term effects and a mediational model. *Journal of Consulting and Clinical Psychology, 74*, 356–366.

Bronfenbrenner, U. (1979). *The ecology of human development: Experiments by nature and design.* Cambridge, MA: Harvard University Press.

Bronfenbrenner, U., & Morris, P. A. (1998). The ecology of developmental processes. In W. Damon & R. M. Lerner (Eds.), *Handbook of child psychology: Vol. 1. Theoretical models of human development* (5th ed., pp. 993–1028). Hoboken, NJ: Wiley.

Brooks-Gunn, J., Duncan, G. J., & Britto, P. R. (1999). Are socioeconomic gradients for children similar to those adults?: Achievement and health of children in the United States. In D. P. Keating & C. Hertzman (Eds.), *Developmental health and the wealth of nations: Social, biological, and educational dynamics* (pp. 94–124). New York: Guilford Press.

Brophy, J. (2010). *Motivating students to learn* (3rd ed.). New York: Routledge.

Brown, G. W. (1974). Meaning, measurement, and stress of life events. In B. S. Dohrenwend & B. P. Dohrenwend (Eds.), *Stressful life events: Their nature and effects.* Oxford, UK: Wiley.

Brown, G. W., & Harris, T. (1978). *Social origins of depression: A study of psychiatric disorder in women.* New York: Free Press.

Brown, K., & Westaway, E. (2011). Agency, capacity, and resilience to environmental change: Lessons from human development, well-being, and disasters. *Annual Review of Environment and Resources, 36*, 321–342.

Buckner, J. C., Mezzacappa, E., & Beardslee, W. R. (2003). Characteristics of resilient youths living in poverty: The role of self-regulatory processes. *Development and Psychopathology, 15*, 139–162.

Buckner, J. C., Mezzacappa, E., & Beardslee, W. R. (2009). Self-regulation and its relations to adaptive functioning in low income youths. *American Journal of Orthopsychiatry, 79*, 19–30.

Buriel, R. (2012). Historical origins of the immigrant paradox for Mexican American students: The cultural integration hypothesis. In C. Garcia Coll

& A. K. Marks (Eds.), *The immigrant paradox in children and adolescents: Is becoming American a developmental risk?* (pp. 37–60). Washington, DC: American Psychological Association.

Burt, K. B., & Masten, A. S. (2010). Development in the transition to adulthood: Vulnerabilities and opportunities. In J. E. Grant & M. N. Potenza (Eds.), *Young adult mental health* (pp. 5–18). New York: Oxford University Press.

Burt, K. B., Obradović, J., Long, J. D., & Masten, A. S. (2008). The interplay of social competence and psychopathology over 20 years: Testing transactional and cascade models. *Child Development, 79,* 359–374.

Burton, L. M., Obeidallah, D. A., & Allison, K. (1996). Ethnographic insights on social context and adolescent development among inner-city African-American teens. In R. Jessor, A. Colby, & R. A. Shweder (Eds.), *Ethnography and human development: Context and meaning in social inquiry* (pp. 395–418). Chicago: University of Chicago Press.

Carlson, S. M., Zelazo, P. D., & Faja, S. (2013). Executive function. In P. D. Zelazo (Ed.), *Oxford handbook of developmental psychology* (pp. 706–743). New York: Oxford University Press.

Carter, C. S., & Porges, S. W. (2013). The biochemistry of love: An oxytocin hypothesis. *EMBO Reports, 14,* 12–16.

Carter, S. C. (2000). *No excuses: Lessons from 21 high-performing, high-poverty schools.* Washington, DC: Heritage Foundation.

Carver, L. J., & Cornew, L. (2011). The development of social information gathering in infancy: A model of neural substrates and developmental mechanisms. In M. de Haan & M. R. Gunnar (Eds.), *Handbook of developmental social neuroscience* (pp. 122–141). New York: Guilford Press.

Casey, E. C., Finsaas, M., Carlson, S. M., Zelazo, P. D., Murphy, B., Durkin, F., et al. (2014). Ready? Set. Go! A collaborative and iterative approach to promoting executive function in homeless and highly mobile preschoolers. In S. Prince-Embury & D. Saklofske (Eds.), *Resilience interventions for youth in diverse populations* (pp. 133–158). New York: Springer.

Caspi, A., McClay, J., Moffitt, T. E., Mill, J., Martin, J., Craig, I. W., et al. (2002). Role of genotype in the cycle of violence in maltreated children. *Science, 297,* 851–854.

Caspi, A., Moffitt, T. E., Morgan, J., Rutter, M., Taylor, A., Arseneault, L., et al. (2004). Maternal expressed emotion predicts children's antisocial behavior problems: Using monozygotic-twin differences to identify environmental effects on behavioral development. *Developmental Psychology, 40,* 149–161.

Cassidy, J., & Shaver, P. (Eds.). (2008). *Handbook of attachment: Theory, research, and clinical applications.* New York: Guilford Press.

Catani, C., Gewirtz, A. H., Wieling, E., Schauer, E., Elbert, T., & Neuner, F. (2010). Tsunami, war, and cumulative risk in the lives of Sri Lankan school children. *Child Development, 81,* 1176–1191.

Catani, C., Kohiladevy, M., Ruf, M., Schauer, E., Elbert, T., & Neuner, F. (2009). Treating children traumatized by war and tsunami: A comparison between exposure therapy and meditation-relaxation in North-East Sri Lanka. *BMC Psychiatry, 9,* 22.

Centers for Disease Control and Prevention. (2012). Youth risk behavior surveillance–United States, 2011. *Morbidity and Mortality Weekly Report, 61*, 1–168. Retrieved from *www.cdc.gov/mmwr/pdf/ss/ss6104.pdf.*

Chaffin, M., Silovsky, J. F., Funderburk, B., Valle, L. A., Brestan, E. V., Balachova, T., et al. (2004). Parent–child interaction therapy with physically abusive parents: Efficacy for reducing future abuse reports. *Journal of Consulting and Clinical Psychology, 72*, 500–510.

Charney, D. (2004). Psychobiological mechanisms of resilience and vulnerability: Implications for successful adaptation to extreme stress. *American Journal of Psychiatry, 161*, 195–216.

Chemtob, C. M., Nomura, Y., Rajendran, K., Yehuda, R., Schwartz, D., & Abramovitz, R. (2010). Impact of maternal posttraumatic stress disorder and depression following exposure to the September 11 attacks on preschool children's behavior. *Child Development, 81*, 1129–1141.

Chong, D. (2001). *The girl in the picture: The story of Kim Phuc, the photograph, and the Vietnam war.* New York: Penguin Books.

Christenson, S. L., Thurlow, M. L., Sinclair, M. F., Lehr, C. A., Kaibel, C. M., Reschly, A. L., et al. (2008). *Check and connect: A comprehensive student engagement intervention manual.* Minneapolis: University of Minnesota, Institute on Community Integration.

Cicchetti, D. (1984). The emergence of developmental psychopathology. *Child Development, 55*, 1–7.

Cicchetti, D. (2006). Development and psychopathology. In D. Cicchetti & D. Cohen (Eds.), *Developmental psychopathology: Vol. 1. Theory and method* (2nd ed., pp. 1–23). Hoboken, NJ: Wiley.

Cicchetti, D. (2010). Resilience under conditions of extreme stress: A multilevel perspective. *World Psychiatry, 9*, 145–154.

Cicchetti, D. (2013). Annual research review: Resilient functioning in maltreated children—past, present, and future perspectives. *Journal of Child Psychology and Psychiatry, 54*, 402–422.

Cicchetti, D., & Curtis, W. J. (2006). The developing brain and neural plasticity: Implications for normality, psychopathology, and resilience. In D. Cicchetti & D. Cohen (Eds.), *Developmental psychopathology: Vol. 2. Developmental neuroscience* (2nd ed., pp. 1–64). Hoboken, NJ: Wiley.

Cicchetti, D., & Garmezy, N. (1993). Editorial: Prospects and promises in the study of resilience. *Development and Psychopathology, 5*, 497–502.

Cicchetti, D., Rappaport, J., Sandler, I. N., & Weissberg, R. P. (Eds.). (2000). *The promotion of wellness in children and adolescents.* Washington, DC: CWLA Press.

Cicchetti, D., & Schneider-Rosen, K. (1986). An organizational approach to childhood depression. In M. Rutter, C. Izard, & P. Read (Eds.), *Depression in young people: Clinical and developmental perspectives* (pp. 71–134). New York: Guilford Press.

Cicchetti, D., Toth, S. L., & Lynch, M. (1995). Bowlby's dream comes full circle: The application of attachment theory to risk and psychopathology. *Advances in Clinical Child Psychology, 17*, 1–75.

Clarke-Stewart, A., & Dunn, J. (2006). *Families count: Effects on child and adolescent development.* New York: Cambridge University Press.

Clewell, B. C., Campbell, P. B., & Perlman, L. (2007). *Good schools in poor neighborhoods: Defying demographics, achieving success*. Washington, DC: Urban Institute Press.

Coddington, R. D. (1972a). The significance of life events as etiologic factors in the diseases of children: I. A survey of professional workers. *Journal of Psychosomatic Research, 16*, 7–18.

Coddington, R. D. (1972b). The significance of life events as etiologic factors in the diseases of children: II. A study of a normal population. *Journal of Psychosomatic Research, 16*, 205–213.

Cohen, J. (2012). Creating a positive school climate: A foundation for resilience. In S. Goldstein & R. B. Brooks (Eds.), *Handbook of resilience in children* (2nd ed., pp. 411–425). New York: Springer.

Collishaw, S., Pickles, A., Messer, J., Rutter, M., Shearer, C., & Maughan, B. (2007). Resilience to adult psychopathology following childhood maltreatment: Evidence from a community sample. *Child Abuse and Neglect, 31*, 211–229.

Comer, J. S., Furr, J. M., Beidas, R. S., Weiner, C. L., & Kendall, P. C. (2008). Children and terrorism-related news: Training parents in coping and media literacy. *Journal of Consulting and Clinical Psychology, 76*, 568–578.

Comer, J. S., & Kendall, P. C. (2007). Terrorism: The psychological impact on youth. *Clinical Psychology: Science and Practice, 14*, 182–212.

Compas, B. E., Jaser, S. S., Dunn, M. J., & Rodriguez, E. M. (2012). Coping with chronic illness in childhood and adolescence. *Annual Review of Clinical Psychology, 8*, 455–480.

Conger, K. J., Rueter, M. A., & Conger, R. D. (2000). The role of economic pressure in the lives of parents and their adolescents: The family stress model. In L. J. Crockett & R. K. Silbereisen (Eds.), *Negotiating adolescence in times of social change* (pp. 201–223). New York: Cambridge University Press.

Conger, R. D., & Conger, K. J. (2002). Resilience in midwestern families: Selected findings from the first decade of a prospective, longitudinal study. *Journal of Marriage and Family, 64*, 361–373.

Conger, R. D., & Elder, G. H., Jr. (1994). *Families in troubled times: Adapting to change in rural America*. Hawthorne, NY: de Gruyter.

Cooper, C. R. (1999). Multiple selves, multiple worlds: Cultural perspectives on individuality and connectedness in adolescent development. In A. S. Masten (Ed.), Cultural processes in child development. *Minnesota Symposia on Child Psychology, 29*, 25–57.

Cornum, R., Matthews, M. D., & Seligman, M. E. P. (2011). Comprehensive soldier fitness: Building resilience in a challenging institutional context. *American Psychologist, 66*, 4–9.

Cortes, L., & Buchanan, M. (2007). The experience of Columbian child soldiers from a resilience perspective. *International Journal for the Advancement of Counselling, 29*, 43–55.

Cowen, E. L., Wyman, P. A., Work, W. C., & Parker, G. R. (1990). The Rochester Child Resilience Project (RCRP): Overview and summary of first year findings. *Development and Psychopathology, 2*, 193–212.

Cozza, S. J., & Lerner, R. M. (Eds.). (2013). Military children and families: Introducing the issue [Special issue]. *Future of Children, 23,* 3–11.

Crawford, E., Wright, M. O., & Masten, A. S. (2006). Resilience and spirituality in youth. In E. C. Roehlkepartain, P. E. King, L. Wagener, & P. L. Benson (Eds.), *The handbook of spiritual development in childhood and adolescence* (pp. 355–370). Thousand Oaks, CA: Sage.

Crick, N. R., & Zahn-Waxler, C. (2003). The development of psychopathology in females and males: Current progress and future challenges. *Development and Psychopathology, 15,* 719–742.

Criddle, J. D. (1998). *To destroy you is no loss: The odyssey of a Cambodian family* (2nd ed.). Auke Bay, AK: East/West Bridge Publishing House.

Cryder, C. H., Kilmer, R. P., Tedeschi, R. G., & Calhoun, L. G. (2006). An exploratory study of posttraumatic growth in children following a natural disaster. *American Journal of Orthopsychiatry, 76,* 65–69.

Cummings, E. M. (2006). Marital conflict and children's functioning. *Social Development, 3,* 16–36.

Cummings, E. M., Davies, P. T., & Campbell, S. B. (2000). *Developmental psychopathology and family process.* New York: Guilford Press.

Cutuli, J. J. (2011). *Context, cortisol, and executive functions among children experiencing homelessness.* Unpublished doctoral dissertation, University of Minnesota, Minneapolis, MN.

Cutuli, J. J., Desjardins, C. D., Herbers, J. E., Long, J. D., Heistad, D., Chan, C., et al. (2013). Academic achievement trajectories of homeless and highly mobile students: Resilience in the context of chronic and acute risk. *Child Development, 84,* 841–857.

Cutuli, J. J., Herbers, J. E., Rinaldi, M., Masten, A. S., & Oberg, C. N. (2010). Asthma and behavior in homeless 4- to 7-year-olds. *Pediatrics, 125,* 145–151.

Dackis, C., & O'Brien, C. (2005). Neurobiology of addiction: Treatment and public policy ramifications. *Nature Neuroscience, 8,* 1431–1436.

Dahl, R. E., & Spear, L. P. (Eds.). (2004). *Adolescent brain development: Vulnerabilities and opportunities* (Vol. 1021). New York: New York Academy of Sciences.

Delahanty, D. L., & Nugent, N. R. (2006). Predicting PTSD prospectively based on prior trauma history and immediate biological responses. *Annals of the New York Academy of Sciences, 1071,* 27–40.

deVries, M. W. (1984). Temperament and infant mortality among the Masai of East Africa. *American Journal of Psychiatry, 141,* 1189–1194.

DeYoung, C. G. (2006). Higher-order factors of the Big Five in a multi-informant sample. *Journal of Personality and Social Psychology, 91,* 1138–1151.

DeYoung, C. G., Cicchetti, D., Rogosch, F. A., Gray, J. R., Eastman, M., & Grigorenko, E. L. (2011). Sources of cognitive exploration: Genetic variation in the prefrontal dopamine system predicts openness/intellect. *Journal of Research in Personality, 45,* 364–371.

Diamond, A., & Lee, K. (2011). Interventions shown to aid executive function development in children 4 to 12 years old. *Science, 333,* 959–964.

Dimitry, L. (2012). A systematic review on the mental health of children and adolescents in areas of armed conflict in the Middle East. *Child: Care, Health, and Development, 38,* 153–161.

DiRago, A. C., & Vaillant, G. E. (2007). Resilience in inner city youth: Childhood predictors of occupational status across the lifespan. *Journal of Youth and Adolescence, 36,* 61–70.

Dishion, T. J., & McMahon, R. J. (1998). Parental monitoring and the prevention of child and adolescent problem behavior: A conceptual and empirical formulation. *Clinical Child and Family Psychology Review, 1,* 61–75.

Doll, B. (2013). Enhancing resilience in classrooms. In S. Goldstein & R. B. Brooks (Eds.), *Handbook of resilience in children* (pp. 399–410). New York: Springer.

Doll, B., LeClair, C., & Kurien, S. (2009). Effective classrooms: Classroom learning environments that foster school success. In T. B. Gutkin & C. R. Reynolds (Eds.), *The handbook of school psychology* (4th ed., pp. 791–807). Hoboken, NJ: Wiley.

Dozier, M., Manni, M., Gordon, M. K., Peloso, E., Gunnar, M. R., Stovall-McClough, K. C., et al. (2006). Foster children's diurnal production of cortisol: An exploration study. *Child Maltreatment, 11,* 189–197.

Dozier, M., Peloso, E., Lewis, E., Laurenceau, J.-P., & Levine, S. (2008). Effects of an attachment-based intervention on the cortisol production of infants and toddlers in foster care. *Developmental Psychopathology, 20,* 845–859.

DuBois, D. L., Holloway, B. E., Valentine, J. C., & Cooper, H. (2002). Effectiveness of mentoring programs for youth: A meta-analytic review. *American Journal of Community Psychology, 30,* 157–197.

Dubow, E. F., Boxer, P., Huesmann, L. R., Landau, S., Dvir, S., Shikaki, K., et al. (2012). Cumulative effects of exposure to violence on posttraumatic stress in Palestinian and Israeli youth. *Journal of Clinical Child and Adolescent Psychology, 41,* 837–844.

Dubowitz, H., & Poole, G. (2012). Child neglect: An overview. *Encyclopedia on early childhood development.* Retrieved from *www.child-encyclopedia.com/pages/PDF/Dubowitz-PoolANGxp1.pdf.*

Duckworth, A. L. (2011). The significance of self-control. *Proceedings of the National Academy of Sciences, 108,* 2639–2640.

DuMont, K., Ehrhard-Dietzel, S., & Kirkland, K. (2012). Averting child maltreatment: Individual, economic, social, and community resources that promote resilient parenting. In M. Ungar (Ed.), *The social ecology of resilience: A handbook of theory and practice* (pp. 199–217). New York: Springer.

Duncan, G. J. (2012). Give us this day our daily breadth. *Child Development, 83,* 6–15.

Duncan, G. J., Ziol-Guest, K. M., & Kalil, A. (2010). Early-childhood poverty and adult attainment, behavior, and health. *Child Development, 81,* 306–325.

Dunn, L. M., & Markwardt, F. C. (1970). *Examiner's manual: Peabody Individual Assessment Test.* Circle Pines, MN: American Guidance Service.

Durbrow, E. H. (1999). Cultural processes in child competence: How rural

Caribbean parents evaluate their children. In A. S. Masten (Ed.), *Cultural processes in child development. Minnesota Symposia on Child Psychology, 29*, 97–121.

Durbrow, E. H., Peña, L. F., Masten, A. S., Sesma, A., & Williamson, I. (2001). Mothers' conceptions of child competence in contexts of poverty: The Philippines, St. Vincent, and the United States. *International Journal of Behavioral Development, 25*, 438–443.

Durlak, J. A. (2009). Prevention programs. In T. B. Gutkin & C. R. Reynolds (Eds.), *The handbook of school psychology* (pp. 905–920). Hoboken, NJ: Wiley.

Durlak, J. A., Weissberg, R. P., & Pachan, M. (2010). A meta-analysis of after-school programs that seek to promote personal and social skills in children and adolescents. *American Journal of Community Psychology, 45*, 294–309.

Dybdahl, R. (2001). Children and mothers in war: An outcome study of a psychosocial intervention program. *Child Development, 72*, 1214–1230.

Earls, M. F., & The Committee on Psychosocial Aspects of Child and Family Health. (2010). Incorporating recognition and management of perinatal and postpartum depression into pediatric practice. *Pediatrics, 126*, 1032–1039.

Eccles, J. S., Barber, B. L., Stone, M., & Hunt, J. (2003). Extracurricular activities and adolescent development. *Journal of Social Issues, 59*, 865–889.

Eccles, J. S., & Roeser, R. W. (2012). School influences on human development. In L. C. Mayes & M. Lewis (Eds.), *The Cambridge handbook of environment in human development* (pp. 259–283). New York: Cambridge University Press.

Edmonds, R. (1979). Effective schools for the urban poor. *Educational Leadership, 37*, 15–24.

Egeland, B., Carlson, E., & Sroufe, L. A. (1993). Resilience as process. *Development and Psychopathology, 5*, 517–528.

Eggerman, M., & Panter-Brick, C. (2010). Suffering, hope, and entrapment: Resilience and cultural values in Afghanistan. *Social Science and Medicine, 71*, 71–83.

Elder, G. H., Jr. (1998). The life course as developmental theory. *Child Development, 69*, 1–12.

Elder, G. H., Jr. (1999). *Children of the great depression: Social change in life experience*. Boulder, CO: Westview Press. (Originally work published in 1974 by University of Chicago Press)

Elder, G. H., Jr., & Conger, R. D. (2000). *Children of the land: Adversity and success in rural America*. Chicago: University of Chicago Press.

Elias, M. J., Zins, J. E., Graczyk, P. A., & Weissberg, R. P. (2003). Implementation, sustainability, and scaling up of social–emotional and academic innovations in public schools. *School Psychology Review, 32*, 303–319.

Elliott, D. S., Menard, S., Rankin, B., Elliott, A., Wilson, W. J., & Huizinga, D. (2006). *Good kids from bad neighborhoods: Successful development in social context*. New York: Cambridge University Press.

Ellis, B. J., Boyce, W. T., Belsky, J., Bakermans-Kranenburg, M. J., & van

IJzendoorn, M. H. (2011). Differential susceptibility to the environment: An evolutionary–neurodevelopmental theory. *Development and Psychopathology, 23*, 7–28.

Epel, E. S., Blackburn, E. H., Lin, J., Dhabhar, F. S., Adler, N. E., Morrow, J. D., et al. (2004). Accelerated telomere shortening in response to life stress. *Proceedings of the National Academy of Sciences of the United States of America, 101*, 17312–17315.

Erikson, E. H. (1963). *Childhood and society* (2nd ed.). New York: Norton.

Erikson, E. H. (1968). *Identity: Youth and crisis.* New York: Norton.

Erikson, K. T. (1976). *Everything in its path: Destruction of community in the Buffalo Creek flood.* New York: Simon & Schuster.

Ertl, V., Pfeiffer, A., Schauer, E., Elbert, T., & Neuner, F. (2011). Community-implemented trauma therapy for former child soldiers in Northern Uganda: A randomized controlled trial. *Journal of the American Medical Association, 306*, 503–512.

Essex, M. J., Shirtcliff, E. A., Burk, L. R., Ruttle, P. L., Klein, M. H., Slattery, M. J., et al. (2011). Influence of early life stress on later hypothalamic–pituitary–adrenal axis functioning and its covariation with mental health symptoms: A study of the allostatic process from childhood into adolescence. *Development and Psychopathology, 23*, 1039–1058.

Eth, S., & Pynoos, R. S. (Eds.). (1985). *Post-traumatic stress disorder in children.* Washington, DC: American Psychiatric Press.

Evans, A. B., Banerjee, M., Meyer, R., Aldana, A., Foust, M., & Rowley, S. (2012). Racial socialization as a mechanism for positive development among African American youth. *Child Development Perspectives, 6*, 251–257.

Evans, G. W., Li, D., & Sepanski Whipple, S. (2013). Cumulative risk and child development. *Psychological Bulletin, 139*, 1342–1396.

Evans, G. W., & Schamberg, M. A. (2009). Childhood poverty, chronic stress, and adult working memory. *Proceedings of the National Academy of Sciences of the United States of America, 106*, 6545–6549.

Fantuzzo, J., & Perlman, S. (2007). The unique impact of out-of-home placement and the mediating effects of child maltreatment and homelessness on early school success. *Child and Youth Services Review, 29*, 941–960.

Feder, A., Charney, D., & Collins, K. (2011). Neurobiology of resilience. In St. M. Southwick, B. T. Litz, D. Charney, & M. J. Friedman (Eds.), *Resilience and mental health: Challenges across the lifespan* (pp. 1–29). New York: Cambridge University Press.

Feder, A., Nestler, E. J., & Charney, D. S. (2009). Psychobiology and molecular genetics of resilience. *Nature Reviews Neuroscience, 10*, 446–457.

Felsman, J. K., & Vaillant, G. E. (1987). Resilient children as adults: A 40-year study. In E. J. Anthony & B. J. Cohler (Eds.), *The invulnerable child* (pp. 289–314). New York: Guilford Press.

Fernando, C., & Ferrari, M. (2011). Spirituality and resilience in children of war in Sri Lanka. *Journal of Spirituality in Mental Health, 13*, 52–77.

Ferrarese, M. J. (1981). *Reflectiveness—impulsivity and competence in children under stress.* Unpublished doctoral dissertation, University of Minnesota, Minneapolis, MN.

Fiese, B. H. (2006). *Family routines and rituals.* New Haven, CT: Yale University Press.

Fiese, B. H., Gundersen, C., Koester, B., & Washington, L. (2011). Household food insecurity: Serious concerns for child development. *Society for Research in Child Development Social Policy Report, 25*(3), 1–19.

Fisher, A., & Rivas, M. E. (2001). *Finding fish.* New York: HarperTorch.

Fisher, P. A., Gunnar, M. R., Dozier, M., Bruce, J., & Pears, K. C. (2006). Effects of therapeutic interventions for foster children on behavioral problems, caregiver attachment, and stress regulatory neural systems. *Annals of the New York Academy of Sciences, 1094,* 215–225.

Fisher, P. A., Van Ryzin, M. J., & Gunnar, M. R. (2011). Mitigating HPA axis dysregulation associated with placement changes in foster care. *Psychoneuroendocrinology, 36,* 531–539.

Fitzmaurice, G. M., Laird, N. M., & Ware, J. H. (2004). *Applied longitudinal analysis.* Hoboken, NJ: Wiley.

Fleming, J. L., Mackrain, M., & LeBuffe, P. A. (2013). Caring for the caregiver: Promoting the resilience of teachers. In S. Goldstein & R. B. Brooks (Eds.), *Handbook of Resilience in Children* (pp. 387–397). New York: Springer.

Flynn, R. J., Dudding, P. M., & Barber, J. G. (Eds.). (2006). *Promoting resilience in child welfare.* Ottawa, Canada: University of Ottawa Press.

Ford, M. E. (1985). The concept of competence: Themes and variations. In J. H. A. Harlowe & R. B. Weinberg (Eds.), *Competence development: Theory and practice in special populations* (pp. 3–49). Springfield, IL: Thomas.

Forgatch, M. S., & DeGarmo, D. S. (1999). Parenting through change: An effective prevention program for single mothers. *Journal of Consulting and Clinical Psychology, 67,* 711–724.

Forgatch, M. S., Plowman, E. J., Gewirtz, A. H., & Stubbs, J. (2010). *Observed family interaction code training manual.* Unpublished manual, University of Minnesota, Minneapolis, MN.

Fox, N. A., Almas, A. N., Degnan, K. A., Nelson, C. A., & Zeanah, C. H. (2011). The effects of severe psychosocial deprivation and foster care intervention on cognitive development at 8 years of age: Findings from the Bucharest Early Intervention Project. *Journal of Child Psychology and Psychiatry, 52,* 919–928.

Fox, S. E., Levitt, P., & Nelson, C. A., III. (2010). How the timing and quality of early experiences influence the development of brain architecture. *Child Development, 81,* 28–40.

Frankl, V. E. (2006). *Man's search for meaning.* Boston: Beacon Press. (Original work published 1959)

Franks, B. A. (2011). Moving targets: A developmental framework for understanding children's changes following disasters. *Journal of Applied Developmental Psychology, 32,* 58–69.

Freud, A., & Burlingham, D. T. (1943). *War and children.* New York: Medical War Books.

Freud, A., & Dann, S. (1951). An experiment in group upbringing. *Psychoanalytic Study of the Child, 6,* 127–168.

Freud, S. (1928). Humor. *International Journal of Psychoanalysis, 9,* 1–6.

Fuligni, A. J., & Telzer, E. H. (2012). The contributions of youth to immigrant families. In A. S. Masten, K. Liebkind, & D. J. Hernandez (Eds.), *Realizing the potential of immigrant youth* (pp. 181–202). New York: Cambridge University Press.

Furr, J. M., Comer, J. S., Edmunds, J. M., & Kendall, P. C. (2010). Disasters and youth: A meta-analytic examination of posttraumatic stress. *Journal of Consulting and Clinical Psychology, 78,* 765–780.

Fushiki, S. (2013). Radiation hazards in children—lessons from Chernobyl, Three Mile Island and Fukushima. *Brain and Development, 35,* 220–227.

Galassi, J. P., & Akos, P. (2007). *Strength-based school counseling: Promoting student development and achievement.* Mahwah, NJ: Erlbaum.

Garcia Coll, C., & Marks, A. K. (Eds.). (2012). *The immigrant paradox in children and adolescents: Is becoming American a developmental risk?* Washington, DC: American Psychological Association.

Garcia Coll, C., Patton, F., Marks, A. K., Dimitrova, R., Yang, R., Suarez, G. A., et al. (2012). Understanding the immigrant paradox in youth: Developmental and contextual considerations. In A. S. Masten, K. Liebkind, & D. J. Hernandez (Eds.), *Realizing the potential of immigrant youth* (pp. 159–180). New York: Cambridge University Press.

Garmezy, N. (1971). Vulnerability research and the issue of primary prevention. *American Journal of Orthopsychiatry, 41,* 101–116.

Garmezy, N. (1974). The study of competence in children at risk for severe psychopathology. In E. J. Anthony & C. Koupernik (Eds.), *The child in his family: Children at psychiatric risk* (Vol. 3, pp. 77–98). New York: Wiley.

Garmezy, N. (1981). Children under stress: Perspectives on antecedents and correlates of vulnerability and resistance to psychopathology. In A. I. Rabin, J. Aronoff, A. M. Barclay, & R. A. Zucker (Eds.), *Further explorations in personality* (pp. 196–269). New York: Wiley.

Garmezy, N. (1982). The case for the single case in research. In A. E. Kazdin & A. H. Tuma (Eds.), *New directions for methodology of social and behavioral sciences: Single-case research designs* (pp. 5–17). San Francisco: Jossey-Bass.

Garmezy, N. (1983). Stressors of childhood. In N. Garmezy & M. Rutter (Eds.), *Stress, coping, and development in children* (pp. 43–84). New York: McGraw-Hill.

Garmezy, N. (1985). Stress-resistant children: The search for protective factors. In J. E. Stevenson (Ed.), *Recent research in developmental psychopathology: Journal of child psychology and psychiatry book supplement, No. 4* (pp. 213–233). Oxford, UK: Pergamon Press.

Garmezy, N., & Crose, J. M. (1948). A comparison of the academic achievement of matched groups of veteran and non-veteran freshman at the University of Iowa. *Journal of Educational Research, 41,* 547–550.

Garmezy, N., & Devine, V. (1984). Project Competence: The Minnesota studies of children vulnerable to psychopathology. In N. F. Watt, E. J. Anthony, L. Wynne, & J. E. Rolf (Eds.), *Children at risk for schizophrenia: A longitudinal perspective* (pp. 289–303). New York: Cambridge University Press.

Garmezy, N., Masten, A. S., & Tellegen, A. (1984). The study of stress and competence in children: A building block for developmental psychopathology. *Child Development, 55*, 97–111.

Garmezy, N., & Rodnick, E. H. (1959). Premormid adjustment and performance in schizophrenia: Implications for interpreting heterogeneity in schizophrenia. *Journal of Nervous and Mental Disease, 129*, 450–466.

Garmezy, N., & Rutter, M. (1985). Acute reactions to stress. In M. Rutter & L. Hersov (Eds.), *Child and adolescent psychiatry: Modern approaches* (2nd ed., pp. 152–176). Oxford, UK: Blackwell Scientific.

Gauvain, M. (2013). Sociocultural contexts of development. In P. D. Zelazo (Ed.), *The Oxford handbook of developmental psychology: Vol. 2. Self and other* (pp. 425–451). New York: Oxford University Press.

Gershoff, E. T., Aber, J. L., Ware, A., & Kotler, J. A. (2010). Exposure to 9/11 among youth and their mothers in New York City: Enduring associations with mental health and sociopolitical attitudes. *Child Development, 81*, 1142–1160.

Gest, S. D., & Davidson, A. J. (2011). A developmental perspective on risk, resilience, and prevention. In M. Underwood & L. Rosen (Eds.), *Social development: Relationships in infancy, childhood, and adolescence* (pp. 427–454). New York: Guilford Press.

Gest, S. D., Reed, M.-G. J., & Masten, A. S. (1999). Measuring developmental changes in exposure to adversity: A life chart and rating scale approach. *Development and Psychopathology, 11*, 171–192.

Gest, S. D., Sesma, A., Jr., Masten, A. S., & Tellegen, A. (2006). Childhood peer reputation as a predictor of competence and symptoms 10 years later. *Journal of Abnormal Child Psychology, 34*, 509–526.

Gettinger, M., & Stoiber, K. (2009). Effective teaching and effective schools. In C. R. Reynolds & T. B. Gutkin (Eds.), *The handbook of school psychology* (4th ed., pp. 769–790). New York: Wiley.

Gewirtz, A., Forgatch, M., & Wieling, E. (2008). Parenting practices as potential mechanisms for child adjustment following mass trauma. *Journal of Marital and Family Therapy, 34*, 177–192.

Gilbert, N., Parton, N., & Skivenes, M. (Eds.). (2011). *Child protection systems: International trends and orientations.* New York: Oxford University Press.

Gleser, G., Green, B., & Winget, C. (1981). *Prolonged psychological effects of disaster: A study of Buffalo Creek.* Maryland Heights, MO: Academic Press.

Glueck, S., & Glueck, E. (1950). *Unraveling juvenile delinquency.* Cambridge, MA: Harvard University Press.

Godeau, E., Vignes, C., Navarro, F., Iachan, R., Ross, J., Pasquier, C., et al. (2005). Effects of a large-scale industrial disaster on rates of symptoms consistent with posttraumatic stress disorders among schoolchildren in Toulouse. *Archives of Pediatrics Adolescent Medicine, 159*, 579–584.

Goldenberg, H., & Goldenberg, I. (2013). *Family therapy: An overview* (8th ed.). Belmont, CA: Brooks/Cole.

Gonzalez, A., Jenkins, J. M., Steiner, M., & Fleming, A. S. (2012). Maternal early life experiences and parenting: The mediating role of cortisol and executive function. *Journal of the American Academy of Child and Adolescent Psychiatry, 51*, 673–682.

Gottesman, I. I., & Hanson, D. R. (2005). Human development: Biological and genetic processes. *Annual Review of Psychology, 56,* 263–286.

Gray, J. R., & Thompson, P. M. (2004). Neurobiology of intelligence: Science and ethics. *Nature Reviews Neuroscience, 5,* 471–482.

Green, B. L., Grace, M. C., Vary, M. G., Kramer, T. L., Gleser, G. C., & Leonard, A. C. (1994). Children of disaster in the second decade: A 17-year follow-up of Buffalo Creek survivors. *Journal of the American Academy of Child and Adolescent Psychiatry, 33,* 71–79.

Greenberg, M. T. (2006). Promoting resilience in children and youth. *Annals of the New York Academy of Sciences, 1094,* 139–150.

Greenberg, M. T., & Harris, A. R. (2012). Nurturing mindfulness in children and youth: Current state of research. *Child Development Perspectives, 6,* 161–166.

Grimm, K. J., Ram, N., & Hamagami, F. (2011). Nonlinear growth curves in developmental research. *Child Development, 82,* 1357–1371.

Gross, C., & Hen, R. (2004). The developmental origins of anxiety. *Nature Reviews Neuroscience, 5,* 545–552.

Gross, J. J. (2007). *Handbook of emotion regulation.* New York: Guilford Press.

Gross, J. J. (2008). Emotion regulation. In M. Lewis, J. M. Haviland-Jones, & L. F. Barrett (Eds.), *Handbook of emotions* (3rd ed., pp. 497–512). New York: Guilford Press.

Grossman, J. B., & Tierney, J. P. (1998). Does mentoring work?: An impact study of the Big Brothers Big Sisters program. *Evaluation Review, 22,* 403–426.

Gruenberg, E. M. (1981). Risk factor research methods. In D. A. Regier & G. Allen (Eds.), *Risk factor research in the major mental disorders.* National Institute of Mental Health (DHHS Publication No. 81-1068, pp. 8–19). Washington, DC: Government Printing Office.

Guerra, N. G., Graham, S., & Tolan, P. H. (2011). Raising healthy children: Translating child development research into practice. *Child Development, 82,* 7–16.

Guerra, S., & Martinez, F. D. (2008). Asthma genetics: From linear to multifactorial approaches. *Annual Review of Medicine, 59,* 327–341.

Gunderson, L. (2010). Ecological and human community resilience in response to natural disasters. *Ecology and Society, 15.* Retrieved from *www.ecologyandsociety.org/vol15/iss2/art18/.*

Gunderson, L. H., Allen, C. R., & Holling, C. S. (Eds.). (2010). *Foundations of ecological resilience.* Washington, DC: Island Press.

Gunderson, L. H., Folke, C., & Janssen, M. (2006). Generating and fostering novelty. *Ecology and Society, 11,* 50. Retrieved from *www.ecologyandsociety.org/vol11/iss1/art50/.*

Gunnar, M., & Quevedo, K. (2007). The neurobiology of stress and development. *Annual Review of Psychology, 58,* 145–173.

Gunnar, M., & Vazquez, D. (2006). Stress neurobiology and developmental psychopathology. In D. Cicchetti & D. Cohen (Eds.), *Developmental psychopathology: Developmental neuroscience* (pp. 533–577). New York: Wiley.

Gunnar, M. R., & Donzella, B. (2002). Social regulation of the cortisol levels in early human development. *Psychoneuroendocrinology, 27,* 199–220.

Gunnar, M. R., & Herrare, A. M. (2013). The neurobiology of stress and development. In P. D. Zelazo (Ed.), *Oxford handbook of developmental psychology*. New York: Oxford University Press.

Hackman, D. A., Farah, M. J., & Meaney, M. J. (2010). Socioeconomic status and the brain: Mechanistic insights from human and animal research. *Nature Reviews Neuroscience, 11*, 651–659.

Halcón, L. L., Robertson, C. L., Savik, K., Johnson, D. R., Spring, M. A., Butcher, J. N., et al. (2004). Trauma and coping in Somali and Oromo refugee youth. *Journal of Adolescent Health, 35*, 17–25.

Han, W.-J. (2012). Bilingualism and academic achievement: Does generation make a difference? In C. Garcia Coll & A. K. Marks (Eds.), *The immigrant paradox in children and adolescents: Is becoming American a developmental risk?* (pp. 235–258). Washington, DC: American Psychological Association.

Harkness, S., & Super, C. M. (2012). The cultural organization of children's environments. In L. C. Mayes & M. Lewis (Eds.), *The Cambridge handbook of environment in human development* (pp. 498–516). New York: Cambridge University Press.

Harter, S. (1978). Effectance motivation reconsidered: Toward a developmental model. *Human Development, 21*, 34–64.

Harter, S. (2012). *The construction of the self: Developmental and sociocultural foundations* (2nd ed.). New York: Guilford Press.

Hauser, R. M., & Featherman, D. L. (1977). *The process of stratification: Trends and analysis*. New York: Academic Press.

Hauser, S. T., Allen, J. P., & Golden, E. (2006). *Out of the woods: Tales of resilient teens*. Cambridge, MA: Harvard University Press.

Havighurst, R. J. (1974). *Developmental tasks and education* (3rd ed.). Philadelphia: McKay.

Hawkins, J. D., Kosterman, R., Catalano, R. F., Hill, K. G., & Abbott, R. D. (2005). Promoting positive adult functioning through social development intervention in childhood: Long-term effects from the Seattle Social Development Project. *Archives of Pediatrics and Adolescent Medicine, 159*, 25–31.

Hayslip, B., Jr., & Smith, G. C. (Eds.). (2012). *Emerging perspectives on resilience in adulthood and later life: Annual review of gerontology and geriatrics* (Vol. 32). New York: Springer.

Heckman, J. J. (2006). Skill formation and the economics of investing in disadvantaged children. *Science, 312*, 1900–1902.

Heckman, J. J., Moon, S. H., Pinto, R., Savelyev, P. A., & Yavitz, A. (2010). The rate of return to the High/Scope Perry Preschool program. *Journal of Public Economics, 94*, 114–128.

Henderson, N. (2012). Resilience in schools and curriculum design. In M. Ungar (Ed.), *The social ecology of resilience: A handbook of theory and practice* (pp. 297–306). New York: Springer.

Herbers, J. E. (2011). *Parent–child relationships in young homeless families: Co-regulation as a predictor of child self-regulation and school adjustment*. Unpublished doctoral dissertation, University of Minnesota, Minneapolis, MN.

Herbers, J. E., Cutuli, J. J., Lafavor, T. L., Vrieze, D., Leibel, C., Obradović, J., et al. (2011). Direct and indirect effects of parenting on the academic functioning of young homeless children. *Early Education and Development, 22,* 77–104.

Herbers, J. E., Cutuli, J. J., Supkoff, L. M., Heistad, D., Chan, C.-K., Hinz, E., et al. (2012). Early reading skills and academic achievement trajectories of students facing poverty, homelessness, and high residential mobility. *Educational Researcher, 41,* 366–374.

Herrfahrdt-Pähle, E., & Pahl-Wostl, C. (2012). Continuity and change in social–ecological systems: The role of institutional resilience. *Ecology and Society, 17*(2). Retrieved from *www.ecologyandsociety.org/vol17/iss2/art8/.*

Hertzman, C., & Boyce, T. (2010). How experience gets under the skin to create gradients in developmental health. *Annual Review of Public Health, 31,* 329–347.

Herzog, J. G. (1984). *Life events as indices of family stress: Relationships with children's current levels of competence.* Unpublished doctoral dissertation, University of Minnesota, Minneapolis, MN.

Hetherington, E. M. (1979). Divorce: A child's perspective. *American Psychologist, 34,* 851–858.

Hill, C., & Kearl, H. (2011). *Crossing the line: Sexual harassment at school.* Washington, DC: American Association of University Women.

Hillman, N. (1987). *Mothers' competence: Correlates and continuity under stress.* Unpublished doctoral dissertation, University of Minnesota, Minneapolis, MN.

Hobfoll, S. E., Watson, P., Bell, C. C., Bryant, R. A., Brymer, M. J., Friedman, M. J., et al. (2007). Five essential elements of immediate and mid-term mass trauma intervention: Empirical evidence. *Psychiatry: Interpersonal and Biological Processes, 70,* 283–315.

Hochberg, Z., Feil, R., Constancia, M., Fraga, M., Junien, C., Carel, J. C., et al. (2011). Child health, developmental plasticity, and epigenetic programming. *Endocrine Reviews, 32,* 159–224.

Holling, C. S. (1973). Resilience and stability of ecological systems. *Annual Review of Ecology and Systematics, 4,* 1–23.

Holmes, T. H., & Rahe, R. H. (1967). The social readjustment rating scale. *Journal of Psychosomatic Research, 11,* 213–218.

Hornik, R., & Gunnar, M. R. (1988). A descriptive analysis of infant social referencing. *Child Development, 59,* 626–634.

Hoven, C. W., Duarte, C. S., Lucas, C. P., Wu, P., Mandell, D. J., Goodwin, R. D., et al. (2005). Psychopathology among New York City public school children 6 months after September 11. *Archives of General Psychiatry, 62,* 545–552.

Howard, K. S., & Brooks-Gunn, J. (2009). The role of home-visiting programs in preventing child abuse and neglect. *The Future of Children, 19,* 119–146.

Howell, J. C. (2010, December). Gang prevention: An overview of research and programs. *Juvenile Justice Bulletin,* 1–22. Washington, DC: U.S. Department of Justice, Office of Juvenile Justice and Delinquency Prevention.

Howell, J. C. (2011). *Gangs in America's communities.* Thousand Oaks, CA: Sage.

Hubbard, J. (1997). *Adaptive functioning and post-traumatic symptoms in adolescent survivors of massive childhood trauma.* Unpublished doctoral dissertation, University of Minnesota, Minneapolis, MN.

Hubbard, J., Realmuto, G. M., Northwood, A. K., & Masten, A. S. (1995). Comorbidity of psychiatric diagnoses with post-traumatic stress disorder in survivors of childhood trauma. *Journal of the American Academy of Child and Adolescent Psychiatry, 34,* 1167–1173.

Hughes, D., Rodriguez, J., Smith, E. P., Johnson, D. J., Stevenson, H. C., & Spicer, P. (2006). Parents' ethnic-racial socialization practices: A review of research and directions for future study. *Developmental Psychology, 42,* 747–770.

Hughes, V. (2012). The roots of resilience. *Nature, 490,* 165–167.

Huizink, A. C., Bartels, M., Rose, R. J., Pulkkinen, L., Eriksson, C. J., & Kaprio, J. (2008). Chernobyl exposure as stressor during pregnancy and hormone levels in adolescent offspring. *Journal of Epidemiology and Community Health, 62*(e5). Retrieved from *http://jech.bmj.com/content/62/4/e5.full.*

Huston, A. C. (Ed.). (1991). *Children in poverty: Child development and public policy.* New York: Cambridge University Press.

Institute of Medicine. (2013, June). *Workshop on "Medical and public health preparedness, response and recovery considerations for children and families."* Meeting conducted at the Forum on Medical and Public Health Preparedness for Catastrophic Events by the Board on Health Sciences Policy, Washington, DC.

Irons, D. E., Iacono, W. G., Oetting, W. S., & McGue, M. (2012). Developmental trajectory and environmental moderation of the effect of *ALDH2* polymorphism on alcohol use. *Alcoholism: Clinical and Experimental Research, 36,* 1882–1891.

Janoff-Bulman, R. (1992). *Shattered assumptions: Towards a new psychology of trauma.* New York: Free Press.

Janoff-Bulman, R., & Frantz, C. (1997). The impact of trauma on meaning: From meaningless world to meaningful life. In M. J. Power & C. R. Brewin (Eds.), *The transformation of meaning in psychological therapies: Integrating theory and practice* (pp. 91–106). Hoboken, NJ: Wiley.

Joëls, M., & Baram, T. Z. (2009). The neuro-symphony of stress. *Nature Reviews Neuroscience, 10,* 459–466.

Jordans, M. J. D., Tol, W. A., Komproe, I. H., & De Jong, J. V. T. M. (2009). Systematic review of evidence and treatment approaches: Psychosocial and mental health care for children in war. *Child and Adolescent Mental Health, 14,* 2–14,

Kağitçibaşi, Ç. (2012). Autonomous–related self and competence: The potential of immigrant youth. In A. S. Masten, K. Liebkind, & D. J. Hernandez (Eds.), *Realizing the potential of immigrant youth* (pp. 281–306). New York: Cambridge University Press.

Karatsoreos, I. N., & McEwen, B. S. (2011). Psychobiological allostasis: Resistance, resilience and vulnerability. *Trends in Cognitive Neuroscience, 15,* 576–584.

Karatsoreos, I. N., & McEwen, B. S. (2013). Annual research review: The neurobiology and physiology of resilience and adaptation across the life course. *Journal of Child Psychology and Psychiatry, 54,* 337–347.

Keating, D. P., & Hertzman, C. (Eds.). (1999). *Developmental health and the wealth of nations: Social, biological, and educational dynamics.* New York: Guilford Press.

Kelly, J. B., & Emery, R. E. (2003). Children's adjustment following divorce: Risk and resilience perspectives. *Family Relations, 52,* 352–362.

Kendall, P. C. (2006). *Coping cat workbook.* Ardmore, PA: Workbook Publishing.

Kendall, P. C., & Hedtke, K. A. (2006). *Cognitive-behavioral therapy for anxious children: Therapist manual.* Ardmore, PA: Workbook Publishing.

Kiernan, K. E., & Mensah, F. K. (2011). Poverty, family resources and children's educational attainment: The mediating rold of parenting. *British Journal of Educational Research, 37,* 317–336.

Kilmer, R. P., & Gil-Rivas, V. (2010). Exploring posttraumatic growth in children impacted by Hurricane Katrina: Correlates of the phenomenon and developmental considerations. *Child Development, 81,* 1211–1227.

Kim-Cohen, J., & Gold, A. L. (2009). Measured gene–environment interactions and mechanisms promoting resilient development. *Current Directions in Psychological Science, 18,* 138–142.

Kim-Cohen, J., & Turkewitz, R. (2012). Resilience and measured gene–environment interactions. *Development and Psychopathology, 24,* 1297–1306.

King, P. E., & Benson, P. L. (2006). Spiritual development and adolescent well-being and thriving. In E. C. Roehlkepartain, P. E. King, L. Wagener, & P. L. Benson (Eds.), *The handbook of spiritual development in childhood and adolescence* (pp. 384–398). Thousand Oaks, CA: Sage.

Kirmayer, L. J., Dandeneau, S., Marshall, E., Phillips, M. K., & Williamson, K. J. (2011). Rethinking resilience from indigenous perspectives. *Canadian Journal of Psychiatry, 56,* 84–91.

Kithakye, M., Morris, A. S., Terranova, A. M., & Myers, S. S. (2010). The Kenyan political conflict and children's adjustment. *Child Development, 81*(4), 1114–1128.

Klasen, F., Oettingen, G., Daniels, J., Post, M., Hoyer, C., & Adam, H. (2010). Posttraumatic resilience in former Ugandan child soldiers. *Child Development, 81,* 1096–1113.

Klein, D. N., Kotov, R., & Bufferd, S. J. (2011). Personality and depression: Explanatory models and review of the evidence. *Annual Review of Clinical Psychology, 7,* 269–295.

Klein, R. A., Kufeldt, K., & Rideout, S. (2006). Resilience theory and its relevance for child welfare practice. In R. J. Flynn, P. M. Dudding, & J. G. Barber (Eds.), *Promoting resilience in child welfare* (pp. 34–51). Ottawa, Canada: University of Ottawa Press.

Kobak, R. (2012). Attachment and early social deprivation: Revisiting Harlow's monkey studies. In A. M. Slater & P. C. Quinn (Eds.), *Developmental psychology: Revisiting the classic studies* (pp. 10–23). London: Sage.

Kobasa, S. C. (1979). Stressful life events, personality, and health: An inquiry into hardiness. *Journal of Personality and Social Psychology, 37,* 1–11.

Kochanska, G., & Knaack, A. (2003). Effortful control as a personality characteristic of young children: Antecedents, correlates, and consequences. *Journal of Personality, 71,* 1087–1112.

Kopp, C. B. (1983). Risk factors in development. In M. M. Haith & J. J. Campos (Eds.), *Handbook of child psychology: Vol. 2. Infancy and developmental psychobiology* (4th ed., pp. 1081–1188). New York: Wiley.

Korol, M., Kramer, T. L., Grace, M. C., & Green, B. L. (2002). Dam break: Long-term follow-up of children exposed to the Buffalo Creek disaster. In A. M. La Greca, W. K. Silverman, E. M. Vernberg, & M. C. Roberts (Eds.), *Helping children cope with disasters and terrorism* (pp. 241–257). Washington, DC: American Psychological Association.

Kouros, C. D., Cummings, E. M., & Davies, P. T. (2010). Early trajectories of interparental conflict and externalizing problems as predictors of social competence in preadolescence. *Developmental Psychopathology, 22,* 527–537.

Kozol, J. (1988). *Rachel and her children.* New York: Random House.

Kronenberg, M. E., Hansel, T. C., Brennan, A. M., Osofsky, H. J., Osofsky, J. D., & Lawrason, B. (2010). Children of Katrina: Lessons learned about postdisaster symptoms and recovery patterns. *Child Development, 81,* 1241–1259.

Kuiper, N. A. (2012). Humor and resiliency: Towards a process model of coping and growth. *Europe's Journal of Psychology, 8,* 475–491.

La Greca, A. M., Lai, B. S., Joormann, J., Auslander, B. B., & Short, M. A. (2013). Children's risk and resilience following a natural disaster: Genetic vulnerability, posttraumatic stress, and depression. *Journal of Affective Disorders, 151,* 860–867.

La Greca, A. M., & Silverman, W. K. (2009). Treatment and prevention of posttraumatic stress reactions in children and adolescents exposed to disasters and terrorism: What is the evidence? *Child Development Perspectives, 3,* 4–10.

La Greca, A. M., Silverman, W. K., Lai, B., & Jaccard, J. (2010). Hurricane-related exposure experiences and stressors, other life events, and social support: Concurrent and prospective impact on children's persistent posttraumatic stress symptoms. *Journal of Consulting and Clinical Psychology, 78,* 794–805.

LaFromboise, T. D., Hoyt, D. R., Oliver, L., & Whitbeck, L. B. (2006). Family, community, and school influences on resilience among American Indian adolescents in the upper midwest. *University of Nebraska–Lincoln Sociology Department, Faculty Publications, Paper 26.*

Lambert, N. M., & Bower, E. M. (1961). *A process for in-school screening of children with emotional handicaps.* Princeton, NJ: Educational Testing Service.

Laub, J. H., & Sampson, R. J. (2003). *Shared beginnings, divergent lives: Delinquent boys to age 70.* Cambridge, MA: Harvard University Press.

Lauer, P. A., Akiba, M., Wilkerson, S. B., Apthorp, H. S., Snow, D., & Martin-Glenn, M. L. (2006). Out-of-school-time programs: A meta-analysis of effects for at-risk students. *Review of Educational Research, 76,* 275–313.

Laufer, A., & Solomon, Z. (2009). Gender differences in PTSD in Israeli youth exposed to terror attacks. *Journal of Interpersonal Violence, 24,* 959–976.

Layne, C. M., Olsen, J. A., Baker, A., Legerski, J., Isakson, B., Pašalić, A., et al. (2010). Unpacking trauma exposure risk factors and differential pathways of influence: Predicting postwar mental distress in Bosnian adolescents. *Child Development, 81,* 1053–1076.

Layne, C. M., Saltzman, W. R., Poppleton, L., Burlingame, G. M., Pašalić, A., Duraković, E., et al. (2008). Effectiveness of a school-based group psychotherapy program for war-exposed adolescents: A randomized controlled trial. *Journal of the American Academy of Child and Adolescent Psychiatry, 47,* 1048–1062.

Lefcourt, H. M. (2002). Humor. In C. R. Snyder & S. J. Shane (Eds.), *Handbook of positive psychology* (pp. 619–631). New York: Oxford University Press.

Lengua, L. J., Long, A. C., Smith, K. I., & Meltzoff, A. N. (2005). Pre-attack symptomatology and temperament as predictors of children's responses to the September 11 terrorist attacks. *Journal of Child Psychology and Psychiatry, 46,* 631–645.

Lengua, L. J., & Wachs, T. D. (2012). Temperament and risk: Resilient and vulnerable responses to adversity. In M. Zentner & R. L. Shiner (Eds.), *Handbook of temperament* (pp. 519–540). New York: Guilford Press.

Lerner, R. M. (2006). Developmental science, developmental systems, and contemporary theories. In R. M. Lerner (Ed.), *Handbook of child psychology: Vol. 1. Theoretical models of human development* (6th ed., pp. 1–17). Hoboken, NJ: Wiley.

Lerner, R. M. (2009). The positive youth development perspective: Theoretical and empirical bases of a strengths-based approach to adolescent development. In C. R. Snyder & S. J. Lopez (Eds.), *Oxford handbook of positive psychology* (pp. 149–163). New York: Oxford University Press.

Lewis, J. M., & Looney, J. G. (1983). *The long struggle: Well-functioning working-class black families.* New York: Brunner/Mazel.

Lewis, M., & Feiring, C. (Eds.). (1998). *Families, risk, and competence.* Mahwah, NJ: Erlbaum.

Lieberman, A. F., & Van Horn, P. (2011). Child–parent psychotherapy: A developmental approach to mental health treatment in infancy and early childhood. In C. H. Zeanah, Jr. (Ed.), *Handbook of infant mental health* (3rd ed., pp. 439–449). New York: Guilford Press.

Linder, H. D. (1985). *A contextual life events interview as a measure of stress: A comparison of questionnaire-based versus interview-based stress indices.* Unpublished doctoral dissertation, University of Minnesota, Minneapolis, MN.

Loman, M. M., & Gunnar, M. R. (2010). Early experience and the development of stress reactivity and regulation in children. *Neuroscience and Behavioral Reviews, 34,* 867–876.

Long, J. V., & Vaillant, G. E. (1984). Natural history of male psychological health: XI. Escape from the underclass. *American Journal of Psychiatry, 141,* 341–346.

Longstaff, P. H., & Yang, S. (2008). Communication management and trust: Their role in building resilience to "surprises" such as natural disasters, pandemic flu, and terrorism. *Ecology and Society, 13*. Retrieved from *www. ecologyandsociety.org/vol13/iss1/art3/*.

Lösel, F., & Farrington, D. P. (2012). Direct and protective and buffering protective factors in the development of youth violence. *American Journal of Preventive Medicine, 43*, S8–S23.

Lundberg, M., & Wuermli, A. (Eds.). (2012). *Children and youth in crisis: Protecting and promoting human development in times of economic shocks*. Washington, DC: World Bank.

Lupien, S. J., Parent, S., Evans, A. C., Tremblay, R. E., Zelazo, P. D., Corbo, C., et al. (2011). Larger amygdala but no change in hippocampal volume in 10-year-old children exposed to maternal depressive symptomology since birth. *Proceedings of the National Academy of Sciences of the United States of America, 108*, 14324–14329.

Luthar, S. S. (1991). Vulnerability and resilience: A study of high-risk adolescents. *Child Development, 62*, 600–616.

Luthar, S. S. (1999). *Poverty and children's adjustment*. Newbury Park, CA: Sage.

Luthar, S. S. (Ed.). (2003). *Resilience and vulnerability: Adaptation in the context of childhood adversities*. New York: Cambridge University Press.

Luthar, S. S. (2006). Resilience in development: A synthesis of research across five decades. In D. Cicchetti & D. J. Cohen (Eds.), *Developmental psychopathology: Vol. 3. Risk, disorder, and adaptation* (2nd ed., pp. 739–795). Hoboken, NJ: Wiley.

Luthar, S. S., Cicchetti, D., & Becker, B. (2000). The construct of resilience: A critical evaluation and guidelines for future work. *Child Development, 71*, 543–562.

Luthar, S. S., Shoum, K. A., & Brown, P. J. (2006). Extracurricular involvement among affluent youth: A scapegoat for "ubiquitous achievement pressures?" *Developmental Psychology, 42*, 583–597.

Magaña-Amato, A. (1993). *Manual for coding expressed emotion from the five-minute speech sample: UCLA Family Project*. Los Angeles: University of California, Los Angeles.

Mahoney, J. L., Larson, R. W., & Eccles, J. S. (2005). *Organized activities as contexts of development: Extracurricular activities, after-school and community programs*. Mahwah, NJ: Erlbaum.

Main, M. (1996). Introduction to the special section on attachment and psychopathology: 2. Overview of the field of attachment. *Journal of Counseling and Clinical Psychology, 64*, 237–243.

Masten, A. S. (1982). *Humor and creative thinking in stress-resistant children*. Unpublished doctoral dissertation, University of Minnesota, Minneapolis, MN.

Masten, A. S. (1986). Humor and competence in school-aged children. *Child Development, 57*, 461–473.

Masten, A. S. (1989). Resilience in development: Implications of the study of successful adaptation for developmental psychopathology. In D. Cicchetti (Ed.), *The emergence of a discipline: Rochester Symposium on Developmental Psychopathology* (Vol. 1, pp. 261–294). Hillsdale, NJ: Erlbaum.

Masten, A. S. (1999). Resilience comes of age: Reflections on the past and outlook for the next generation of research. In M. D. Glantz & J. L. Johnson (Eds.), *Resilience and development: Positive life adaptations* (pp. 281–296). New York: Plenum.

Masten, A. S. (2001). Ordinary magic: Resilience processes in development. *American Psychologist, 56*, 227–238.

Masten, A. S. (2003). Commentary: Developmental psychopathology as a unifying context for mental health and education models, research, and practice in schools. *School Psychology Review, 32*, 169–173.

Masten, A. S. (2004). Regulatory processes, risk, and resilience in adolescent development. *Annals of the New York Academy of Sciences, 1021*, 310–319.

Masten, A. S. (2006a). Developmental psychopathology: Pathways to the future. *International Journal of Behavioral Development, 30*, 47–54.

Masten, A. S. (2006b). Promoting resilience in development: A general framework for systems of care. In R. J. Flynn, P. Dudding, & J. G. Barber (Eds.), *Promoting resilience in child welfare* (pp. 3–17). Ottawa, Canada: University of Ottawa Press.

Masten, A. S. (2007). Resilience in developing systems: Progress and promise as the fourth wave rises. *Development and Psychopathology, 19*, 921–930.

Masten, A. S. (2011). Resilience in children threatened by extreme adversity: Frameworks for research, practice, and translational synergy. *Development and Psychopathology, 23*, 141–154.

Masten, A. S. (2012a). Resilience in children: Vintage Rutter and beyond. In A. Slater & P. Quinn (Eds.), *Developmental psychology: Revisiting the classic studies* (pp. 204–221). London: Sage.

Masten, A. S. (2012b). Risk and resilience in the educational success of homeless and highly mobile children: Introduction to the special section. *Educational Researcher, 41*, 363–365.

Masten, A. S. (2013a). Competence, risk and resilience in military families: Conceptual commentary. *Clinical Child and Family Psychology Review, 16*, 278–281.

Masten, A. S. (2013b). Risk and resilience in development. In P. D. Zelazo (Ed.), *Oxford handbook of developmental psychology: Vol. 2. Self and other* (pp. 579–607). New York: Oxford University Press.

Masten, A. S. (2014). Global perspectives on resilience in children and youth. *Child Development, 85*, 6–20.

Masten, A. S., Best, K. M., & Garmezy, N. (1990). Resilience and development: Contributions from the study of children who overcome adversity. *Development and Psychopathology, 2*, 425–444.

Masten, A. S., Burt, K. B., & Coatsworth, J. D. (2006). Competence and psychopathology in development. In D. Cicchetti & D. Cohen (Eds.), *Developmental psychopathology: Vol. 3. Risk, disorder and psychopathology* (2nd ed., pp. 696–738). New York: Wiley.

Masten, A. S., Burt, K. B., Roisman, G. I., Obradović, J., Long, J. D., & Tellegen, A. (2004). Resources and resilience in the transition to adulthood: Continuity and change. *Development and Psychopathology, 16*, 1071–1094.

Masten, A. S., & Cicchetti, D. (Eds.). (2010a). Developmental cascades: Part 1 [Special issue]. *Development and Psychopathology, 22*(3), 491–715.

Masten, A. S., & Cicchetti, D. (Eds.). (2010b). Developmental cascades: Part 2 [Special issue]. *Development and Psychopathology, 22*(4), 717–983.

Masten, A. S., & Cicchetti, D. (Eds.). (2010c). Editorial: Developmental cascades: Part 1 [Special issue]. *Development and Psychopathology, 22*, 491–495.

Masten, A. S., & Cicchetti, D. (2012). Risk and resilience in development and psychopathology: The legacy of Norman Garmezy. *Development and Psychopathology, 24*, 333–334.

Masten, A. S., & Coatsworth, J. D. (1995). Competence, resilience, and psychopathology. In D. Cicchetti & D. J. Cohen (Eds.), *Developmental psychopathology: Vol. 2. Risk, disorder, and adaptation* (pp. 715–752). New York: Wiley.

Masten, A. S., & Coatsworth, J. D. (1998). The development of competence in favorable and unfavorable environments: Lessons from research on successful children. *American Psychologist, 53*, 205–220.

Masten, A. S., Coatsworth, J. D., Neemann, J., Gest, S. D., Tellegen, A., & Garmezy, N. (1995). The structure and coherence of competence from childhood through adolescence. *Child Development, 66*, 1635–1659.

Masten, A. S., Desjardins, C. D., McCormick, C. M., Kuo, S. I.-C., & Long, J. D. (2010). The significance of childhood competence and problems for adults success in work: A developmental cascade analysis. *Development and Psychopathology, 22*, 679–694.

Masten, A. S., Garmezy, N., Tellegen, A., Pellegrini, D. S., Larkin, K., & Larsen, A. (1988). Competence and stress in school children: The moderating effects of individual and family qualities. *Journal of Child Psychology and Psychiatry, 29*, 745–764.

Masten, A. S., Herbers, J., Cutuli, J., & Lafavor, T. (2008). Promoting competence and resilience in the school context. *Professional School Counseling, 12*, 76–84.

Masten, A. S., Herbers, J. E., Desjardins, C. D., Cutuli, J. J., McCormick, C. M., Sapienza, J. K., et al. (2012). Executive function skills and school success in young children experiencing homelessness. *Educational Researcher, 41*, 375–384.

Masten, A. S., Hubbard, J. J., Gest, S. D., Tellegen, A., Garmezy, N., & Ramirez, M. (1999). Competence in the context of adversity: Pathways to resilience and maladaptation from childhood to late adolescence. *Development and Psychopathology, 11*, 143–169.

Masten, A. S., Liebkind, K., & Hernandez, D. J. (2012a). Introduction. In A. S. Masten, K. Liebkind, & D. J. Hernandez (Eds.), *Realizing the potential of immigrant youth* (pp. 1–15). New York: Cambridge University Press.

Masten, A. S., Liebkind, K., & Hernandez, D. J. (Eds.). (2012b). *Realizing the potential of immigrant youth*. New York: Cambridge University Press.

Masten, A. S., Long, J. D., Kuo, S. I.-C., McCormick, C. M., & Desjardins, C. D. (2009). Developmental models of strategic intervention. *International Journal of Developmental Science, 3*, 282–291.

Masten, A. S., Miliotis, D., Graham-Bermann, S., Ramirez, M., & Neeman, J. (1993). Children in homeless families: Risks to mental health and development. *Journal of Consulting and Clinical Psychology, 61*, 335–343.

Masten, A. S., & Monn, A. R. (2015). Child and family resilience: A call for integrated science, practice, and professional training. *Family Relations, 64*, 5–21.

Masten, A. S., Morison, P., & Pellegrini, D. S. (1985). A revised class play method of peer assessment. *Developmental Psychology, 21*, 523–533.

Masten, A. S., & Narayan, A. J. (2012). Child development in the context of disaster, war and terrorism: Pathways of risk and resilience. *Annual Review of Psychology, 63*, 227–257.

Masten, A. S., Narayan, A. J., Silverman, W. K., & Osofsky, J. D. (2015). Children in war and disaster. In R. M. Lerner (Ed.), M. H. Bornstein, & T. Leventhal (Vol. Eds.), *Handbook of child psychology and developmental science: Vol. 4. Ecological settings and processes in developmental systems* (7th ed., pp. 704–745). New York: Wiley.

Masten, A. S., Neemann, J., & Andenas, S. (1994). Life events and adjustment in adolescents: The significance of event independence, desirability, and chronicity. *Journal of Research on Adolescence, 4*, 71–97.

Masten, A. S., & Obradović, J. (2006). Competence and resilience in development. *Annals of the New York Academy of Sciences, 1094*, 13–27.

Masten, A. S., & Obradović, J. (2008). Disaster preparation and recovery: Lessons from research on resilience in human development. *Ecology and Society, 13*. Retrieved from www.ecologyandsociety.org/vol13/iss1/art9/.

Masten, A. S., Obradović, J., & Burt, K. B. (2006). Resilience in emerging adulthood: Developmental perspectives on continuity and transformation. In J. J. Arnett & J. L. Tanner (Eds.), *Emerging adults in America: Coming of age in the 21st century* (pp. 173–190). Washington, DC: American Psychological Association Press.

Masten, A. S., & O'Connor, M. J. (1989). Vulnerability, stress, and resilience in the early development of a high risk child. *Journal of the American Academy of Child and Adolescent Psychiatry, 28*, 274–278.

Masten, A. S., & Osofsky, J. D. (2010). Disasters and their impact on child development: Introduction to the special section. *Child Development, 81*, 1029–1039.

Masten, A. S., Roisman, G. I., Long, J. D., Burt, K. B., Obradović, J., Riley, J. R., et al. (2005). Developmental cascades: Linking academic achievement and externalizing and internalizing symptoms over 20 years. *Developmental Psychology, 41*, 733–746.

Masten, A. S., & Sesma, A., Jr. (1999). Risk and resilience among children homeless in Minneapolis. *Children, 47*, 24.

Masten, A. S., Sesma, A., Si-Asar, R., Lawrence, C., Miliotis, D., & Dionne, J. A. (1997). Educational risks for children experiencing homelessness. *Journal of School Psychology, 35*, 27–46.

Masten, A. S., & Shaffer, A. (2006). How families matter in child development: Reflections from research on risk and resilience. In A. Clarke-Stewart & J. Dunn (Eds.), *Families count: Effects on child and adolescent development* (pp. 5–25). New York: Cambridge University Press.

Masten, A. S., & Tellegen, A. (2012). Resilience in developmental psychopathology: Contributions of the Project Competence Longitudinal Study. *Development and Psychopathology, 24,* 345–361.

Masten, A. S., & Wright, M. O. (2010). Resilience over the lifespan: Developmental perspectives on resistance, recovery, and transformation. In J. W. Reich, A. J. Zautra, & J. S. Hall (Eds.), *Handbook of adult resilience* (pp. 213–237). New York: Guilford Press.

McCormick, C. M., Kuo, S. I.-C., & Masten, A. S. (2011). Developmental tasks across the lifespan. In K. L. Fingerman, C. Berg, T. C. Antonucci, & J. Smith (Eds.), *The handbook of lifespan development* (pp. 117–140). New York: Springer.

McCubbin, H. I., & Patterson, J. M. (1982). Family adaptation to crises. In H. I. McCubbin, A. E. Cauble, & J. M. Patterson (Eds.), *Family stress, coping, and social support* (pp. 26–47). Springfield, IL: Charles C. Thomas.

McCubbin, H. I., & Patterson, J. M. (1983). The family stress process: The double ABCX model of family adjustment and adaptation. *Marriage and Family Review, 6,* 7–37.

McDermott, B. M., Lee, E. M., Judd, M., & Gibbon, P. (2005). Posttraumatic stress disorder and general psychopathology in children and adolescents following a wildfire disaster. *Canadian Journal of Psychiatry, 50,* 137–143.

McDermott, J. M., Westerlund, A., Zeanah, C. H., Nelson, C. A., & Fox, N. A. (2012). Early adversity and neural correlates of executive function: Implications for academic adjustment. *Developmental Cognitive Neuroscience, 2,* S59–S66.

McEwen, B. S., & Gianaros, P. J. (2011). Stress- and allostasis-induced brain plasticity. *Annual Review of Medicine, 62,* 431–445.

McEwen, B. S., & Stellar, E. (1993). Stress and the individual: Mechanisms leading to disease. *Archives of Internal Medicine, 153,* 2093–2101.

McFarlane, A. C. (1987). Posttraumatic phenomena in a longitudinal study of children following a natural disaster. *Journal of the American Academy of Child and Adolescent Psychiatry, 26,* 764–769.

McFarlane, A. C., Policansky, S. K., & Irwin, C. (1987). A longitudinal study of the psychological morbidity in children due to a natural disaster. *Psychological Medicine, 17,* 727–738.

McFarlane, A. C., & Van Hooff, M. (2009). Impact of childhood exposure to a natural disaster on adult mental health: 20-year longitudinal follow-up study. *British Journal of Psychiatry, 195,* 142–148.

McGhee, P. (Ed.). (1989). *Humor and children's development: A guide to practical applications.* New York: Haworth Press.

McGhee, P. (2010). *Humor: The lighter path to resilience and health.* Bloomington, IN: AuthorHouse.

McGhee, P. E., & Chapman, A. J. (1980). *Children's humor.* Chichester, UK: Wiley.

McGloin, J. M., & Widom, C. S. (2001). Resilience among abused and neglected children grown up. *Development and Psychopathology, 13,* 1021–1038.

McLoyd, V. C. (1998). Socioeconomic disadvantage and child development. *American Psychologist, 53,* 185–204.

Mead, M. (2001). *Coming of age in Samoa.* New York: Perennial. (Original work published 1928)

Meaney, M. J. (2010). Epigenetics and the biological definition of gene × environment interactions. *Child Development, 81,* 41–79.

Meyer-Lindenberg, A., Domes, G., Kirsch, P., & Heinrichs, M. (2011). Oxytocin and vasopressin in the human brain: Social neuropeptides for translational medicine. *Nature, 12,* 524–538.

Miliotis, D., Sesma, A., Jr., & Masten, A. S. (1999). Parenting as a protective process for school success in children from homeless families. *Early Education and Development, 10,* 111–133.

Miller, G., Chen, E., & Cole, S. (2009). Health psychology: Developing biologically plausible models linking the social world and physical health. *Annual Review of Psychology, 60,* 501–524.

Miller, P. M. (2011). A critical analysis of the research on student homelessness. *Review of Educational Research, 81,* 308–337.

Minuchin, S., & Minuchin, S. (1974). *Families and family therapy.* Cambridge, MA: Harvard University Press.

Mischel, W., Ayduk, O., Berman, M. G., Casey, B. J., Gotlib, I. H., Jonides, J., et al. (2011). "Willpower" over the life span: Decomposing self-regulation. *Social Cognitive and Affective Neuroscience, 6,* 252–256.

Miyake, A., Friedman, N. P., Emerson, M. J., Witzki, A. H., Howerter, A., & Wager, T. D. (2000). The unity and diversity of exeuctive functions and their contributions to complex "frontal lobe" tasks: A latent variable analysis. *Cognitive Psychology, 41,* 49–100.

Moffitt, T. E., Arseneault, L., Belsky, D., Dickson, N., Hancox, R. J., Harrington, H., et al. (2011). A gradient of childhood self-control predicts health, wealth, and public safety. *Proceedings of the National Academy of Sciences of the United States of America, 108,* 2693–2698.

Morison, P., & Masten, A. S. (1991). Peer reputation in middle childhood as a predictor of adaptation in adolescence: A seven-year follow-up. *Child Development, 62,* 991–1007.

Motti-Stefanidi, F., Berry, J., Chryssochoou, X., Sam, D. L., & Phinney, J. (2012). Positive immigrant youth adaptation in context: Developmental, acculturation, and social–psychological perspectives. In A. S. Masten, K. Liebkind, & D. J. Hernandez (Eds.), *Realizing the potential of immigrant youth* (pp. 116–158). New York: Cambridge University Press.

Munro, E. (2011). *The Munro review of child protection: Final report. A child-centered system.* Paper presented to Parliament by the Secretary of State for Education by Command of Her Majesty.

Murray, L. (2010). *Breaking night: A memoir of forgiveness, survival, and my journey from homeless to Harvard.* New York: Hyperion.

Murry, V. M., Berkel, C., Gaylord-Harden, N. K., Copeland-Linder, N., & Nation, M. (2011). Neighborhood poverty and adolescent development. *Journal of Research on Adolescents, 21,* 114–128.

Muthén, B., & Muthén, L. (2000). Integrating person-centered and variable-centered analysis: Growth mixture modeling with latent trajectory classes. *Alcoholism: Clinical and Experimental Research, 24,* 882–891.

Nagin, D. S. (1999). Analyzing developmental trajectories: A semiparametric group-based approach. *Psychological Methods, 4,* 139–157.

Narayan, A. J., Herbers, J. E., Plowman, E. J., Gewirtz, A. H., & Masten, A. S. (2012). Expressed emotion in homeless families: A methodological study of the five-minute speech sample. *Journal of Family Psychology, 26,* 648–653.

Nation, M., Crusto, C., Wandersman, A., Kumpfer, K. L., Seybolt, D., Morrissey-Kane, E., et al. (2003). What works in prevention: Principles of effective prevention programs. *American Psychologist, 58,* 449–456.

National Commission on Children and Disasters. (2010). *National Commission on Children and Disasters: 2010 report to the President and Congress.* AHRQ Publication No. 10-M037, October 2010. Rockville, MD: Agency for Healthcare Research and Quality.

National Research Council and Institute of Medicine. (2002). *Community programs to promote youth development.* Washington, DC: National Academies Press.

National Research Council and Institute of Medicine. (2004). *Engaging schools: Fostering high school students' motivation to learn.* Committee on Increasing High School Students' Engagement and Motivation to Learn. Board on Children, Youth, and Familes. Washington, DC: National Academies Press.

National Research Council and Institute of Medicine. (2010). *Student mobility: Exploring the impact of frequent moves on achievement: Summary of a workshop.* Washington, DC: National Academies Press.

Nelson, C. A., Zeanah, C. H., Fox, N. A., Marshall, P. J., Smyke, A. T., & Guthrie, D. (2007). Cognitive recovery in socially deprived young children: The Bucharest Early Intervention Project. *Science, 318,* 1937–1940.

Neuner, F., Catani, C., Ruf, M., Schauer, E., Schauer, M., & Elbert, T. (2008). Narrative exposure therapy for the treatment of traumatized children and adolescents (KidNET): From neurocognitive theory to field intervention. *Refugee Mental Health, 17,* 641–664.

Nichols, W. C. (2013). Roads to understanding family resilience: 1920s to the twenty-first century. In D. S. Becvar (Ed.), *Handbook of family resilience* (pp. 1–16). New York: Springer.

Norris, F., Friedman, M. J., & Watson, P. (2002). 60,000 disaster victims speak: Part II. Summary and implications of the disaster mental health research. *Psychiatry, 65,* 240–260.

Norris, F., Friedman, M. J., Watson, P., Byrne, C. M., Diaz, E., & Kaniasty, K. (2002). 60,000 disaster victims speak: Part I. An empirical review of the empirical literature, 1981–2001. *Psychiatry, 65,* 207–239.

Norris, F., Stevens, S., Pfefferbaum, B., Wyche, K., & Pfefferbaum, R. (2008). Community resilience as a metaphor, theory, set of capacities, and strategy for disaster readiness. *American Journal of Community Psychology, 41,* 127–150.

Norris, F. H., Sherrieb, K., & Pfefferbaum, B. (2011). Community resilience: Concepts, assessment, and implications for intervention. In S. M. Southwick, B. T. Litz, D. Charney, & M. J. Friedman (Eds.), *Resilience and mental health: Challenges across the lifespan* (pp. 162–175). New York: Cambridge University Press.

Obradović, J. (2010). Effortful control and adaptive functioning of homeless children: Variable-focused and person-focused analyses. *Journal of Applied Developmental Psychology, 31,* 109–117.

Obradović, J. (2012). How can the study of physiological reactivity contribute to our understanding of adversity and resilience processes in development? *Development and Psychopathology, 24,* 371–387.

Obradović, J., & Boyce, W. T. (2009). Individual differences in behavioral, physiological, and genetic sensitivities to contexts: Implications for development and adaptation. *Developmental Neuroscience, 31,* 300–308.

Obradović, J., Bush, N. R., & Boyce, W. T. (2011). The interactive effect of marital conflict and stress reactivity on externalizing and internalizing symptoms: The role of laboratory stressors. *Development and Psychopathology, 23,* 101–114.

Obradović, J., Bush, N. R., Stamperdahl, J., Adler, N. E., & Boyce, W. T. (2010). Biological sensitivity to context: The interactive effects of stress reactivity and family adversity on socioemotional behavior and school readiness. *Child Development, 81,* 270–289.

Obradović, J., Long, J. D., Cutuli, J. J., Chan, C., Hinz, E., Heistad, D., et al. (2009). Academic achievement of homeless and highly mobile children in an urban school district: Longitudinal evidence on risk, growth, and resilience. *Development and Psychopathology, 21,* 493–518.

Obradović, J., & Masten, A. S. (2007). Developmental antecedents of young adult civic engagement. *Applied Developmental Science, 11,* 1–29.

Obradović, J., Shaffer, A., & Masten, A. S. (2012). Risk and adversity in developmental psychopathology: Progress and future directions. In L. C. Mayes & M. Lewis (Eds.), *The Cambridge handbook of environment in human development: A handbook of theory and measurement* (pp. 35–37). New York: Cambridge University Press.

Ogbu, J. U. (1981). Origins of human competence: A cultural–ecological perspective. *Child Development, 52,* 413–429.

Okada, H., Kuhn, C., Feillet, H., & Bach, J.-F. (2010). The "hygiene hypothesis" for autoimmune and allergic diseases: An update. *Clinical and Experimental Immunology, 160,* 1–9.

Olds, D. L. (2006). The nurse–family partnership: An evidence-based preventive intervention. *Infant Mental Health Journal, 27,* 5–25.

Olson, D. H. (2000). Circumplex model of marital and family systems. *Journal of Family Therapy, 22,* 144–167.

Olson, D. H., & Gorall, D. M. (2003). Circumplex model of marital and family systems. In F. Walsh (Ed.), *Normal family processes* (3rd ed., pp. 514–547). New York: Guilford Press.

Osofsky, J. D., Osofsky, H. J., & Harris, W. W. (2007). Katrina's children: Social policy considerations for children in disasters. *Special Policy Report, 21,* 3–18.

Otto, M. W., Henin, A., Hirshfeld-Becker, D. R., Pollack, M. H., Biederman, J., & Rosenbaum, J. F. (2007). Posttraumatic stress disorder symptoms following media exposure to tragic events: Impact of 9/11 on children at risk for anxiety disorders. *Journal of Anxiety Disorders, 21,* 888–902.

Overton, W. F. (2013). A new paradigm for developmental science: Relationism and relational–developmental systems. *Applied Developmental Science, 17,* 94–107.

Panter-Brick, C., Goodman, A., Tol, W., & Eggerman, M. (2011). Mental health and childhood adversities: A longitudinal study in Kabul, Afghanistan. *Journal of the American Academy of Child and Adolescent Psychiatry, 50,* 349–363.

Panter-Brick, C., & Leckman, J. F. (2013). Editorial commentary: Resilience in child development—interconnected pathways to well-being. *Journal of Child Psychology and Psychiatry, 54,* 333–336.

Park, N. (2011). Military children and families: Strengths and challenges during peace and war. *American Psychologist, 66,* 65–72.

Patterson, G. R., Forgatch, M. S., & DeGarmo, D. S. (2010). Cascading effects following intervention. *Developmental Psychopathology, 22,* 941–970.

Patterson, G. R., Reid, J. B., & Dishion, T. J. (1992). *Antisocial boys.* Eugene, OR: Castalia.

Patterson, J. M. (2002). Integrating family resilience and family stress theory. *Journal of Marriage and Family, 64,* 349–360.

Pellegrini, D. S. (1985). Social cognition and competence in middle childhood. *Child Development, 56,* 253–264.

Pellegrini, D. S., Masten, A. S., Garmezy, N., & Ferrarese, M. J. (1987). Correlates of social and academic competence in middle childhood. *Journal of Child Psychology and Psychiatry, 28,* 699–714.

Peltonen, K., & Punamäki, R. (2010). Preventive interventions among children exposed to trauma of armed conflict: A literature review. *Aggressive Behavior, 36,* 95–116.

Pfefferbaum, B., Nixon, S. J., Tivis, R. D., Doughty, D. E., Pynoos, R. S., Gurwitch, R. H., et al. (2001). Television exposure in children after a terrorist incident. *Psychiatry: Interpersonal and Biological Processes, 64,* 202–211.

Pfefferbaum, B., Seale, T. W., Brandt, E. N., Pfefferbaum, R., Doughty, D. E., & Rainwater, R. M. (2003). Media exposure in children one hundred miles from a terrorist bombing. *Annals of Clinical Psychiatry, 15,* 1–8.

Phillips, D., Prince, S., & Schiebelhut, L. (2004). Elementary school children's responses 3 months after the September 11 terrorist attacks: A study in Washington, DC. *American Journal of Orthopsychiatry, 74,* 509–528.

Phillips, D. I. W. (2007). Programming of the stress response: A fundamental mechanism underlying the long-term effects of the fetal environment? *Journal of Internal Medicine, 261,* 453–460.

Pianta, R. C. (2006). Schools, schooling, and developmental psychopathology. In D. Cicchetti & D. J. Cohen (Eds.), *Developmental psychopathology: Vol. 1. Theory and method* (2nd ed., pp. 494–529). Hoboken, NJ: Wiley.

Pilling, D. (1990). *Escape from disadvantage.* Bristol, PA: Falmer Press.

Pine, D. S., Costello, J., & Masten, A. (2005). Trauma, proximity, and developmental psychopathology: The effects of war and terrorism on children. *Neuropsychopharmacology, 30,* 1781–1792.

Plowman, E. J., Narayan, A. J., Masten, A. S., Desjardins, D., & Herbers, J. E. (2012, February). *Everything but the kitchen sink?: Using second-order confirmatory factor analysis to inform measurement of parenting quality.* Poster presentation at the Developmental Methodology Theme Meeting of the Society for Research on Child Development, Tampa, FL.

Pluess, M., & Belsky, J. (2013). Vantage sensitivity: Individual differences in response to positive experiences. *Psychological Bulletin, 139,* 901–916.

Pop-Jordanova, N., & Gucev, Z. (2009). Game-based peripheral biofeedback for stress assessment in children. *Pediatrics International, 52,* 428–431.

Porges, S. W. (2011). *The polyvagal theory: Neurophysiological foundations of emotions, attachment, communication, and self-regulation.* New York: Norton.

Pratt, L. V. (1976). *Family structure and effective health behavior: The energized family.* Boston: Houghton Mifflin.

Qouta, S., Punamäki, R., & El Sarraj, E. (2008). Child development and family mental health in war and military violence: The Palestinian experience. *International Journal of Behavioral Development, 32,* 310–321.

Raby, K. L., & Roisman, G. I. (2013). Gene–environment interplay and risk and resilience during childhood. *Encyclopedia of Early Childhood Development.* Retrieved from *www.child-encyclopedia.com/documents/Raby-RoismanANGxp1.pdf.*

Raver, C. C., Blair, C., & Willoughby, M. (2013). Poverty as a predictor of 4-year-olds' executive function: New perspectives on models of differential susceptibility. *Developmental Psychology, 49,* 292–304.

Raver, C. C., Li-Grining, C., Bub, K., Jones, S. M., Zhai, F., & Pressler, E. (2011). CSRP's impact on low-income preschoolers' preacademic skills: Self-regulation as a mediating mechanism. *Child Development, 82,* 362–378.

Realmuto, G. M., Masten, A. S., Carole, L. F., Hubbard, J., Groteluschen, A., & Chhun, B. (1992). Adolescent survivors of massive childhood trauma in Cambodia: Life events and current symptoms. *Journal of Traumatic Stress, 5,* 589–599.

Reed, R. V., Fazel, M., Jones, L., Panter-Brick, C., & Stein, A. (2012). Mental health of displaced refugee children resettled in low-income and middle-income countries: Risk and protective factors. *Lancet, 379,* 250–265.

Reich, J. W., Zautra, A. J., & Hall, J. S. (Eds.). (2010). *Handbook of adult resilience.* New York: Guilford Press.

Repetti, R. L., Robles, T. F., & Reynolds, B. (2011). Allostatic processes in the family. *Development and Psychopathology, 23,* 921–938.

Resilience Alliance. (2002). Resilience. Retrieved July 5, 2013, from *www.resilience.org/index.php/resilience.*

Reynolds, A. J., Temple, J. A., White, B. A. B., Ou, S.-R., & Robertson, D. L. (2011). Age 26 cost-benefit analysis of the Child–Parent Center early education program. *Child Development, 82,* 379–404.

Riggs, N. R., Jahromi, L. B., Razza, R. P., Dillworth-Bart, J. E., & Mueller, U. (2006). Executive function and the promotion of social–emotional competence. *Journal of Applied Developmental Psychology, 27,* 300–309.

Riley, J. R. (2004). *Demonstrating the art of factor analysis: Bridging the gap between the world of the factor analyst and the world of the developmental researcher.* Unpublished doctoral dissertation, University of Minnesota, Minneapolis, MN.

Roisman, G. I., Masten, A. S., Coatsworth, J. D., & Tellegen, A. (2004). Salient and emerging developmental tasks in the transition to adulthood. *Child Development, 75,* 123–133.

Rothbart, M. K. (2011). *Becoming who we are: Temperament and personality in development.* New York: Guilford Press.

Ruf, M., Schauer, M, Neuner, F., Catani, C., Schauer, E., & Elbert, T. (2010). Narrative exposure therapy for 7–16-year-olds: A randomized control trial with traumatized refugee children. *Journal of Traumatic Stress, 23,* 437–445.

Russo, S. J., Murrough, J. W., Han, M.-H., Charney, D. S., & Nestler, E. J. (2012). Neurobiology of resilience. *Nature Neuroscience, 15,* 1475–1484.

Rutter, M. (1979). Protective factors in children's responses to stress and disadvantage. In M. W. Kent & J. E. Rolf (Eds.), *Primary prevention of psychopathology: Vol. 3. Social competence in children* (pp. 49–74). Hanover, NH: University Press of New England.

Rutter, M. (1983). Stress, coping, and development: Some issues and some questions. In N. Garmezy & M. Rutter (Eds.), *Stress, coping, and development in children* (pp. 1–41). New York: McGraw-Hill.

Rutter, M. (1987). Psychosocial resilience and protective mechanisms. *American Journal of Orthopsychiatry, 57,* 316–331.

Rutter, M. (1989). Isle of Wight revisited: Twenty-five years of child psychiatric epidemiology. *Journal of the American Academy of Child and Adolescent Psychiatry, 28,* 633–653.

Rutter, M. (1990). Psychosocial resilience and protective mechanisms. In J. Rolf, A. S. Masten, D. Cicchetti, K. H. Nuechterlein, & S. Weintraub (Eds.), *Risk and protective factors in the development of psychopathology* (pp. 181–214). New York: Cambridge University Press.

Rutter, M. (2006). Implications of resilience concepts for scientific understanding. *Annals of the New York Academy of Sciences, 1094,* 1–12.

Rutter, M. (2009). Understanding and testing risk mechanisms for mental disorders. *Journal of Child Psychology and Psychiatry, 50,* 44–52.

Rutter, M. (2012a). Achievements and challenges in the biology of environmental effects. *Proceedings of the National Academy of Sciences, 109,* 17149–17153.

Rutter, M. (2012b). Resilience as a dynamic concept. *Development and Psychopathology, 24,* 335–344.

Rutter, M. (2013). Annual research review: Resilience—clinical implications. *Journal of Child Psychology and Psychiatry, 54,* 474–487.

Rutter, M., & the English and Romanian Adoptees (ERA) Study Team. (1998). Developmental catch-up and deficit, following adoption after severe global early privation. *Journal of Child Psychology and Psychiatry, 39,* 465–476.

Rutter, M., & Maughan, B. (2002). School effectiveness findings 1979–2002. *Journal of School Psychology, 40,* 451–475.

Rutter, M., Sonuga-Barke, E. J, Beckett, C., Castle, J., Kreppner, J., Kumsta, R., et al. (2010). Deprivation-specific psychological patterns: Effects of institutional deprivation. *Monographs of the Society for Research in Child Development, 75*(1, Serial No. 295).

Rutter, M., Sonuga-Barke, E. J., & Castle, J. (2010). Investigating the impact of early institutional deprivation on development: Background and research strategy of the English and Romanian Adoptees (ERA) study. *Monographs of the Society for Research in Child Development, 75*, 1–20.

Ryan, R. M., & Deci, E. L. (2000). Self-determination theory and the facilitation of intrinsic motivation, social development, and well-being. *American Psychologist, 55*, 68–78.

Saltzman, W., Lester, P., Beardslee, W., Layne, C., Woodward, K., & Nash, W. (2011). Mechanisms of risk and resilience in military families: Theoretical and empirical basis of a family-focused resilience enhancement program. *Clinical Child and Family Psychology Review, 14*, 213–230.

Sameroff, A. J. (2006). Identifying risk and protective factors for healthy child development. In A. Clark-Stewart & J. Dunn (Eds.), *Families count: Effects on child and adolescent development* (pp. 53–76). Cambridge, UK: Cambridge University Press.

Sameroff, A. J., & Chandler, M. J. (1975). Reproductive risk and the continuum of caretaking casualty. In F. D. Horowitz, E. M. Hethterington, S. Scarr-Salapatek, & G. M. Siegel (Eds.), *Review of child development research* (Vol. 4, pp. 187–243). Chicago: University of Chicago Press.

Sameroff, A. J., & Fiese, B. H. (2000). Transactional regulation: The developmental ecology of early intervention. In J. P. Shonkoff & S. J. Meisels (Eds.), *Handbook of early childhood intervention* (2nd ed., pp. 135–159). Cambridge, UK: Cambridge University Press.

Sameroff, A. J., & Seifer, R. (1983). Familial risk and child competence. *Child Development, 54*, 1254–1268.

Sameroff, A. J., Seifer, R., Barocas, R., Zax, M., & Greenspan, S. (1987). Intelligence quotient scores of 4-year-old children: Social–environmental risk factors. *Pediatrics, 79*, 343–350.

Sameroff, A. J., Seifer, R., & Bartko, W. T. (1997). Environmental perspectives on adaptation during childhood and adolescence. In S. S. Luthar, J. A. Burack, D. Cicchetti, & J. R. Weisz (Eds.), *Developmental psychopathology: Perspectives on adjustment, risk, and disorder* (pp. 507–526). New York: Cambridge University Press.

Samuels, J., Shinn, M., & Buckner, J. C. (2010). *Homeless children: Update on research, policy, programs, and opportunities.* Washington, DC: U.S. Department of Health and Human Services, Office of the Assistant Secretary for Planning and Evaluation.

Sanders, M. R. (2012). Development, evaluation, and multinational dissemination of the Triple P-Positive Parenting Program. *Annual Review of Clinical Psychology, 8*, 345–379.

Sandler, I., Schoenfelder, E., Wolchik, S., & MacKinnon, D. (2011). Long-term impact of prevention programs to promote effective parenting: Lasting effects but uncertain processes. *Annual Review of Psychology, 62*, 299–329.

Sandoval, J., & Brock, S. E. (2009). Managing crisis: Prevention, intervention, and treatment. In T. B. Gutkin & C. R. Reynolds (Eds.), *The handbook of school psychology* (4th ed., pp. 886–904). Hoboken, NJ: Wiley.

Sapienza, J. K., & Masten, A. S. (2011). Understanding and promoting resilience in children and youth. *Current Opinion in Psychiatry, 24*, 267–273.

Sattler, J. M. (1988). *Assessment of children* (3rd ed., Rev. ed.). San Diego, CA: Author.

Saylor, C. F., Cowart, B. L., Lipovsky, J. A., Jackson, C., & Finch, A. J. (2003). Media exposure to September 11. *American Behavioral Scientist, 46*, 1622–1642.

Scales, P. C., Benson, P. L., Leffert, N., & Blyth, D. A. (2000). Contribution of developmental assets to the prediction of thriving among adolescents. *Applied Developmental Science, 4*, 27–46.

Scales, P. C., Benson, P. L., Roehlkepartain, E. C., Sesma, A., Jr., & van Dulmen, M. (2006). The role of developmental assets in predicting academic achievement: A longitudinal study. *Journal of Adolesence, 291*, 691–708.

Schiff, M., Pat-Horenczyk, R., Benbenishty, R., Brom, D., Baum, N., & Astor, R. A. (2012). High school students' posttraumatic symptoms, substance abuse and involvement in violence in the aftermath of war. *Social Science and Medicine, 75*, 1321–1328.

Schoon, I. (2006). *Risk and resilience: Adaptations in changing times.* New York: Cambridge University Press.

Schorr, L. B., & Schorr, D. (1989). *Within our reach: Breaking the cycle of disadvantage.* New York: Doubleday.

Schulz, L. C. (2010). The Dutch Hunger Winter and the developmental origins of health and disease. *Proceedings of the National Academy of Sciences of the United States of America, 107*, 16757–16758.

Schuster, M. A., Stein, B. D., Jaycox, L. H., Collins, R. L., Marshall, G. N., Elliott, M. N., et al. (2001). A national survey of stress reactions after the September 11, 2001, terrorist attacks. *New England Journal of Medicine, 345*, 1507–1512.

Serafica, F. C., & Vargas, L. A. (2006). Cultural diversity in the development of child psychopathology. In D. Cicchetti & D. J. Cohen (Eds.), *Developmental psychopathology: Vol. 1. Theory and method* (2nd ed., pp. 588–626). Hoboken, NJ: Wiley.

Sesma, A., Mannes, M., & Scales, P. C. (2013). Positive adaptation, resilience and the developmental assets framework. In S. Goldstein & R. B. Brooks (Eds.), *Handbook of resilience in children* (pp. 427–442). New York: Springer.

Šešo-Šimić, Ð., Sedmak, G., Hof, P. R., & Šimić, G. (2010). Recent advances in the neurobiology of attachment behavior. *Translational Neuroscience, 1*, 148–159.

Shaffer, A., Burt, K. B., Obradović, J., Herbers, J. E., & Masten, A. S. (2009). Intergenerational continuity in parenting quality: The mediating role of social competence. *Developmental Psychology, 45*, 1227–1240.

Shaffer, A., Coffino, B., Boelcke-Stennes, K., & Masten, A. S. (2007). From urban girls to resilient women: Studying adaptation across development in the context of adversity. In B. J. R. Leadbeater & N. Way (Eds.), *Urban girls revisited: Building strengths* (pp. 53–72). New York: New York University Press.

Shapiro, S. L. (2009). Meditation and positive psychology. In C. R. Snyder & S. J. Lopez (Eds.), *Oxford handbook of positive psychology* (2nd ed., pp. 601–610). New York: Oxford University Press.

Shiner, R. L. (1998). How shall we speak of children's personalities in middle childhood?: A preliminary taxonomy. *Psychological Bulletin, 124*, 308–332.

Shiner, R. L. (2000). Linking childhood personality with adaptation: Evidence for continuity and change across time into late adolescence. *Journal of Personality and Social Psychology, 78*, 310–325.

Shiner, R. L., & Masten, A. S. (2008). Personality in childhood: A bridge from early temperament to adult outcomes. *International Journal of Developmental Science, 2*, 158–175.

Shiner, R. L., & Masten, A. S. (2012). Childhood personality as a harbinger of competence and resilience in adulthood. *Development and Psychopathology, 24*, 507–528.

Shiner, R. L., Masten, A. S., & Roberts, J. M. (2003). Childhood personality foreshadows adult personality and life outcomes two decades later. *Journal of Personality, 71*, 1145–1170.

Shiner, R. L., Masten, A. S., & Tellegen, A. (2002). A developmental perspective on personality in emerging adulthood: Childhood antecedents and concurrent adaptation. *Journal of Personality and Social Psychology, 83*, 1165.

Shonkoff, J. P. (2011). Protecting brains, not simply stimulating minds. *Science, 333*, 982–983.

Shonkoff, J. P., Boyce, W. T., & McEwen, B. S. (2009). Neuroscience, molecular biology, and the childhood roots of health disparities. *Journal of the American Medical Association, 301*, 2252–2259.

Shonkoff, J. P., & Phillips, D. A. (Eds.). (2000). *From neurons to neighborhoods: The science of early childhood development.* Washington, DC: National Academy Press.

Sigal, A. B., Wolchik, S. A., Tein, J.-Y., & Sandler, I. N. (2012). Enhancing youth outcomes following parental divorce: A longitudinal study of the effects of the New Beginnings Program on educational and occupational goals. *Journal of Clinical Child and Adolescent Psychology, 41*, 150–165.

Sirin, S. R., & Gupta, T. (2012). Muslim, American, and immigrant: Integration despite challenges. In A. S. Masten, K. Liebkind, & D. J. Hernandez (Eds.), *Realizing the potential of immigrant youth* (pp. 253–279). New York: Cambridge University Press.

Skinner, E. A., & Zimmer-Gembeck, M. J. (2007). The development of coping. *Annual Review of Psychology, 58*, 119–144.

Smart, E., & Stewart, C. (2013). *My story.* New York: St. Martin's Press.

Smeeding, T. M., Robson, K., Wing, C., & Gershuny, J. I. (2012). Income poverty and income support for minority and immigrant households with children in rich countries. In A. S. Masten, K. Liebkind, & D. J. Hernandez (Eds.), *Realizing the potential of immigrant youth* (pp. 63–89). New York: Cambridge University Press.

Somerville, L. H., & Casey, B. J. (2010). Developmental neurobiology of cognitive control and motivational systems. *Current Opinion in Neurobiology, 20*, 236–241.

Sorce, J. F., Emde, R. N., Campos, J. J., & Klinnert, M. D. (1985). Maternal emotional signaling: Its effect on the visual cliff behavior of 1-year-olds. *Developmental Psychology, 21*, 195–200.

Southwick, S. M., Litz, B. T., Charney, D., & Friedman, M. J. (Eds.). (2011). *Resilience and mental health: Challenges across the lifespan.* New York: Cambridge University Press.

Southwick, S. M., Vythilingam, M., & Charney, D. S. (2005). The psychobiology of depression and resilience to stress: Implications for prevention and treatment. *Annual Review of Clinical Psychology, 1*, 255–291.

Spencer, M. B., Harpalani, V., Cassidy, E., Jacobs, C. Y., Donde, S., Goss, T. N., et al. (2006). Understanding vulnerability and resilience from a normative developmental perspective: Implications for racially and ethnically diverse youth. In D. Cicchetti & D. J. Cohen (Eds.), *Developmental psychopathology: Vol. 1. Theory and method* (2nd ed., pp. 627–672). Hoboken, NJ: Wiley.

Spivack, G., & Swift, M. (1967). *The Devereux Elementary School Behavior Rating Scale.* Devon, PA: Devereux Foundation.

Sprung, M. (2008). Unwanted intrusive thoughts and cognitive functioning in kindergarten and young elementary school-age children following Hurricane Katrina. *Journal of Child Clinical and Adolescent Psychology, 37*, 575–587.

Sroufe, L. A. (1979). The coherence of individual development: Early care, attachment, and subsequent developmental issues. *American Psychologist, 34*, 834–841.

Sroufe, L. A. (2005). Attachment and development: A prospective, longitudinal study from birth to adulthood. *Attachment and Human Development, 7*, 349–367.

Sroufe, L. A., Carlson, E. A., Levy, A. K., & Egeland, B. (1999). Implications of attachment theory for developmental psychopathology. *Development and Psychopathology, 11*, 1–13.

Sroufe, L. A., Egeland, B., Carlson, E. A., & Collins, A. W. (2005). *The development of the person: The Minnesota study of risk and adaptation from birth to adulthood.* New York: Guilford Press.

Stattin, H., & Kerr, M. (2000). Parental monitoring: A reinterpretation. *Child Development, 71*, 1072–1085.

Steinberg, L. (2001). We know some things: Parent–adolescent relationships in retrospect and prospect. *Journal of Research on Adolescence, 11*, 1–19.

Steinberg, L., Dahl, R., Keating, D., Kupfer, D. J., Masten, A. S., & Pine, D. S. (2006). Psychopathology in adolescence: Integrating affective neuroscience with the study of context. In D. Cicchetti & D. Cohen (Eds.), *Developmental psychopathology: Vol. 2. Developmental neuroscience* (2nd ed., pp. 710–741). New York: Wiley.

Sterling, P., & Eyer, J. (1988). Allostasis: A new paradigm to explain arousal pathology. In S. Fisher & J. Reason (Eds.), *Handbook of life stress, cognition and health* (pp. 629–649). Oxford, UK: Wiley.

Stern, A. M., & Markel, H. (2005). The history of vaccines and immunizations: Familiar patterns, new challenges. *Health Affairs, 24,* 611–621.

Stevens, H. E., Leckman, J. F., Coplan, J. D., & Suomi, S. J. (2009). Risk and resilience: Early manipulation of macaque social experience and persistent behavioral and neurophysiological outcomes. *Journal of the American Academy of Child and Adolescent Psychiatry, 48,* 114–127.

Stroud, K. C., & Reynolds, C. R. (2009). Assessment of learning strategies and related constructs in children and adolescents. In T. B. Gutkin & C. R. Reynolds (Eds.), *The handbook of school psychology* (4th ed., pp. 739–765). Hoboken, NJ: Wiley.

Suomi, S. J. (1999). Attachment in rhesus monkeys. In J. Cassidy & P. R. Shaver (Eds.), *Handbook of attachment: Theory, research, and clinical applications* (pp. 181–197). New York: Guilford Press.

Suomi, S. J. (2006). Risk, resilience, and gene × environment interactions in rhesus monkeys. *Annals of the New York Academy of Sciences, 1094,* 52–62.

Suomi, S. J. (2011). Risk, resilience, and gene–environment interplay in primates. *Journal of the Canadian Academy of Child and Adolescent Psychiatry, 20,* 289–297.

Szanton, S. L., & Gill, J. M. (2010). Facilitating resilience using a society-to-cells framework: A theory of nursing essentials applied to research and practice. *Advances in Nursing Science, 33,* 329–343.

Tang, A., Reeb-Sutherland, B. C., Romeo, R. D., & McEwen, B. S. (2014). On the causes of early life experience effects: Evaluating the role of mom. *Frontiers in Neuroendocrinology, 35,* 245–251.

Tangney, J. P., Baumeister, R. F., & Boone, A. L. (2008). High self-control predicts good adjustment, less pathology, better grades, and interpersonal success. *Journal of Personality, 72,* 271–324.

Tarter, R. E., & Vanyukov, M. (1999). Re-visiting the validity of the construct of resilience. In M. D. Glantz & J. L. Johnson (Eds.), *Resilience and development: Positive life adaptations* (pp. 85–100). New York: Springer.

Tellegen, A. (1982). *Brief manual of the Multidimensional Personality Questionnaire.* Unpublished manuscript, University of Minnesota.

Terr, L. C., Bloch, D. A., Michel, B. A., Shi, H., Reinhardt, J. A., & Metayer, S. (1999). Children's symptoms on the wake of *Challenger*: A field study of distant-traumatic effects and an outline of related conditions. *American Journal of Psychiatry, 156,* 1536–1544.

Terranova, A. M., Boxer, P., & Morris, A. S. (2009). Factors influencing the course of posttraumatic stress following a natural disaster: Children's reactions to Hurricane Katrina. *Journal of Applied Developmental Psychology, 30,* 344–355.

Theron, L. C., & Engelbrecht, P. (2012). Caring teachers: Teacher-youth transactions to promote resilience. In M. Ungar (Ed.), *The social ecology of resilience: A handbook of theory and practice* (pp. 265–280). New York: Springer.

Theron, L. C., Theron, A. M. C., & Malindi, M. J. (2013). Toward an African definition of resilience: A rural South African community's view of resilient Basotho youth. *Journal of Black Psychology, 39,* 63–87.

Thomas, R., & Zimmer-Gembeck, M. J. (2011). Accumulating evidence for parent–child interaction therapy in the prevention of child maltreatment. *Child Development, 82*, 177–192.

Thompson, R. A. (2000). The legacy of early attachments. *Child Development, 71*, 145–152.

Tol, W. A., Komproe, I. H., Jordans, M. J. D., Gross, A. L., Susanty, D., Macy, R. D., et al. (2010). Mediators and moderators of a psychosocial intervention for children affected by political violence. *Journal of Consulting and Clinical Psychology, 78*, 818–828.

Toth, S. L., & Cicchetti, D. (1999). Developmental psychopathology and child psychotherapy. In S. Russ & R. Ollendick (Eds.), *Handbook of psychotherapies with children and families* (pp. 15–44). New York: Plenum Press.

Toth, S. L., & Gravener, J. (2012). Bridging research and practice: Relational interventions for maltreated children. *Child and Adolescent Mental Health, 17*, 131–138.

Toth, S. L., & Manley, J. T. (2011). Bridging research and practice: Challenges and successes in implementing evidence-based preventive intervention strategies for child maltreatment. *Child Abuse and Neglect, 35*, 633–636.

Tough, P. (2009). *Whatever it takes: Geoffrey Canada's question to change Harlem and America*. New York: Houghton Mifflin Harcourt (Mariner Books).

Tronick, E., & Beeghly, M. (2011). Infants' meaning-making and the development of mental health problems. *American Psychologist, 66*, 107–119.

Troy, A. S., & Mauss, I. B. (2011). Resilience in the face of stress: Emotion regulation as a protective factor. In S. M. Southwick, B. T. Litz, D. Charney, & M. J. Friedman (Eds.), *Resilience and mental health: Challenges across the lifespan* (pp. 30–44). Cambridge, UK: Cambridge University Press.

Turnbaugh, P. J., Ley, R. E., Hamady, M., Fraser-Liggett, C. M., Knight, R., & Gordon, J. I. (2007). The human microbiome project. *Nature, 449*, 804–810.

Tyrka, A. R., Price, L. H., Kao, H.-T., Porton, B., Marsella, S. A., & Carpenter, L. L. (2010). Childhood maltreatment and telomere shortening: Preliminary support for an effect of early stress on cellular aging. *Biological Psychiatry, 67*, 531–534.

Ungar, M. (2008). Resilience across cultures. *British Journal of Social Work, 38*, 218–235.

Ungar, M. (2011). The social ecology of resilience: Addressing contextual and cultural ambiguity of a nascent construct. *American Journal of Orthopsychiatry, 81*, 1–17.

Ungar, M. (Ed.). (2012). *The social ecology of resilience: A handbook of theory and practice*. New York: Springer.

Ungar, M., Ghazinour, M., & Richter, J. (2013). What is resilience within the social ecology of human development? *Journal of Child Psychology and Psychiatry, 54*, 348–366.

Ungar, M., & Liebenberg, L. (2005). The International Resilience Project. In M. Ungar (Ed.), *Handbook for working with children and youth: Pathways to resilience across cultures and contexts* (pp. 211–225). Thousand Oaks, CA: Sage.

United States Department of Agriculture Food and Nutrition Service

(2013, September). *National School Lunch Program.* "Factsheet" downloaded March 23, 2014, from *http://www.fns.usda.gov/sites/default/files/ NSLPFactSheet.pdf*

Verkuyten, M. (2012). Understanding ethnic minority identity. In A. S. Masten, K. Liebkind, & D. J. Hernandez (Eds.), *Realizing the potential of immigrant youth* (pp. 230–252). New York: Cambridge University Press.

Vigil, J. M., Geary, D. C., Granger, D. A., & Flinn, M. V. (2010). Sex differences in salivary cortisol, alpha-amylase, and psychological functioning following Hurricane Katrina. *Child Development, 81,* 1228–1240.

von Bertalanffy, L. (1968). *General system theory: Foundation, development, application.* New York: Braziller.

von Mutius, E., & Radon, K. (2008). Living on a farm: Impact on asthma induction and clinical course. *Immunology and Allergy Clinics of North America, 28,* 631–647.

Walden, T. A., & Ogan, T. A. (1988). The development of social referencing. *Child Development, 59,* 1230–1240.

Walker, S. P., Wachs, T. D., Gardner, J. M., Lozoff, B., Wasserman, G. A., Pollitt, E., et al. (2007). Child development: Risk factors for adverse outcomes in developing countries. *Lancet, 369,* 145–157.

Walker, S. P., Wachs, T. D., Grantham-McGregor, S., Black, M. M., Nelson, C. A., Huffman, S. L., et al. (2011). Inequality in early childhood: Risk and protective factors for early child development. *Lancet, 378,* 1325–1338.

Walsh, F. (2006). *Strengthening family resilience* (2nd ed.). New York: Guilford Press.

Walsh, F. (Ed.). (2011). *Family processes: Growing diversity and complexity.* New York: Guilford Press.

Waters, E., & Sroufe, L. A. (1983). Social competence as a developmental construct. *Developmental Review, 3,* 79–97.

Watt, N. F., Anthony, E. J., Wynne, L. C., & Rolf, J. E. (Eds.). (1984). *Children at risk for schizophrenia: A longitudinal perspective.* New York: Cambridge University Press.

Wechsler, D. (1958). *The measurement and appraisal of adult intelligence.* Baltimore: Williams & Wilkins.

Weems, C. F., Pina, A. A., Costa, N. M., Watts, S. E., Taylor, L. K., & Cannon, M. F. (2007). Predisaster trait anxiety and negative affect predict posttraumatic stress in youths after Hurricane Katrina. *Journal of Consulting and Clinical Psychology, 75,* 154–159.

Werner, E. E. (1993). Risk, resilience, and recovery: Perspectives from the Kauai Longitudinal Study. *Development and Psychopathology, 5,* 503–515.

Werner, E. E., & Smith, R. S. (1982). *Vulnerable but invincible: A study of resilient children.* New York: McGraw-Hill.

Werner, E. E., & Smith, R. S. (1992). *Overcoming the odds: High risk children from birth to adulthood.* Ithaca, NY: Cornell University Press.

Werner, E. E., & Smith, R. S. (2001). *Journeys from childhood to midlife: Risk, resilience, and recovery.* Ithaca, NY: Cornell University Press.

Whitbeck, L. B., Hoyt, D. R., Chen, X., & Stubben, J. D. (2002). Predictors of gang involvement among American Indian adolescents. *Journal of Gang Research 10*, 11–26.

White, J. L., & Cones, J. H., III. (1999). *Black man emerging: Facing the past and seizing a future in America.* New York: Freeman.

White, R. W. (1959). Motivation reconsidered: The concept of competence. *Psychological Review, 66*, 297–333.

Wickrama, K. A. S., & Kaspar, V. (2007). Family context of mental health risk in tsunami-exposed adolescents: Findings from a pilot study in Sri Lanka. *Social Science and Medicine, 64*, 713–723.

Williams, K. R., & Guerra, N. G. (2007). Prevalence and predictors of internet bullying. *Journal of Adolescent Health, 41*, S14–S21.

Wolchik, S. A., Sandler, I. N., Millsap, R. E., Plummer, B. A., Greene, S. M., Anderson, E. R., et al. (2002). Six-year follow-up of preventive interventions for children of divorce. *Journal of the American Medical Association, 288*, 1874–1881.

Wolmer, L., Hamiel, D., & Laor, N. (2011). Preventing children's posttraumatic stress after disaster with teacher-based intervention: A controlled study. *Journal of the American Academy of Child and Adolescent Psychiatry, 50*, 340–348.e2.

Wright, M. O'D., Crawford, F., & Sebastian, K. (2007). Positive resolution of childhood sexual abuse experiences: The role of coping, benefit-finding and meaning-making. *Journal of Family Violence, 22*, 597–608.

Wright, M. O'D., Masten, A. S., & Narayan, A. J. (2013). Resilience processes in development: Four waves of research on positive adaptation in the context of adversity. In S. Goldstein & R. B. Brooks (Eds.), *Handbook of resilience in children* (pp. 15–37). New York: Springer.

Wyman, P. A. (2003). Emerging perspectives on context specificity of children's adaptation and resilience: Evidence from a decade of research with urban children in adversity. In S. S. Luthar (Ed.), *Resilience and vulnerability: Adaptation in the context of childhood adversities* (pp. 293–317). New York: Cambridge University Press.

Yates, T. M., & Grey, I. K. (2012). Adapting to aging out: Profiles of risk and resilience among emancipated foster youth. *Development and Psychopathology, 24*, 475–492.

Yehuda, R., Bell, A., Bierer, L. M., & Schmiedler, J. (2008). Maternal, not paternal, PTSD related to increased risk for PTSD in offspring of holocaust survivors. *Journal of Psychiatric Research, 42*, 1104–1111.

Yehuda, R., & Bierer, L. M. (2009). The relevance of epigenetics to PTSD: Implications for the DSM-V. *Journal of Traumatic Stress, 22*, 427–434.

Yehuda, R., Teicher, M. H., Seckl, J. R., Grossman, R. A., Morris, A., & Bierer, L. M. (2007). Parental posttraumatic stress disorder as a vulnerability factor for low cortisol trait in offspring of holocaust survivors. *Archives of General Psychiatry, 64*, 1040–1048.

Yoshikawa, H., Aber, J. L., & Beardslee, W. R. (2012). The effects of poverty on the mental, emotional, and behavioral health of children and youth: Implications for prevention. *American Psychologist, 67*, 272–284.

Zeanah, C. H., Shauffer, C., & Dozier, M. (2011). Foster care for young children: Why it must be developmentally informed. *Journal of the American Academy of Child and Adolescent Psychiatry, 50,* 1199–1201.

Zeanah, C. H., Smyke, A. T., & Settles, L. D. (2006). Orphanages as a developmental context for early childhood. In K. McCartney & D. Phillips (Eds.), *Blackwell handbook of early childhood development* (pp. 424–454). Malden, MA: Blackwell.

Zelazo, P. D. (2013). Developmental psychology: A new synthesis. In P. D. Zelazo (Ed.), *The Oxford handbook of developmental psychology: Vol. 1. Body and mind* (pp. 3–12). New York: Oxford University Press.

Zelazo, P. D., & Bauer, P. J. (Eds.). (2013). National Institutes of Health Toolbox Cognition Battery (NIH Toolbox CB): Validation for children between 3 and 15 years. *Monographs of the Society for Research in Child Development, 78*(4), 1–172.

Zelazo, P. D., & Carlson, S. M. (2012). Hot and cool executive function in childhood and adolescence: Development and plasticity. *Child Development Perspectives, 6,* 354–360.

Zelazo, P. D., & Lyons, K. E. (2011). Mindfulness training in childhood. *Human Development, 54,* 61–65.

Zhang, R. Y., Labonté, B., Wen, X. L., Turecki, G., & Meaney, M. J. (2013). Epigenetic mechanisms for the early environmental regulation of hippocampal glucocorticoid receptor gene expression in rodents and humans. *Neuropsychopharmacology Reviews, 38,* 111–123.

Zigler, E., & Styfco, S. J. (2010). *The hidden history of Head Start.* New York: Oxford University Press.

Zipes, J. (2012). *The irresistible fairy tail: The cultural and social history of a genre.* Princeton, NJ: Princeton University Press.

Zolli, A., & Healy, A. M. (2012). *Resilience: Why things bounce back.* New York: Free Press.

INDEX

Page numbers followed by *f* indicate figures; followed by *t* indicate tables

363